Fifth Edition

Dimensional Analysis for Meds:

Refocusing on Essential Metric Calculations

Anna M. Curren

RN. Royal Victoria Hospital, Montreal, Quebec, Canada

BN. Public Health, Dalhousie University, Halifax, Nova Scotia, Canada

MA. Education Instructional Design, California State University

LL.D (Hon). Memorial University of Newfoundland, St. John's

Formerly Associate Professor of Nursing
Long Beach Community College
Long Beach, California

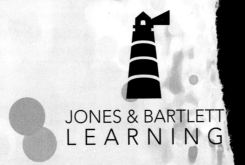

JONES & BARTLETT
LEARNING

World Headquarters
Jones & Bartlett Learning
5 Wall Street
Burlington, MA 01803
978-443-5000
info@jblearning.com
www.jblearning.com

Jones & Bartlett Learning books and products are available through most bookstores and online booksellers. To contact Jones & Bartlett Learning directly, call 800-832-0034, fax 978-443-8000, or visit our website, www.jblearning.com.

Substantial discounts on bulk quantities of Jones & Bartlett Learning publications are available to corporations, professional associations, and other qualified organizations. For details and specific discount information, contact the special sales department at Jones & Bartlett Learning via the above contact information or send an email to specialsales@jblearning.com.

Composition: S4Carlisle Publishing Services
Cover Design: Michael O'Donnell
Text Design: Michael O'Donnell
Rights Specialist: John Rusk
Media Development Editor: Troy Liston
Cover Image (Title Page, Section Opener, Chapter Opener):
   © Oxygen/Getty Images
Printing and Binding: LSC Communications
Cover Printing: LSC Communications

tial metric

nes & Bartlett

k.)

truction

513--dc23

The Pedagogy

Dimensional Analysis for Meds: Refocusing on Essential Metric Calculations, Fifth Edition has been carefully written and thoroughly tested to allow all dosage content and considerations to proceed from simple to complex. This text takes an interactive approach and addresses different learning styles, thereby ensuring that all students can successfully master **all basic dosage calculations**. The following pedagogical aids help to reinforce key concepts and appear in most chapters.

OBJECTIVES

Each chapter opens with a list of Objectives, which provide instructors and students with a summary of the content and concepts to be presented in the chapter. These objectives serve as a checklist to help guide students and focus their study.

KEY POINTS

Key Points reinforce safety considerations related to dimensional analysis and the administration of prescription medications. Each Key Point is easily identified by a key icon.

EXAMPLES

Examples provide real-world scenarios related to solving calculations in a clinical setting.

PROBLEMS

Practice Problems allow students to demonstrate their knowledge of key concepts presented throughout the text. Answers are provided after each problem set so they can check their work.

SUMMARY SELF-TESTS

Summary Self-Tests allow students to test their comprehension of key concepts at the end of each chapter. Answers are provided at the end of each self-test set so they can check their work.

Contents

Preface

The preface is an introduction written by an author to explain a text's content. I welcome this opportunity.

The most important content in *Dimensional Analysis for Meds* begins in **Chapter 1** with the **Metric System**. My personal estimate is that **98%** of all dosage calculations **involve metric measures**. That's a conservative estimate—the real percentage is probably even higher. By the time the student completes **Chapter 10, calculating metric dosages will have become automatic** for the learner. In these pivotal 10 chapters, students learn to read oral and parenteral dosage labels, and calculate a wide range of ordered dosages. For parenteral dosages, this includes the measurement of dosages using appropriate-sized syringe calibrations.

The **Refresher Math** needed later for IV calculations using dimensional analysis is presented in **Section 2**, primarily to reassure learners that they are capable of doing it. Students are referred back to this content for review when they reach the topic of **dimensional analysis** in **Chapter 11**, where they will use the math for the first time in IV calculations.

The decision to include dimensional analysis as the **ONLY calculation method** is quite deliberate. This approach **reduces multiple IV factor entries to a single common-fraction equation**. Neither ratio and proportion nor the formula method, both of which involve multiple calculation steps, can make this claim and make calculations as easy and reliably correct.

Additional text chapters, primarily on safe medication administration, pediatric dosage calculations based on body weight and body surface area, and other pediatric considerations in medication administration are included, wrapping up this concise 20-chapter text.

Letter for the Learner

Welcome to our journey together through *Dimensional Analysis for Meds*. Many students have written me over the years to tell me how much they enjoyed learning from my text, and I anticipate you will enjoy it, too.

First things first: Put aside any worry that you have over your math skills. Your admission to your current nursing or technical program guarantees that you have the ability to succeed. Clinical math is NOT complicated, and you WILL be successful. While math lends itself best to a printed text, you can also successfully use an online instructional version.

HERE ARE YOUR MOST IMPORTANT GUIDELINES FOR SUCCESS

1. The first requirement is to locate a clear writing surface, and to gather lots of scratch paper, pencils, pens, and a calculator.
2. Record your answers both in the text and on paper, which will make checking multiple answers much easier.
3. Programmed learning proceeds in small steps. Do exactly as the text instructs you to do, and no more. Jumping ahead may cause confusion.
4. All chapters allow you to proceed at your own speed, and you may be surprised at how quickly you move ahead.
5. Keep *Dimensional Analysis for Meds* in your professional library. You may move to different clinical areas in your career, and a quick refresher of contents may be helpful.

There is nothing quite like finishing a lesson and feeling like you've nailed it, and you are going to do just that using this text! So settle down, and enjoy your clinical dosage journey with me.

—Anna M. Curren

Instructor Guidelines

The content of *Dimensional Analysis for Meds (DAFM), Fifth Edition* has been carefully organized from simple to complex, concentrating most heavily on essential metric system concepts and calculations. This is reflected in our new subtitle: *Refocusing on Essential Metric Calculations. DAFM* has moved much faster than most texts to keep pace with clinical reality, and all essentials have been covered in this revised edition. Its 19 chapters have been designed for assignment in chronological order, 1 through 19.

The obvious problem in all learning is, How do I get students to do their homework? The author recommends administering a short, **graded quiz** at the start of the lecture following the first chapter assignment. Tell the students **in advance** that you will give this quiz. It takes only minutes to do, and you can have the students self-correct it, or hand off their test paper to someone in front, behind, or to one side to correct it as you give the answers. Collect the **already graded papers** and you have established a winning learning curve.

Most importantly, you can use **any** of the examples or problems in the text for testing, because it is **impossible** for students to memorize them. Once established, this routine is effective and enjoyable for all.

DAFM has been and is used extensively in programs ranging from PN/LPN to BSN, and its content has been specifically tailored to relate to both student audiences. It is easily understandable for beginning learners, and respectful of advanced learner needs to move more quickly. Educator and student feedback on their use of *DAFM* has been particularly helpful to the author over its years of publication, and once again we solicit your participation in this evaluation process. All emails to info@jblearning.com will be promptly forwarded to the author for her consideration and/or comment.

Pretest

If you can complete the Pretest with 100% accuracy, you are off to an exceptional start. But don't be alarmed if you make some errors.

The Refresher Math section in this text is designed to bring your math skills up to date. **Regardless of your math proficiency, it's important that you complete the entire Refresher Math Section**. It includes memory cues and shortcuts for simplifying and solving many of the clinical calculations that are included in the entire text, and you will need to be familiar with these strategies.

Identify the decimal fraction with the greatest value in each set.

1. (a) 4.4   (b) 2.85   (c) 5.3   _____

2. (a) 6.3   (b) 5.73   (c) 4.4   _____

3. (a) 0.18   (b) 0.62   (c) 0.35   _____

4. (a) 0.2   (b) 0.125   (c) 0.3   _____

5. (a) 0.15   (b) 0.11   (c) 0.14   _____

6. (a) 4.27   (b) 4.31   (c) 4.09   _____

7. If tablets with a strength of 0.2 mg are available and 0.6 mg is ordered, how many tablets must you give? _____

8. If tablets are labeled 0.8 mg and 0.4 mg is ordered, how many tablets must you give?

_____

9. If the available tablets have a strength of 1.25 mg and 2.5 mg is ordered, how many tablets must you give? _____

10. If 0.125 mg is ordered and the tablets available are labeled 0.25 mg, how many tablets must you give? _____

Express these numbers to the nearest tenth.

11. 2.17   = _____

12. 0.15   = _____

13. 3.77   = _____

14. 4.62   = _____

15. 11.74   = _____

16. 5.26   = _____

Express these numbers to the nearest hundredth.

17. 1.357   = _____

18. 7.413   = _____

19. 10.105   = _____

20. 3.775   = _____

21. 0.176   = _____

Multiply these decimals. Express your answers to the nearest tenth.

22. 0.7×1.2 = _____

23. 1.8×2.6 = _____

24. $5.1 \times 0.25 \times 1.1$ = _____

25. 3.3×3.75 = _____

Divide these fractions. Express your answers to the nearest hundredth.

26. $16.3 \div 3.2$ = _____

27. $15.1 \div 1.1$ = _____

28. $2 \div 0.75$ = _____

29. $4.17 \div 2.7$ = _____

Define the following terms.

30. Numerator

_____

_____

31. Denominator

_____

_____

32. Greatest common denominator

_____

_____

Solve these equations. Express your answers to the nearest tenth.

33. $\dfrac{1}{4} \times \dfrac{2}{3}$ = _____

34. $\dfrac{240}{170} \times \dfrac{135}{300}$ = _____

35. $\dfrac{0.2}{1.75} \times \dfrac{1.5}{0.2}$ = _____

36. $\dfrac{2.1}{3.6} \times \dfrac{1.7}{1.3}$ = _____

37. $\dfrac{0.26}{0.2} \times \dfrac{3.3}{1.2}$ = _____

38. $\dfrac{50}{1} \times \dfrac{60}{240} \times \dfrac{1}{900} \times \dfrac{400}{1}$ = _____

39. $\dfrac{50}{40} \times \dfrac{450}{40} \times \dfrac{1}{900} \times \dfrac{114}{1}$ = _____

ANSWERS

1. c

2. a

3. b

4. c

5. a

6. b

7. 3 tab

8. ½ tab

9. 2 tab

10. ½ tab

11. 2.2

12. 0.2

13. 3.8

14. 4.6

15. 11.7

16. 5.3

17. 1.36

18. 7.41

19. 10.11

20. 3.78

21. 0.18

22. 0.8

23. 4.7

24. 1.4

25. 12.4

26. 5.09

27. 13.73

28. 2.67

29. 1.54

30. The top number in a common fraction

31. The bottom number in a common fraction

32. The greatest number that can be divided into two numbers to reduce them to their lowest terms (values)

33. 0.2

34. 0 6

35. 0.9

36. 0.8

37. 3.6

38. 5.6

39. 1.5

Dedication

ROGER C. HAERR

Roger is a Director of the San Diego County Bar Association, and is recognized by Best of the Bar®, Top Lawyer®, and the Legal 500®. Roger rose to my challenge of obtaining reversion rights to *Dimensional Analysis for Meds* when my former publisher elected not to publish new editions of this popular text. It would take an entire book to describe the path that Roger and I took during our successful search for the perfect new publisher of the fifth edition: Jones & Bartlett Learning.

JONATHAN KIRSCH

Jon is the ultimate legal authority on everything about books of all kinds. He is an author and columnist himself, and his law practice in Los Angeles is dedicated to helping authors and fellow attorneys with every conceivable legal question. Jon is proud that his shelves are lined with the books of authors whom he has gracefully assisted, a shelf on which this fifth edition of *Dimensional Analysis for Meds* will be proudly displayed.

WILLIAM R. FREEMAN, MD

Distinguished Professor of Ophthalmology and Director of La Jolla, California's Jacobs Retina Center, Dr. Freeman's research into and treatment during my 6-year successful battle with wet macular degeneration has made it possible for me to continue writing. Dr. Freeman asked for a dedication, which will give you a good idea of how refreshing the treatment of an incurable eye disease can be with the perfect doctor.

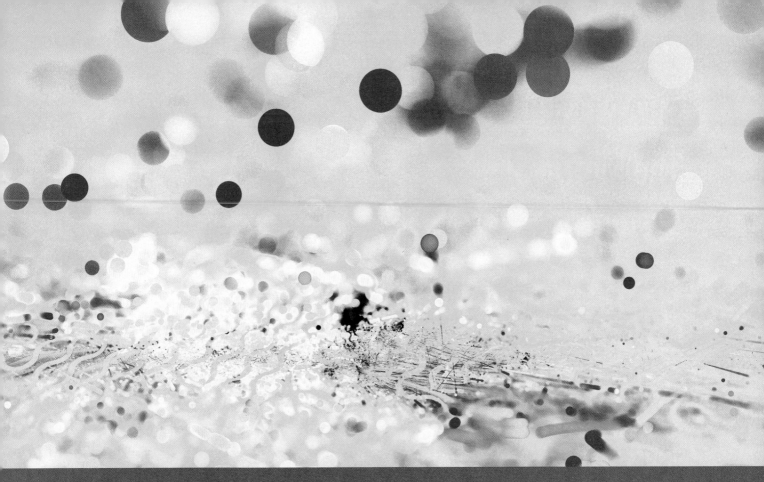

SECTION 1
The Metric System and Additional Drug Measures

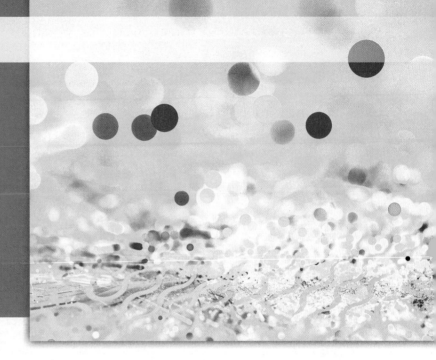

CHAPTER 1
The Metric/SI System

OBJECTIVES

The learner will:

1. Identify the relative value of decimal numbers.

2. List the commonly used units of measure in the metric system.

3. Express metric weights and volumes using correct notation rules.

4. Convert metric weights and volumes within the system.

PREREQUISITE

Sixth Grade Math

INTRODUCTION

You will all have at least some familiarity with the metric system. Canada went completely metric in 1975, but the United States did not, so miles for distance, pounds and ounces for weight, and gallons for volume are still in common use in the United States.

Invented in France in 1875 as the **Systemé International (SI)**, the metric system is **a decimal system**, in which all units of measure for weight, volume, or length **relate to each other**.

This is incredibly important in the physical sciences, commerce, **and dosage calculations**, because **values can be changed from one unit to another by simply moving a decimal point**, and **multiple-step calculations can be reduced to a single equation**.

Clinical medicine and drug dosages went metric decades ago, and 98% of all clinical calculations you do will involve the metric system.

Both the U.S. and Canadian currencies of dollars and cents are decimal systems.

So, since you already know **how to count money**, you already know **how to recognize the value of decimal numbers in drug dosages**. That said, a quick refresher in the relative value of decimal numbers commonly seen in dosages is the logical place to start your introduction to the metric system.

RELATIVE VALUE OF DECIMAL NUMBERS

The whole numbers in dosages have the same relative value as dollars, and decimal fractions have the same value as cents: **The greater the number, the greater the value**.

The range of drug dosages, which includes decimal fractions, stretches from millions on the whole number side, to thousandths on the decimal side. Refer to the decimal scale in **Figure 1-1**, and locate the decimal point, which is slightly to the right on this scale. Notice the whole numbers on the left of the scale, which rise in value from ones (units) to millions, which is the largest whole-number drug dosage in current use.

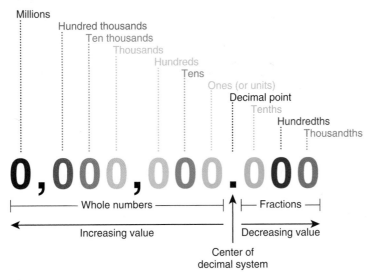

Figure 1-1

🔑 The first determiner of the relative value of decimals is the presence of whole numbers. The greater the whole number, the greater the value.

EXAMPLE 1   10.1 is greater than 9.15

EXAMPLE 2   3.2 is greater than 2.99

EXAMPLE 3   7.01 is greater than 6.99

PROBLEMS 1-1

Choose the greatest value in each set.

1. (a) 3.5   (b) 2.7   (c) 4.2   _____

2. (a) 6.15   (b) 5.95   (c) 4.54   _____

3. (a) 12.02   (b) 10.19   (c) 11.04   _____

4. (a) 2.5   (b) 1.75   (c) 0.75   _____

5.	(a) 4.3	(b) 2.75	(c) 5.1	_____
6.	(a) 6.15	(b) 7.4	(c) 5.95	_____
7.	(a) 7.25	(b) 8.1	(c) 9.37	_____
8.	(a) 4.25	(b) 5.1	(c) 3.75	_____
9.	(a) 9.4	(b) 8.75	(c) 7.4	_____
10.	(a) 5.1	(b) 6.33	(c) 4.2	_____

Answers **1.** c   **2.** a   **3.** a   **4.** a   **5.** c   **6.** b   **7.** c   **8.** b   **9.** a   **10.** b

If, however, the whole numbers are the same—for example, **10.**2 and **10.**7—or if there are no whole numbers—for example, **0.**25 and **0.**35—**then the fraction will determine the relative value.** Let's take a closer look at the fractional side of the scale (refer to **Figure 1-2**).

It is necessary to **consider only three figures after the decimal point on the fractional side**, because drug dosages measured as decimal fractions do not contain more than three digits, for example, 0.125 mg. Notice that a **zero is used to replace the whole number** in this decimal fraction and in all dosages that do not contain a whole number.

> 🔑 If a decimal fraction is not preceded by a whole number, a zero is used in front of the decimal point to emphasize that the number is a fraction.

EXAMPLE 4   **0.**125   **0.**1   **0.**45

Look again at Figure 1-2. The numbers to the right of the decimal point represent **tenths**, **hundredths**, and **thousandths**, in that order. When you see a decimal fraction in which the **whole numbers are the same**, or if there are **no whole numbers**, stop and look first at the number representing **tenths**.

> 🔑 The fraction with the greater number representing tenths has the greater value.

EXAMPLE 5   0.3 is greater than 0.27

EXAMPLE 6   0.4 is greater than 0.29

EXAMPLE 7   1.2 is greater than 1.19

EXAMPLE 8   3.5 is greater than 3.2

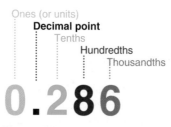

Ones (or units)
Decimal point
Tenths
Hundredths
Thousandths

0.286

Figure 1-2

PROBLEMS 1-2

Choose the greatest value in each set.

1. (a) 0.4   (b) 0.2   (c) 0.5   _____

2. (a) 2.73   (b) 2.61   (c) 2.87   _____

3. (a) 0.19   (b) 0.61   (c) 0.34   _____

4. (a) 3.5   (b) 3.75   (c) 3.25   _____

5. (a) 0.3   (b) 0.25   (c) 0.4   _____

6. (a) 1.35   (b) 1.29   (c) 1.4   _____

7. (a) 2.5   (b) 2.7   (c) 2.35   _____

8. (a) 4.51   (b) 4.75   (c) 4.8   _____

9. (a) 0.8   (b) 0.3   (c) 0.4   _____

10. (a) 2.1   (b) 2.05   (c) 2.15   _____

Answers 1. c   2. c   3. b   4. b   5. c   6. c   7. b   8. c   9. a   10. c

If in decimal fractions the numbers representing **the tenths are identical**—for example, 0.25 and 0.27—then **the number representing the hundredths will determine the relative value**.

⚷ When the tenths are identical, the fraction with the greater number representing hundredths will have the greater value.

EXAMPLE 9   0.**27** is greater than 0.**25**

EXAMPLE 10   0.**15** is greater than 0.1 (0.1 is the same as 0.**10**)

⚷ Extra zeros on the end of decimal fractions are omitted in drug dosages because they can easily be misread and lead to errors.

EXAMPLE 11   2.25 is greater than 2.2 (same as 2.20)

EXAMPLE 12   9.77 is greater than 9.7 (same as 9.70)

PROBLEMS 1-3

Choose the greatest value in each set.

1. (a) 0.12   (b) 0.15   (c) 0.17   _____

2. (a) 1.2   (b) 1.24   (c) 1.23   _____

3. (a) 0.37   (b) 0.3   (c) 0.36   _____

4. (a) 3.27   (b) 3.25   (c) 3.21   _____

5. (a) 0.16   (b) 0.11   (c) 0.19   _____

6. (a) 4.23   (b) 4.2   (c) 4.09   _____

7. (a) 3.27   (b) 3.21   (c) 3.29   _____

8. (a) 2.75   (b) 2.73   (c) 2.78   _____

9. (a) 0.31   (b) 0.37   (c) 0.33   _____

10. (a) 0.43   (b) 0.45   (c) 0.44   _____

Answers 1. c   2. b   3. a   4. a   5. c   6. a   7. c   8. c   9. b   10. b

PROBLEM 1-4

Which fraction has the greater value?

(a) 0.125   (b) 0.25   _____

Answer: If you chose 0.125, you have just made a serious drug dosage error. Look again at the numbers representing the tenths, and you will see that 0.**25** is greater than 0.**1**25. Remember that extra zeros are omitted in decimal fraction dosages because they can lead to errors. In this fraction, 0.25 is the same as 0.250, which is exactly double the value of 0.125. **Check the tenths carefully, regardless of the total of numbers after the decimal point.**

EXAMPLE 13 0.15 (same as 0.150) is greater than 0.125

EXAMPLE 14 0.3 (same as 0.30) is greater than 0.15

EXAMPLE 15 0.75 (same as 0.750) is greater than 0.325

EXAMPLE 16 0.8 (same as 0.80) is greater than 0.16

⚬┬ The number of figures on the right of the decimal point is not an indication of relative value. Always look at the figure representing the tenths first, and if these are identical, check the hundredths to determine which has the greater value.

This completes your introduction to the relative value of decimals. The key points just reviewed will cover all situations in dosage calculations in which you have to recognize greater and lesser values. Test yourself more extensively on this information in the following problems.

PROBLEMS 1-5

Choose the greatest value in each set.

1. (a) 0.24   (b) 0.5   (c) 0.125   _____

2. (a) 0.4   (b) 0.45   (c) 0.5   _____

3. (a) 7.5   (b) 6.25   (c) 4.75   _____

4. (a) 0.3   (b) 0.25   (c) 0.35   _____

5. (a) 1.125   (b) 1.75   (c) 1.5   _____

6. (a) 4.5   (b) 4.75   (c) 4.25   _____

7. (a) 0.1   (b) 0.01   (c) 0.04   _____

8. (a) 5.75   (b) 6.25   (c) 6.5   _____

9. (a) 0.6   (b) 0.16   (c) 0.06   _____

10. (a) 3.55   (b) 2.95   (c) 3.7   _____

Answers 1. b   **2.** c   **3.** a   **4.** c   **5.** b   **6.** b   **7.** a   **8.** c   **9.** a   **10.** c

BASIC UNITS OF THE METRIC/SI SYSTEM

Three types of metric measures are in common clinical use: those for **length**, **volume** (or capacity), and **weight**. The basic units of these measures are:

Length: meter

Volume: liter

Weight: gram

Memorize the basic units if you do not already know them.

In addition to the basic units, **there are both larger and smaller units of measure** for length, volume, and weight. Let's compare this concept with something familiar. The pound is a unit of weight that we use every day. A smaller unit of measure is the ounce; a larger unit, the ton. **However, all of these units measure weight**.

In the same way, there are smaller and larger units than the basic meter, liter, and gram. In the metric system, however, there is one very important advantage: **All other units, whether larger or smaller than the basic units, have the name of the basic unit incorporated in them**. So, when you see a unit of metric measure, there is no doubt what it is measuring: **meter—length**, **liter—volume**, and **gram—weight**.

PROBLEMS 1-6

Identify the metric measures with their appropriate category of weight, length, or volume.

1. milligram   _____

2. centimeter   _____

3. milliliter   _____

4. millimeter   _____

5. kilogram   _____

6. microgram _____

7. kilometer   _____

8. kiloliter   _____

Answers 1. weight   **2.** length   **3.** volume   **4.** length   **5.** weight   **6.** weight   **7.** length   **8.** volume

METRIC/SI PREFIXES

Prefixes are used in combination with the names of the basic units to identify larger and smaller units of measure. The same prefixes are used with all three measures. Therefore, there is a kilo**meter**, kilo**gram**, and a kilo**liter**.

> ⛏ Identical prefixes are used to identify units that are larger or smaller than the basic metric measures.

Prefixes also change the value of each of the basic units by the same amount. For example, the prefix "kilo" identifies a unit of measure that is larger than (or multiplies) the basic unit by 1000.

$$1 \text{ kilometer} = 1000 \text{ meters}$$

$$1 \text{ kilogram} = 1000 \text{ grams}$$

$$1 \text{ kiloliter} = 1000 \text{ liters}$$

Kilo is the **only** prefix you will be using in the clinical setting that identifies a measure **larger** than the basic unit. Kilograms are frequently used as a measure for body weight, especially for infants and children.

You will see only three measures **smaller** than the basic unit in common clinical use. The prefixes for these are:

milli (as in milligram) for weight

micro (as in microgram) for weight

centi (as in centimeter) for length

Therefore, you will actually be working with only four prefixes: **kilo**, which identifies a larger unit of measure than the basic unit; and **milli**, **micro**, and **centi**, which identify smaller units than the basic unit.

METRIC/SI ABBREVIATIONS

In clinical use, units of metric measure are abbreviated.

> ⛏ The basic units are abbreviated to their first initial and printed in small (lowercase) letters, with the exception of liter, which is capitalized (uppercase).

meter is abbreviated **m**

gram is abbreviated **g**

liter is abbreviated **L**

O— The abbreviations for the prefixes used in combination with the basic units are all printed using small letters.

kilo is **k** (as in kilogram—kg)

milli is **m** (as in milligram—mg)

micro is **mc** (as in microgram—mcg)

centi is **c** (as in centimeter—cm)

In combination, liter remains capitalized. Therefore, milliliter is **mL** and kiloliter is **kL**.

PROBLEMS 1-7

Abbreviate the following metric units.

1. microgram _____

2. liter _____

3. kilogram _____

4. milliliter _____

5. centimeter _____

6. milligram _____

7. meter _____

8. kiloliter _____

9. millimeter _____

10. gram _____

Answers **1.** mcg **2.** L **3.** kg **4.** mL **5.** cm **6.** mg **7.** m **8.** kL **9.** mm **10.** g

METRIC/SI NOTATION RULES

To remember the rules of metric **notation**, in which **a unit of measure is expressed with a quantity**, it is helpful to memorize some prototypes (examples) that incorporate all the rules. For the metric system, the notations for one-half, one, and one and one-half milliliters incorporate all the official notation rules.

Prototype notations: **0.5 mL**   **1 mL**   **1.5 mL**

RULE 1: The quantity is written in Arabic numerals: 1, 2, 3, 4, and so forth.

Example 1 0.5   1   1.5

RULE 2: The numerals representing the quantity are placed in front of the abbreviations.

Example 2 0.5 mL   1 mL   1.5 mL   (**not** mL 0.5, mL 1, mL 1.5)

RULE 3: A full space is used between the numeral and the abbreviation.

    Example 3   0.5 mL   1 mL   1.5 mL   (**not** 0.5mL, 1mL, 1.5mL)

RULE 4: Fractional parts of a unit are expressed as decimal fractions.

    Example 4   0.5 mL   1.5 mL   (**not** ½ mL, 1½ mL)

RULE 5: A zero is placed in front of the decimal when it is not preceded by a whole number to emphasize the decimal point.

    Example 5   0.5 mL   (**not** .5 mL)

RULE 6: Excess zeros following a decimal fraction are eliminated.

    Example 6   0.5 mL   1 mL   1.5 mL   (**no**t 0.50 mL, 1.0 mL, 1.50 mL)

PROBLEMS 1-8

Write the metric measures using official abbreviations and notation rules.

1. two grams   _____

2. five hundred milliliters   _____

3. five-tenths of a liter   _____

4. two-tenths of a milligram   _____

5. five-hundredths of a gram   _____

6. two and five-tenths kilograms   _____

7. one hundred micrograms   _____

8. two and three-tenths milliliters   _____

9. seven-tenths of a milliliter   _____

10. three-tenths of a milligram   _____

11. two and four-tenths liters   _____

12. seventeen and five-tenths kilograms   _____

13. nine-hundredths of a milligram   _____

14. ten and two-tenths micrograms   _____

15. four-hundredths of a gram   _____

Answers 1. 2 g   **2.** 500 mL   **3.** 0.5 L   **4.** 0.2 mg   **5.** 0.05 g   **6.** 2.5 kg   **7.** 100 mcg   **8.** 2.3 mL
9. 0.7 mL   **10.** 0.3 mg   **11.** 2.4 L   **12.** 17.5 kg   **13.** 0.09 mg   **14.** 10.2 mcg   **15.** 0.04 g

CONVERSION BETWEEN METRIC/SI UNITS

When you administer medications, you will be routinely **converting units of measure within the metric system**—for example, g to mg and mg to mcg. Learning the relative value of the units with which you will be working is the first prerequisite for accurate conversions.

There are only four metric **weights** commonly used in medicine. From **greater** to **lesser** value, these are:

kg	=	kilogram
g	=	gram
mg	=	milligram
mcg	=	microgram

Only two units of **volume** are frequently used. From **greater** to **lesser** value, these are:

L	=	liter
mL	=	milliliter

Each of these clinical metric measures differs from the next by 1000.

1 kg	=	1000 g
1 g	=	1000 mg
1 mg	=	1000 mcg
1 L	=	1000 mL

Once again, from greater to lesser value, the units are, for weight, kg—g—mg—mcg, and for volume, L—mL. Each unit differs in value from the next by 1000, and **all conversions will be between touching units of measure**—for example, g to mg, mg to mcg, and L to mL.

PROBLEMS 1-9

Choose true (T) or false (F) for each conversion.

1. T	F	1000 mL	=	1000 L
2. T	F	1000 mg	=	1 g
3. T	F	1000 g	=	1 kg
4. T	F	1000 mg	=	1 mcg
5. T	F	1000 mcg	=	1 g
6. T	F	1 kg	=	1000 g
7. T	F	1 mg	=	1000 g

8. T	F	1000 mcg	=	1 mg
9. T	F	1 g	=	100 mcg
10. T	F	1000 L	=	1 kL

Answers 1. F   2. T   3. T   4. F   5. F   6. T   7. F   8. T   9. F   10. T

Because the metric system is a decimal system, **conversions between the units are accomplished by moving the decimal point**. Also, because each unit of measure in clinical use differs from the next by 1000, if you know one conversion, you know them all.

How far do you move the decimal point? There is an unforgettable memory cue that you can use with **all** metric conversions. There are **three zeros in 1000**. The decimal point moves **three places**, the **same number of places as the zeros** in the conversion.

> 🔑 In metric conversions between touching units of clinical measures differing by 1000, the decimal point is moved three places, the same as the number of zeros in 1000.

CONVERTING TO A SMALLER UNIT OF METRIC MEASURE

If you are converting to a **smaller** unit of measure—for example, g to mg or L to mL—the **quantity must get larger**. The decimal point must move three places to the **right**.

EXAMPLE 1   0.5 g = _____ mg

You are converting to smaller units of measure, from **g to mg**, so the quantity will be **larger**. Move the decimal point **three places to the right**. To do this, you must **add two zeros** to the end of the quantity, and **eliminate the zero in front** of it. The larger 500 mg quantity indicates that you have moved the decimal point in the correct direction.

$$0.5 \text{ g} = .500. \text{ mg} \qquad \text{Move the decimal three places to the right}$$

Answer: 0.5 g = 500 mg

EXAMPLE 2   2.5 L = _____ mL

You are converting to smaller units of measure, so the quantity will be **larger**. Move the decimal point **three places to the right**. To do this, you must **add two zeros**. The larger 2500 mL quantity indicates that you have moved the decimal point in the correct direction.

$$2.5 \text{ L} = 2.500. \text{ mL}$$

Answer: 2.5 L = 2500 mL

PROBLEMS 1-10

Convert the metric measures.

1. 7 mg   = _____ mcg

2. 1.7 L   = _____ mL

3. 3.2 g   = _____ mg

4. 0.03 kg   = _____ g

5. 0.4 mg   = _____ mcg

6. 1.5 mg   = _____ mcg

7. 0.7 g   = _____ mg

8. 0.3 L   = _____ mL

9. 7 kg   = _____ g

10. 0.01 mg   = _____ mcg

Answers 1. 7000 mcg   **2.** 1700 mL   **3.** 3200 mg   **4.** 30 g   **5.** 400 mcg   **6.** 1500 mcg   **7.** 700 mg
8. 300 mL   **9.** 7000 g   **10.** 10 mcg

CONVERTING TO A LARGER UNIT OF METRIC MEASURE

In metric conversions from **smaller to larger units** of measurement, such as mL to L and mcg to mg, the quantity will be **smaller**. The decimal point is moved **three places to the left**.

EXAMPLE 1   200 mL = _____ L

You are converting to a larger unit of measure, **mL** to **L**, so the quantity will be **smaller**. Move the decimal point **three places to the left**.

.200. mL = .200 L

Eliminate the two unnecessary zeros at the end of the quantity (to make it .2), then add a zero in front of the decimal point to correctly write the dosage as 0.2 L.

Answer: 200 mL = 0.2 L

EXAMPLE 2   1500 mcg = _____mg

You are converting to a larger unit of measure, so the quantity will be smaller. Move the decimal point **three places to the left**. **Place a decimal point in front of** the 5, and **eliminate the two zeros** after the 5.

1.500. mcg = 1.500 mg

Answer: 1500 mcg = 1.5 mg

EXAMPLE 3   300 mcg = _____ mg

You are converting to a larger unit of measure, **mcg** to **mg**, so the quantity will be **smaller**. Move the decimal point **three places to the left**.

.300. mcg = .300 mg

Eliminate two zeros from the end of this decimal fraction (to make it .3), and place a zero in front of the decimal point to complete the decimal fraction.

Answer: 300 mcg = 0.3 mg

PROBLEMS 1-11

Convert the metric measures.

1. 3500 mL = _____ L

2. 520 mg = _____ g

3. 1800 mcg = _____ mg

4. 750 mL = _____ L

5. 150 mg = _____ g

6. 250 mcg = _____ mg

7. 1200 mg = _____ g

8. 600 mL = _____ L

9. 100 mg = _____ g

10. 950 mcg = _____ mg

Answers **1.** 3.5 L **2.** 0.52 g **3.** 1.8 mg **4.** 0.75 L **5.** 0.15 g **6.** 0.25 mg **7.** 1.2 g **8.** 0.6 L **9.** 0.1 g **10.** 0.95 mg

COMMON ERRORS IN METRIC/SI DOSAGES

Most errors in the metric system occur because orders are not written using correct notation rules, or they are not transcribed correctly. **Errors usually involve decimal fractions**. Even though you have just finished learning metric notation rules, let's review the most common errors.

One error is the **failure to enter a zero in front of a decimal point**—for example, .2 mg instead of 0.2 mg. Regardless of the presence of a zero in front of the decimal in a written order, one must be added when the order is transcribed to a medication administration record.

⚷ Fractional dosages in the metric system are transcribed with a zero in front of the decimal point.

Another common error is to **include zeros where they should not be**—for example, to write 2.**0** mg instead of 2 mg or to write .**20** mg instead of 0.2 mg. Each error can be misread as 20 mg, a dosage greatly in excess of the intended dosage.

⚷ Eliminate unnecessary zeros when transcribing metric dosages.

Errors are also more likely to occur in **calculations that include decimal fractions**. The presence of a decimal fraction in a calculation raises a warning flag, indicating that you should slow down and double-check all math. **Use your reasoning powers**. If a decimal is misplaced, the answer will be a minimum of 10 times too large or 10 times too small. **Question quantities that seem unreasonable**. A 1.5 mL intramuscular (IM) injection dosage makes sense, but a 0.15 mL or 15 mL does not, and this is the type of error you might see.

⚷ Question orders and calculations that seem unreasonably large or small.

Other potential sources of errors are **conversions within the metric system**. Errors in conversions can be eliminated by thinking **three**. All conversions between the g, mg, mcg, mL, and L measures are accomplished by moving the decimal point **three** places—always and forever. There are not many things for which you can use the words "always" and "forever," but converting between these units of measure in the metric system is one of those rare instances.

> 🔑 Conversions between g, mg, mcg, mL, and L units of measure in metric measures require moving the decimal point three places.

Be constantly mindful of these problem areas to become a safe clinical practitioner.

SUMMARY

This concludes the refresher on the metric system. The important points to remember from this chapter are:

- If a decimal fraction contains a whole number, the value of the whole number is the first determiner of relative value.

- If a fraction does not include a whole number, a zero is placed in front of the decimal point to emphasize that it is a fractional dosage.

- If there is no whole number, or if the whole numbers are the same, the number representing the tenths in the decimal fraction will be the next determiner of relative value.

- If the tenths in decimal fractions are identical, the number representing hundredths will determine relative value.

- The meter (m), liter (L), and gram (g) are the basic units of metric measure.

- Only the abbreviation for liter, L, is capitalized.

- Larger and smaller units than the basics are identified by the use of prefixes.

- The prefixes are printed using small (lowercase) letters.

- The one larger unit you will be seeing is the kilo, whose prefix is k.

- The smaller units you will be seeing are milli (m), micro (mc), and centi (c).

- Each prefix changes the value of a basic unit by the same amount.

- Converting from one unit to another within the system is accomplished by moving a decimal point.

- When you convert from larger to smaller units of measurement, the quantity will increase.

- To convert from larger to smaller units, move the decimal point to the right.

- When you convert from smaller to larger units of measurement, the quantity will be smaller.

- To convert from smaller to larger units, move the decimal point to the left.

- Conversions from g to mg, mg to mcg, and mL to L all require moving the decimal point three places.

- Fractional dosages are transcribed with a zero in front of the decimal point.

- Unnecessary zeros are eliminated from dosages.

SUMMARY SELF-TEST

List the basic units of measure of the metric system and the measure they are used for.

1. _____ _____

   _____ _____

   _____ _____

Identify the official metric/SI abbreviations.

2. (a) L
   (b) g
   (c) kL
   (d) mgm
   (e) mg
   (f) kg
   (g) ml
   (h) G

   _____

Use official metric abbreviations and notation rules to express these as numerals.

3. six-hundredths of a milligram   _____

4. three hundred and ten milliliters   _____

5. three-tenths of a kilogram   _____

6. four-tenths of a milliliter   _____

7. one and five-tenths grams   _____

8. one-hundredth of a gram   _____

9. four thousand milliliters   _____

10. one and two-tenths milligrams   _____

List the four commonly used clinical units of weight and the two of volume from greater to lesser value.

11. Weight _____ _____ _____ _____

    Volume _____ _____

Convert the metric measures.

12. 160 mg   = _____ g

13. 10 kg   = _____ g

14. 1500 mcg   = _____ mg

15. 750 mg   = _____ g

16. 200 mL   = _____ L

17. 0.3 g   = _____ mg

18. 0.05 g   = _____ mg

19. 0.15 g   = _____ mg

20. 1.2 L   = _____ mL

21. 1800 mL   = _____ L

22. 2 mg   = _____ mcg

23. 900 mcg   = _____ mg

24. 2.1 L   = _____ mL

25. 475 mL   = _____ L

26. 0.9 L   = _____ mL

27. 300 mg   = _____ g

28. 2.5 mg   = _____ mcg

29. 1 kL   = _____ L

30. 3 L   = _____ mL

31. 2 L   = _____ mL

32. 0.7 mg   = _____ mcg

33. 4 g   = _____ mg

34. 1000 mL   = _____ L

35. 2500 mL   = _____ L

36. 1000 mg   = _____ g

37. 0.2 mg   = _____ mcg

38. 2000 g   = _____ kg

39. 1.4 g   = _____ mg

40. 2.5 L   = _____ mL

Answers

1. gram, weight;
   liter, volume;
   meter, length
2. a, b, c, e, f
3. 0.06 mg
4. 310 mL
5. 0.3 kg
6. 0.4 mL
7. 1.5 g
8. 0.01 g
9. 4000 mL

10. 1.2 mg
11. kg, g, mg, mcg;
    L, mL
12. 0.16 g
13. 10,000 g
14. 1.5 mg
15. 0.75 g
16. 0.2 L
17. 300 mg
18. 50 mg
19. 150 mg

20. 1200 mL
21. 1.8 L
22. 2000 mcg
23. 0.9 mg
24. 2100 mL
25. 0.475 L
26. 900 mL
27. 0.3 g
28. 2500 mcg
29. 1000 L
30. 3000 mL

31. 2000 mL
32. 700 mcg
33. 4000 mg
34. 1 L
35. 2.5 L
36. 1 g
37. 200 mcg
38. 2 kg
39. 1400 mg
40. 2500 mL

CHAPTER 2

Additional Drug Measures: Units, Percentage, Milliequivalent, Ratio, and Household

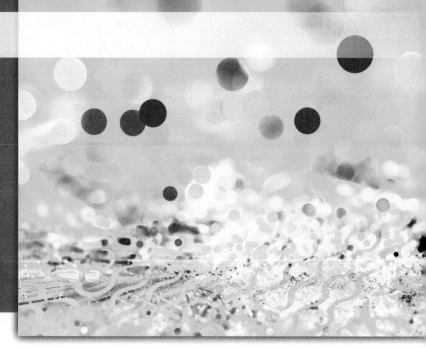

OBJECTIVES

The learner will recognize dosages:

1. Measured in units.

2. Measured as percentages.

3. Using ratio strengths.

4. In milliequivalents.

5. In household measures.

INTRODUCTION

Although metric measures predominate in medications, there are several other measures frequently used, particularly in parenteral (injectable) solutions, that are important for you to know. In addition, you must be familiar with several measures in the household system because you may occasionally see these.

INTERNATIONAL UNITS (units)

A unit **measures a drug in terms of its action**, not its physical weight. The word "units" is **not abbreviated; it is written in lowercase using Arabic numerals in front of the measure, with a space between**—for example, 2000 units or 1,000,000 units. **Commas are not usually used in a quantity unless it has at least five numbers**—for example, 45,000 units. A number of drugs are measured in international units; insulin, penicillin, and heparin are commonly seen examples. Antibiotics, such as penicillin, have dosages in the hundredths of thousands and millions, and heparin has dosages in the thousandths.

PROBLEMS 2-1

Express the unit dosages in numerals.

1. two hundred and fifty thousand units   _____

2. ten units   _____

3. five thousand units   _____

4. forty-four units   _____

5. forty thousand units   _____

6. one million units   _____

7. one thousand units   _____

8. twenty-five hundred units   _____

9. thirty-four units   _____

10. one hundred units   _____

Answers 1. 250,000 units   **2.** 10 units   **3.** 5000 units   **4.** 44 units   **5.** 40,000 units   **6.** 1,000,000 units
7. 1000 units   **8.** 2500 units   **9.** 34 units   **10.** 100 units

PERCENTAGE (%)

Percentage strengths are used extensively in intravenous solutions, and somewhat less commonly for a variety of other medications, including eye and topical (for external use) ointments. **Percentage (%) means parts per hundred. The greater the percentage strength, the stronger the solution or ointment**; for example, 3% is stronger than 1%. Fractional percentages are expressed as decimal fractions—for example, 0.45%. Notice that, unlike other written dosages, percentages are generally written with **no space between the quantity and percentage sign**.

⚷ In solutions, percent represents the number of grams of drug per 100 mL of solution.

EXAMPLE 1   100 mL of a 1% solution will contain 1 g of drug.

EXAMPLE 2   100 mL of a 2.5% solution will contain 2.5 g of drug.

EXAMPLE 3   100 mL of a 10% solution will contain 10 g of drug.

EXAMPLE 4   100 mL of a 0.9% solution will contain 0.9 g of drug.

⚷ These examples are included to point out that percentage solutions contain a significant amount of drug or other solute, and that reading percentage labels requires the same care as that used with other drug dosages.

MILLIEQUIVALENT (mEq)

Milliequivalents (**mEq**) is **an expression of the number of grams of a drug contained in 1 mL of a normal solution**. This is a definition that is quite understandable to a pharmacist or chemist, but you need not memorize it. Milliequivalent dosages are also written using **Arabic numerals**, with a space between the **abbreviation that follows**—for example, 30 mEq. You will see milliequivalents used in a variety of oral and parenteral solutions, potassium chloride being a common intravenous example.

PROBLEMS 2-2

Express the milliequivalent dosages in numerals.

1. sixty milliequivalents   _____

2. fifteen milliequivalents   _____

3. forty milliequivalents   _____

4. one milliequivalent   _____

5. fifty milliequivalents   _____

6. eighty milliequivalents   _____

7. fifty-five milliequivalents   _____

8. seventy milliequivalents   _____

9. thirty milliequivalents   _____

10. twenty milliequivalents   _____

Answers 1. 60 mEq **2.** 15 mEq **3.** 40 mEq **4.** 1 mEq **5.** 50 mEq **6.** 80 mEq **7.** 55 mEq **8.** 70 mEq **9.** 30 mEq **10.** 20 mEq

---

RATIO

Ratio strengths are used primarily in solutions. They represent **parts of drug per parts of solution**—for example, 1 : 1000 (one part drug to 1000 parts solution).

> **EXAMPLE 1**   A 1 : 100 strength solution has 1 part drug in 100 parts solution.

> **EXAMPLE 2**   A 1 : 5 solution contains 1 part drug in 5 parts solution.

> **EXAMPLE 3**   A solution that is 1 part drug in 2 parts solution would be written 1 : 2.

🔑 The less solution a drug is dissolved in, the stronger the solution.

For example, a ratio strength of 1 : 10 (1 part drug to 10 parts solution) is much stronger than a 1 : 100 (1 part drug in 100 parts solution).

Ratio strengths are always expressed in their **simplest terms**. For example, 2 : 10 would be incorrect because it can be reduced to 1 : 5. Notice that ratio dosages are written separated by a colon, with a space between both numbers and the colon. Dosages using ratio strengths are not common, but you do need to know what they represent.

PROBLEMS 2-3

Express as ratios.

1. 1 part drug to 200 parts solution _____

2. 1 part drug to 4 parts solution _____

3. 1 part drug to 7 parts solution _____

Identify the strongest solution.

4. (a) 1 : 20   (b) 1 : 200   (c) 1 : 2

5. (a) 1 : 50   (b) 1 : 20   (c) 1 : 100

6. (a) 1 : 1000   (b) 1 : 5000   (c) 1 : 2000

Answers 1. 1 : 200   **2.** 1 : 4   **3.** 1 : 7   **4.** c   **5.** b   **6.** a

HOUSEHOLD

Household measures are most often used in the home care setting, and their clinical use is becoming less frequent. The measures you may occasionally see include the **ounce**, **tablespoon**, and **teaspoon**. Abbreviations and/or names for all of these measures, except the drop, **still appear on many disposable medication cups**, and care must be taken not to confuse them with metric dosages. It is quite possible that these measures will be eliminated in the future because the healthcare industry has been moving rapidly to improve dosage labeling and medication abbreviation guidelines to reduce the possibility of errors.

The various abbreviations for household dosages and their metric equivalents are in **Table 2-1**.

TABLE 2-1 Household Measures		
Household Measure	**Abbreviation**	**Metric Equivalent**
ounce	oz	30 mL
tablespoon	T, TBS, tbs	15 mL
teaspoon	t, TSP, tsp	5 mL
dram	dr	4 mL
drop	gtt	

Because metric and household measures are calibrated on the disposable paper and plastic medication cups used in clinical settings, take a moment to read them now on the medication cups provided in **Figure 2-1**.

When measuring liquid dosages using these medication cups, be careful to **line up the correct calibration set you are measuring**.

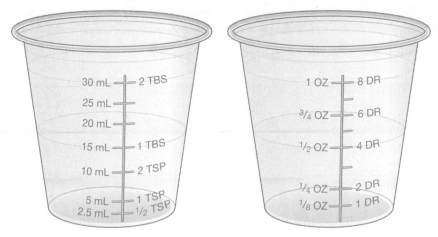

Figure 2-1

🗝 Accurate measurement of solution dosages using a medication cup requires that they be poured and read at eye level.

🗝 The volume of a drop depends on the size of the dropper being used.

A drop is so inaccurate a measure that medication droppers are now an integral part of small-volume liquid medication preparations. The use of drops is largely restricted to eye and ear drop use. One exception is in small-volume pediatric liquid medications, which are prepared with **integral medicine droppers that are calibrated by volume, or by actual dosage**.

SUMMARY

This concludes your introduction to the additional measures you will see used in dosages and in solutions. The important points to remember from this chapter are:

- International units measure a drug by its action, rather than by its weight.
- There is no abbreviation for units; it is written in full, units, in lowercase letters.
- Percentage (%) strengths are frequently used in solutions and ointments.
- Percent represents grams of drug per 100 mL of solution.
- The greater the percentage strength, the stronger the solution.
- Milliequivalent is abbreviated mEq and is frequently used in solution measurements.
- Ratio strengths represent parts of drug per parts of solution.
- The smaller the volume of solution, the greater the ratio strength.
- T or tbs is the abbreviation for tablespoon (15 mL), and t or tsp for teaspoon (5 mL).
- The abbreviation gtt is used for drop, and oz for ounce.

SUMMARY SELF-TEST

Express the dosages using the official symbols/abbreviations.

1. three hundred thousand units   _____

2. forty-five units   _____

3. ten percent   _____

4. two and a half percent   _____

5. forty milliequivalents   _____

6. a one in two thousand ratio   _____

7. a one in ten ratio   _____

8. one percent   _____

9. one drop   _____

10. two thousand units   _____

11. five milliequivalents   _____

12. nine-tenths percent   _____

13. ten units   _____

14. a one in two ratio   _____

15. five percent   _____

16. twenty milliequivalents   _____

17. fourteen units   _____

18. twenty percent   _____

19. two million units   _____

20. one hundred thousand units   _____

Answers

1. 300,000 units	**6.** 1 : 2000	**11.** 5 mEq	**16.** 20 mEq
2. 45 units	**7.** 1 : 10	**12.** 0.9%	**17.** 14 units
3. 10%	**8.** 1%	**13.** 10 units	**18.** 20%
4. 2.5%	**9.** 1 gtt	**14.** 1 : 2	**19.** 2,000,000 units
5. 40 mEq	**10.** 2000 units	**15.** 5%	**20.** 100,000 units

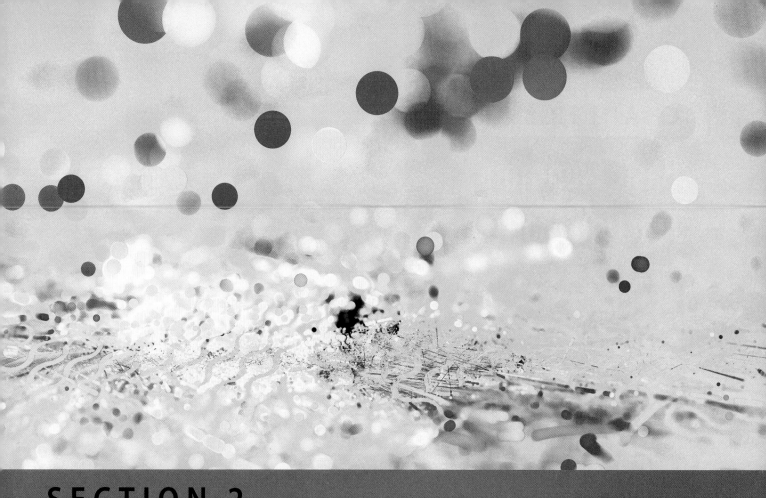

SECTION 2
Refresher Math

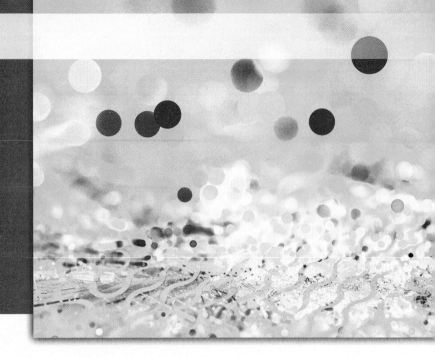

CHAPTER 3

Basic Common Fraction Math

OBJECTIVES

The learner will:

1. Multiply decimal fractions.

2. Divide decimal fractions.

3. Define product, numerator, and denominator.

4. Simplify common fractions containing decimal numbers.

5. Reduce fractions using common denominators.

6. Reduce common fractions that end in zeros.

7. Express answers to the nearest tenth and hundredth.

8. Use a calculator to multiply and divide.

INTRODUCTION

In a later chapter, you will learn how to enter multiple drug dosage information into a single common fraction equation to calculate an unknown, X, using dimensional analysis. However, since many drugs include **decimal dosages**, the logical place to start is by revisiting the math of decimal fraction numbers. This chapter will also introduce you to several ways to simplify decimal numbers in equations.

MULTIPLICATION OF DECIMALS

The main precaution in multiplication of decimals is the **placement of the decimal point in the answer**, which is called the **product**.

🔑 The decimal point in the product of decimal fractions is placed the same number of places to the left in the product as the total of numbers following the decimal points in the fractions multiplied.

EXAMPLE 1   Multiply 0.35 by 0.5

It is safer to begin by lining up the numbers to be multiplied on the right side. Then, disregard the decimals during multiplication.

$$
\begin{array}{r}
0.35 \\
\times\ \underline{0.5} \\
175
\end{array}
$$

The product/answer is 175; 0.35 has two numbers after the decimal and 0.5 has one. Place the decimal point three places to the left in the product to make it .175, then add a zero (0) in front of the decimal to emphasize the fraction.

Answer: 0.175

EXAMPLE 2   Multiply 1.61 by 0.2

$$
\begin{array}{r}
1.61 \\
\times\ \underline{0.2} \\
322
\end{array}
$$ Line up the numbers on the right

The product is 322; 1.61 has two numbers after the decimal point and 0.2 has one. Place the decimal point three places to the left in the product so that 322 becomes .322, then add a zero in front of the decimal to emphasize the fraction.

Answer: 0.322

🔑 If the product contains insufficient numbers for correct placement of the decimal point, add as many zeros as necessary to the left of the product to correct this.

EXAMPLE 3   Multiply 1.5 by 0.06

$$
\begin{array}{r}
1.5 \\
\times\ \underline{0.06} \\
90
\end{array}
$$ Line up the numbers on the right

The product is 90; 1.5 has one number after the decimal point and 0.06 has two. To place the decimal three places to the left in the product, a zero must be added, making it .090. Eliminate the extra zero from the end of the fraction, and add a zero in front of the decimal point.

Answer: 0.09

EXAMPLE 4   Multiply 0.21 by 0.32

$$
\begin{array}{r}
0.21 \\
\times\ \underline{0.32} \\
42 \\
\underline{63} \\
672
\end{array}
$$

Indent second-number multiplication
Add the totals

In this example, 0.21 has two numbers after the decimal point and 0.32 also has two. Add a zero in front of 672 to allow correct placement of the decimal point, making it .0672, then add a zero in front of the fraction to emphasize it.

Answer: 0.0672

EXAMPLE 5   Multiply 0.12 by 0.2

$$
\begin{array}{r}
0.12 \\
\times\ \underline{0.2} \\
24
\end{array}
$$

In this example, there are a total of three numbers after the decimal points in 0.12 and 0.2. Add a zero in front of 24 for correct decimal placement, making it .024, then add a zero in front of .024 to emphasize the fraction.

Answer: 0.024

PROBLEMS 3-1

Multiply the decimal fractions without using a calculator.

1. 0.45×0.2 = _____

2. 0.35×0.12 = _____

3. 1.3×0.05 = _____

4. 0.7×0.04 = _____

5. 0.4×0.17 = _____

6. 2.14×0.03 = _____

7. 1.4×0.4 = _____

8. 3.3×1.2 = _____

9. 2.7×2.2 = _____

10. 2.1×0.3 = _____

Answers 1. 0.09   **2.** 0.042   **3.** 0.065   **4.** 0.028   **5.** 0.068   **6.** 0.0642   **7.** 0.56   **8.** 3.96   **9.** 5.94   **10.** 0.63

DIVISION OF DECIMAL FRACTIONS

Let's start by reviewing the terminology of common fraction division, as well as **three important precalculator** steps that may make final manual division easier: **elimination of decimal points**, **reduction of the fractions**, and **reduction of numbers ending in zero**. The following is a sample of a common fraction division seen in dosages.

EXAMPLE 1 $\dfrac{0.25}{0.125} = \dfrac{\text{numerator}}{\text{denominator}}$

You'll recall that the **top number** in a common fraction is called the **numerator**, whereas the **bottom number** is called the **denominator**. If you have trouble remembering which is which, think of **D**, for **down**, for **denominator**. The denominator is on the bottom.

With this basic terminology reviewed, we are now ready to look at preliminary math steps that can be used to simplify a fraction or actually solve an equation and eliminate the need for calculator division.

ELIMINATION OF DECIMAL POINTS

Decimal points can be eliminated from numbers in a decimal fraction without changing its value, if they are moved the same number of places in one numerator and one denominator.

> 🔑 To eliminate the decimal points from decimal fractions, move them the same number of places to the right in a numerator and a denominator until they are eliminated from both. Zeros may have to be added to accomplish this.

EXAMPLE 1 $\dfrac{0.25}{0.125}$ becomes $\dfrac{250}{125}$

The decimal point must be moved three places to the right in the denominator 0.125 to make it 125. Therefore, it must be moved three places to the right in the numerator 0.25, which requires the addition of one zero to make it 250.

EXAMPLE 2 $\dfrac{0.3}{0.15}$ becomes $\dfrac{30}{15}$

The decimal point must be moved two places in 0.15 to make it 15, so it must be moved two places in 0.3, which requires the addition of one zero to become 30.

EXAMPLE 3 $\dfrac{1.5}{2}$ becomes $\dfrac{15}{20}$

Move the decimal point one place in 1.5 to make it 15; add one zero to 2 to make it 20.

EXAMPLE 4 $\dfrac{4.5}{0.95}$ becomes $\dfrac{450}{95}$

> 🔑 Eliminating the decimal points from a decimal fraction before final division does not alter the value of the fraction, or the answer obtained in the final division.

PROBLEMS 3-2

Eliminate the decimal points from these common fractions.

1. $\dfrac{17.5}{2}$ = _____

2. $\dfrac{0.5}{25}$ = _____

3. $\dfrac{6.3}{0.6}$ = _____

4. $\dfrac{3.76}{0.4}$ = _____

5. $\dfrac{8.4}{0.7}$ = _____

6. $\dfrac{0.1}{0.05}$ = _____

7. $\dfrac{0.9}{0.03}$ = _____

8. $\dfrac{10.75}{2.5}$ = _____

9. $\dfrac{0.4}{0.04}$ = _____

10. $\dfrac{1.2}{0.4}$ = _____

Answers 1. $\dfrac{175}{20}$ 2. $\dfrac{5}{250}$ 3. $\dfrac{63}{6}$ 4. $\dfrac{376}{40}$ 5. $\dfrac{84}{7}$ 6. $\dfrac{10}{5}$ 7. $\dfrac{90}{3}$ 8. $\dfrac{1075}{250}$ 9. $\dfrac{40}{4}$ 10. $\dfrac{12}{4}$

REDUCTION OF FRACTIONS

Once the decimal points are eliminated, a second simplification step is to reduce the numbers as far as possible using common denominators/divisors, the largest number that will divide both the numerator and the denominator.

> **O—** To further reduce fractions, divide numbers by their greatest common denominator—the largest number that will divide into both the numerator and the denominator.

The **greatest common denominator** is usually 2, 3, 4, 5, **or multiples of these numbers**, such as 6, 8, 25, and so on.

EXAMPLE 1 $\dfrac{175}{20}$ The greatest common denominator is 5.

$$\dfrac{\cancel{175}}{\cancel{20}} = \dfrac{35}{4}$$

EXAMPLE 2 $\dfrac{63}{6}$ The greatest common denominator is 3.

$$\dfrac{\cancel{63}}{\cancel{6}} = \dfrac{21}{2}$$

EXAMPLE 3 $\dfrac{1075}{250}$ The greatest common denominator is 25.

$$\dfrac{\cancel{1075}}{\cancel{250}} = \dfrac{43}{10}$$

There is a second way you could have reduced the fraction in this example, and it is equally as correct: Divide by 5, then by 5 again.

$$\dfrac{\cancel{1075}}{\cancel{250}} = \dfrac{\cancel{215}}{\cancel{50}} = \dfrac{43}{10}$$

⚷ If the greatest common denominator is difficult to determine, reduce several times by using smaller common denominators.

EXAMPLE 4 $\dfrac{376}{40} = \dfrac{47}{5}$ Divide by 8.

Or divide by 4, then 2: $\dfrac{\cancel{376}}{\cancel{40}} = \dfrac{\cancel{94}}{\cancel{10}} = \dfrac{47}{5}$

Or divide by 2, then 2, then 2: $\dfrac{\cancel{376}}{\cancel{40}} = \dfrac{\cancel{188}}{\cancel{20}} = \dfrac{\cancel{94}}{\cancel{10}} = \dfrac{47}{5}$

Remember that **simple numbers are easiest to work with**, and the time spent in extra reductions may be well worth the payoff in safety.

PROBLEMS 3-3

Reduce the fractions in preparation for final division.

1. $\dfrac{84}{8}$ = _____

2. $\dfrac{20}{16}$ = _____

3. $\dfrac{250}{325}$ = _____

4. $\dfrac{96}{34}$ = _____

5. $\dfrac{175}{20}$ = _____

6. $\dfrac{40}{14}$ = _____

7. $\dfrac{82}{28}$ = _____

8. $\dfrac{100}{75}$ = _____

9. $\dfrac{50}{75}$ = _____

10. $\dfrac{60}{88}$ = _____

Answers 1. $\dfrac{21}{2}$ 2. $\dfrac{5}{4}$ 3. $\dfrac{10}{13}$ 4. $\dfrac{48}{17}$ 5. $\dfrac{35}{4}$ 6. $\dfrac{20}{7}$ 7. $\dfrac{41}{14}$ 8. $\dfrac{4}{3}$ 9. $\dfrac{2}{3}$ 10. $\dfrac{15}{22}$

REDUCTION OF NUMBERS ENDING IN ZERO

The third type of simplification is not solely related to decimal fractions, but is best covered at this time. It concerns reductions in a common fraction when both the numerator and the denominator end with zeros.

> **O—** Numbers that end in a zero or zeros may be reduced by crossing off the same number of zeros in both the numerator and the denominator.

EXAMPLE 1 $\dfrac{800}{250}$

In this fraction, the numerator, 800, has two zeros, but the denominator, 250, has one zero. The number of zeros crossed off must be the same in both numerator and denominator, so only one zero can be eliminated from each.

$$\frac{80\cancel{0}}{25\cancel{0}} = \frac{80}{25}$$

$$\text{Reduce by } 5 = \frac{16}{5}$$

EXAMPLE 2 $\dfrac{24\cancel{00}}{20\cancel{00}} = \dfrac{24}{20}$

$$\text{Reduce by } 4 = \frac{6}{5}$$

Two zeros can be eliminated from the denominator and the numerator in this fraction.

EXAMPLE 3 $\dfrac{15\cancel{000}}{30\cancel{000}} = \dfrac{15}{30}$

$$\text{Reduce by } 15 = \frac{1}{2}$$

In this fraction, three zeros can be eliminated.

PROBLEMS 3-4

Reduce the fractions to their lowest terms.

1. $\dfrac{50}{250}$ = _____

2. $\dfrac{120}{50}$ = _____

3. $\dfrac{2500}{1500}$ = _____

4. $\dfrac{1,000,000}{750,000}$ = _____

5. $\dfrac{800}{150}$ = _____

6. $\dfrac{110}{100}$ = _____

7. $\dfrac{200,000}{150,000}$ = _____

8. $\dfrac{1000}{800}$ = _____

9. $\dfrac{60}{40}$ = _____

10. $\dfrac{150}{200}$ = _____

Answers 1. $\dfrac{1}{5}$ 2. $\dfrac{12}{5}$ 3. $\dfrac{5}{3}$ 4. $\dfrac{4}{3}$ 5. $\dfrac{16}{3}$ 6. $\dfrac{11}{10}$ 7. $\dfrac{4}{3}$ 8. $\dfrac{5}{4}$ 9. $\dfrac{3}{2}$ 10. $\dfrac{3}{4}$

USING A CALCULATOR

It's okay to use a calculator for final divisions throughout the text. So, this is a good time to consider safety tips when using one.

Calculators vary in how addition, subtraction, division, and multiplication must be entered, and in the number of fractional numbers displayed after the decimal point. The first precaution in calculator use is to ensure you **know how to use the one available to you**. If you have to use a calculator regularly, it would be wise to buy and use your own.

The next precaution—and this is critical—is to enter decimal numbers correctly, which includes **entering the decimal points**. This is not as easy to remember as it sounds, and this is a step where dosage calculation errors can occur.

EXPRESSING TO THE NEAREST TENTH

When a fraction is reduced as much as possible, it is ready for final division. This will be done using a calculator to **divide the numerator by the denominator**.

🔑 To express an answer to the nearest tenth, carry the division to hundredths (two places after the decimal). When the number representing hundredths is 5 or larger, increase the number representing tenths by 1.

EXAMPLE 1 $\dfrac{0.35}{0.4}$ = 0.35 ÷ 0.4 = 0.87

Answer: 0.9

The number representing hundredths is 7, so the number representing tenths is increased by 1: 0.87 becomes 0.9.

EXAMPLE 2 $\dfrac{0.5}{0.3}$ = 0.5 ÷ 0.3 = 1.66 = **1.7**

The number representing hundredths, 6, is larger than 5, so 1.66 becomes 1.7.

EXAMPLE 3 $\dfrac{0.16}{0.3} = 0.53 = \mathbf{0.5}$

The number representing hundredths, 3, is less than 5, so the number representing tenths, 5, remains unchanged.

EXAMPLE 4 $\dfrac{0.2}{0.3} = 0.66 = \mathbf{0.7}$

EXAMPLE 5   An answer of 1.42 remains **1.4**

EXAMPLE 6   An answer of 1.86 becomes **1.9**

PROBLEMS 3-5

Use a calculator to divide the common fractions. Express answers to the nearest tenth.

1. $\dfrac{5.1}{2.3}$ = _____

2. $\dfrac{0.9}{0.7}$ = _____

3. $\dfrac{3.7}{2}$ = _____

4. $\dfrac{6}{1.3}$ = _____

5. $\dfrac{1.5}{2.1}$ = _____

6. $\dfrac{2.7}{1.1}$ = _____

7. $\dfrac{4.2}{5}$ = _____

8. $\dfrac{0.5}{2.5}$ = _____

9. $\dfrac{5.2}{0.91}$ = _____

10. $\dfrac{2.4}{2.7}$ = _____

Answers 1. 2.2   **2.** 1.3   **3.** 1.9   **4.** 4.6   **5.** 0.7   **6.** 2.5   **7.** 0.8   **8.** 0.2   **9.** 5.7   **10.** 0.9

EXPRESSING TO THE NEAREST HUNDREDTH

Some drugs are administered in dosages carried to the nearest hundredth. This is common in pediatric dosages, and in drugs that alter a vital function of the body—for example, heart rate.

> To express an answer to the nearest hundredth, the division is carried to thousandths (three places after the decimal point). When the number representing thousandths is 5 or larger, the number representing hundredths is increased by 1.

EXAMPLE 1   0.736 becomes **0.74**

The number representing thousandths, 6, is larger than 5, so the number representing hundredths, 3, is increased by 1 to become 4.

EXAMPLE 2   0.777 becomes **0.78**

EXAMPLE 3   0.373 remains **0.37**

The number representing thousandths, 3, is less than 5, so the number representing hundredths, 7, remains unchanged.

EXAMPLE 4   0.934 remains **0.93**

PROBLEMS 3-6

Express the numbers to the nearest hundredth.

1. 0.175   = _____

2. 0.344   = _____

3. 1.853   = _____

4. 0.306   = _____

5. 3.015   = _____

6. 2.154   = _____

7. 1.081   = _____

8. 1.327   = _____

9. 0.739   = _____

10. 0.733   = _____

11. 2.072   = _____

12. 0.089   = _____

Answers 1. 0.18   **2.** 0.34   **3.** 1.85   **4.** 0.31   **5.** 3.02   **6.** 2.15   **7.** 1.08   **8.** 1.33   **9.** 0.74   **10.** 0.73
11. 2.07   **12.** 0.09

SUMMARY

This concludes the chapter on multiplication and division of decimals. The important points to remember from this chapter are:

- When decimal fractions are multiplied manually, the decimal point is placed the same number of places to the left in the product as the total of numbers after the decimal points in the fractions multiplied.

- Zeros must be placed in front of a product if it contains insufficient numbers for the correct placement of the decimal point.

- Excess trailing zeros are eliminated in dosages.

- To simplify fractions for final division, the preliminary steps of eliminating decimal points, reducing the numbers by common denominators, and reducing numbers ending in zeros can be used.

- To express to tenths, increase the answer by 1 if the number representing the hundredths is 5 or larger.

- To express to hundredths, increase the answer by 1 if the number representing the thousandths is 5 or larger.

- Practice using a calculator until proficiency is achieved.

- All calculator entries and answers must be double-checked.

- Disregard calculator running totals because they can cause confusion.

SUMMARY SELF-TEST

Use the shortcuts that you just learned to initially simplify the numbers in the following test problems. Use a calculator only for final divisions.

Multiply the decimals.

1. 1.49×0.05 = _____

2. 0.15×3.04 = _____

3. 0.025×3.5 = _____

4. 0.55×2.5 = _____

5. 1.3×2.7 = _____

6. 5.3×1.02 = _____

7. 0.35×1.2 = _____

8. 4.32×0.05 = _____

9. 0.2×0.02 = _____

10. 0.4×1.75 = _____

11. You are to administer four tablets with a dosage strength of
    0.04 mg each. What total dosage are you giving?   _____

12. You have given 2½ (2.5) tablets with a strength of 1.25 mg
    per tablet. What total dosage is this?   _____

13. The tablets your patient is to receive are labeled 0.1 mg, and you are
    to give 3½ (3.5) tablets. What total dosage is this?   _____

14. You gave your patient 3 tablets labeled 0.75 mg each, and he was
    to receive a total of 2.25 mg. Did he receive the correct dosage?   _____

15. The tablets available for your patient are labeled 12.5 mg, and you are
    to give 4½ (4.5) tablets. What total dosage will this be?   _____

16. Your patient is to receive a dosage of 4.5 mg. The tablets available are labeled 3.5 mg,
    and there are 2½ tablets in his medication drawer. Is this a correct dosage?   _____

Divide the fractions. Express answers to the nearest tenth.

17. $\dfrac{1.3}{0.7}$ = _____

18. $\dfrac{1.9}{3.2}$ = _____

19. $\dfrac{32.5}{9}$ = _____

20. $\dfrac{0.04}{0.1}$ = _____

21. $\dfrac{1.45}{1.2}$ = _____

22. $\dfrac{250}{1000}$ = _____

23. $\dfrac{0.8}{0.09}$ = _____

24. $\dfrac{2,000,000}{1,500,000}$ = _____

25. $\dfrac{4.1}{2.05}$ = _____

26. $\dfrac{7.3}{12}$ = _____

27. $\dfrac{150,000}{120,000}$ = _____

28. $\dfrac{0.15}{0.08}$ = _____

29. $\dfrac{2700}{900}$ = _____

30. $\dfrac{0.25}{0.15}$ = _____

Divide the fractions. Express answers to the nearest hundredth.

31. $\dfrac{900}{1700}$ = _____

32. $\dfrac{0.125}{0.3}$ = _____

33. $\dfrac{1450}{1500}$ = _____

34. $\dfrac{65}{175}$ = _____

35. $\dfrac{0.6}{1.35}$ = _____

36. $\dfrac{0.04}{0.12}$ = _____

37. $\dfrac{750}{10,000}$ = _____

38. $\dfrac{0.65}{0.8}$ = _____

39. $\dfrac{3.01}{4.2}$ = _____

40. $\dfrac{4.5}{6.1}$ = _____

41. $\dfrac{0.13}{0.25}$ = _____

42. $\dfrac{0.25}{0.7}$ = _____

43. $\dfrac{3.3}{5.1}$ = _____

44. $\dfrac{0.19}{0.7}$ = _____

45. $\dfrac{1.1}{1.3}$ = _____

46. $\dfrac{3}{4.1}$ = _____

47. $\dfrac{62}{240}$ = _____

48. $\dfrac{280,000}{300,000}$ = _____

49. $\dfrac{115}{255}$ = _____

50. $\dfrac{10}{14.3}$ = _____

Answers

1. 0.0745	**14.** Yes	**27.** 1.3	**40.** 0.74
2. 0.456	**15.** 56.25 mg	**28.** 1.9	**41.** 0.52
3. 0.0875	**16.** No	**29.** 3	**42.** 0.36
4. 1.375	**17.** 1.9	**30.** 1.7	**43.** 0.65
5. 3.51	**18.** 0.6	**31.** 0.53	**44.** 0.27
6. 5.406	**19.** 3.6	**32.** 0.42	**45.** 0.85
7. 0.42	**20.** 0.4	**33.** 0.97	**46.** 0.73
8. 0.216	**21.** 1.2	**34.** 0.37	**47.** 0.26
9. 0.004	**22.** 0.3	**35.** 0.44	**48.** 0.93
10. 0.7	**23.** 8.9	**36.** 0.33	**49.** 0.45
11. 0.16 mg	**24.** 1.3	**37.** 0.08	**50.** 0.7
12. 3.125 mg	**25.** 2	**38.** 0.81	
13. 0.35 mg	**26.** 0.6	**39.** 0.72	

CHAPTER 4

Solving for X in Common Fraction Equations

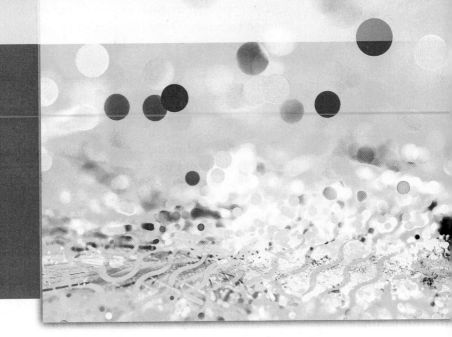

OBJECTIVES

The learner will solve equations containing:

1. Whole numbers.

2. Decimal numbers.

3. Multiple numbers.

INTRODUCTION

Later in the text, you will be introduced to **intravenous calculations** that will contain **a number of common fraction entries**, and to **dimensional analysis**, which you will use to set these equations up. However, this is the point in your instruction where the **math of common fractions** is most appropriately practiced. **This will make you at ease** with solving for the **unknown X** in IV calculations when we get to those later.

A number of the examples and problems included in this chapter represent actual IV calculations, but an equal number are random dosages included for practice. This should be encouraging for you. As you are being consistently reminded, **math in dosages is nothing to be afraid of**. Just enjoy the exercises, and you will have all the math skills you need.

The majority of clinical drug dosage calculations involve solving an equation containing one to five common fractions. Two examples are:

$$\frac{2}{5} \times \frac{3}{4}$$

and

$$\frac{20}{1} \times \frac{1000}{60{,}000} \times \frac{1200}{1} \times \frac{1}{60}$$

Two options are available to solve common fraction equations: calculator use throughout, or initial fraction reduction followed by calculator use for final division. Both options are presented in this chapter, and you may use whichever you wish, or whichever your instructor requires.

🔑 In common fraction calculations, the numerators are multiplied, then divided by the product of the denominators.

It is important that you do the calculations for each example and then compare them with the math provided. **Just reading the examples will not teach you the calculation skills you need.** The examples and problems provided incorporate all the content covered in previous chapters. They represent the full range of calculations you will be doing on a continuing basis.

🔑 Calculator solution of equations is most safely done by concentrating only on the entries being made, not the numbers that register and change throughout the calculation.

WHOLE-NUMBER EQUATIONS

EXAMPLE 1   **Option 1: Initial Reduction of Fractions**

$$\frac{2}{5} \times \frac{3}{4}$$

$$\frac{^1\cancel{2}}{5} \times \frac{3}{\cancel{4}_2}$$ Divide the numerator, 2, and the denominator, 4, by 2 (to become 1 and 2).

$$3 \div 5 \div 2$$ Use the calculator to divide the remaining numerator, 3, by the remaining denominators, 5 and 2.

$$= 0.3$$

Answer: 0.3 (tenth)

Option 2: Calculator Use Throughout

$$\frac{2}{5} \times \frac{3}{4}$$

$$2 \times 3 \div 5 \div 4$$ Multiply the numerators, 2 and 3; then divide by the denominators, 5 then 4, in continuous entries.

$$= 0.3$$

Answer: 0.3 (tenth)

🔑 Initial reduction of fractions in an equation can simplify final calculator entries, especially if the numbers are large, or contain decimal fractions or zeros.

EXAMPLE 2   **Option 1: Initial Reduction of Fractions**

$$\frac{250}{175} \times \frac{150}{325}$$

$$\frac{\overset{10}{\cancel{250}}}{\underset{7}{\cancel{175}}} \times \frac{\overset{6}{\cancel{150}}}{\underset{13}{\cancel{325}}}$$

Divide the numerator, 250, and the denominator, 175, by 25 (to become 10 and 7); divide the numerator, 150, and denominator, 325, by 25 (to become 6 and 13).

$10 \times 6 \div 7 \div 13$ Use the calculator to multiply the numerators, 10 and 6; then divide by the denominators, 7 and 13.

$= 0.659$

Answer: 0.7 (tenth) or 0.66 (hundredth)

Option 2: Calculator Use Throughout

$$\frac{250}{175} \times \frac{150}{325}$$

$250 \times 150 \div 175 \div 325$ Multiply the numerators, 250 and 150; then divide by the denominators, 175 and 325.

$= 0.659$

Answer: 0.7 (tenth) or 0.66 (hundredth)

EXAMPLE 3   **Option 1: Initial Reduction of Fractions**

$$\frac{7}{50} \times \frac{25}{3} \times \frac{120}{32}$$

$$\frac{7}{\underset{2}{\cancel{50}}} \times \frac{\overset{1}{\cancel{25}}}{3} \times \frac{\overset{15}{\cancel{120}}}{\underset{4}{\cancel{32}}}$$ Divide 25 and 50 by 25; then divide 120 and 32 by 8.

$7 \times 15 \div 2 \div 3 \div 4$

$= 4.375$

Answer: 4.4 (tenth) or 4.38 (hundredth)

Option 2: Calculator Use Throughout

$$\frac{7}{50} \times \frac{25}{3} \times \frac{120}{32}$$

$7 \times 25 \times 120 \div 50 \div 3 \div 32$ Multiply the numerators, 7, 25, and 120; then divide by the denominators, 50, 3, and 32.

$= 4.375$

Answer: 4.4 (tenth) or 4.38 (hundredth)

EXAMPLE 4   **Option 1: Initial Reduction of Fractions**

$$\frac{20}{1} \times \frac{1000}{60,000} \times \frac{1200}{1} \times \frac{1}{60}$$

$$\frac{\overset{1}{\cancel{20}}}{1} \times \frac{\overset{1}{\cancel{1000}}}{\underset{3}{\cancel{60,000}}} \times \frac{\overset{20}{\cancel{1200}}}{1} \times \frac{1}{\underset{1}{\cancel{60}}}$$

$20 \div 3$

$= 6.666$

Answer: 6.7 (tenth) or **6.67 (hundredth)**

Option 2: Calculator Use Throughout

$$\frac{20}{1} \times \frac{1000}{60,000} \times \frac{1200}{1} \times \frac{1}{60}$$

$20 \times 1000 \times 1200 \div 60,000 \div 60$

$= 6.666$

Answer: 6.7 (tenth) or **6.67 (hundredth)**

EXAMPLE 5   **Option 1: Initial Reduction of Fractions**

$$\frac{2000}{1500} \times \frac{2500}{3000}$$

$$\frac{\overset{2}{\cancel{2000}}}{\underset{3}{\cancel{1500}}} \times \frac{\overset{5}{\cancel{2500}}}{\underset{3}{\cancel{3000}}}$$

$2 \times 5 \div 3 \div 3$

$= 1.111$

Answer: 1.1 (tenth) or **1.11 (hundredth)**

Option 2: Calculator Use Throughout

$$\frac{2000}{1500} \times \frac{2500}{3000}$$

$2000 \times 2500 \div 1500 \div 3000$

$= 1.111$

Answer: 1.1 (tenth) or **1.11 (hundredth)**

PROBLEMS 4-1

Solve the equations. Express answers to the nearest tenth and hundredth. You may use a calculator.

1. $\dfrac{3}{8} \times \dfrac{6}{3}$ = _____ _____

2. $\dfrac{3}{4} \times \dfrac{10}{2}$ = _____ _____

3. $\dfrac{3}{5} \times \dfrac{1050}{40}$ = _____ _____

4. $\dfrac{10}{1} \times \dfrac{750}{40,000} \times \dfrac{1000}{1} \times \dfrac{1}{60}$ = _____ _____

5. $\dfrac{12}{1} \times \dfrac{500}{2700} \times \dfrac{2000}{1} \times \dfrac{1}{60}$ = _____ _____

6. $\dfrac{1500}{750} \times \dfrac{350}{600}$ = _____ _____

7. $\dfrac{1000}{2700} \times \dfrac{1300}{500} \times \dfrac{70}{50}$ = _____ _____

8. $\dfrac{15}{1} \times \dfrac{2500}{20,000} \times \dfrac{1000}{1} \times \dfrac{1}{60}$ = _____ _____

9. $\dfrac{8}{1} \times \dfrac{1000}{5000} \times \dfrac{100}{1} \times \dfrac{1}{60}$ = _____ _____

10. $\dfrac{750}{500} \times \dfrac{250}{300}$ = _____ _____

Answers **1.** 0.8; 0.75 **2.** 3.8; 3.75 **3.** 15.8; 15.75 **4.** 3.1; 3.13 **5.** 74.1; 74.07 **6.** 1.2; 1.17 **7.** 1.3; 1.35 **8.** 31.3; 31.25 **9.** 2.7; 2.67 **10.** 1.3; 1.25

DECIMAL-FRACTION EQUATIONS

Decimal-fraction equations raise an instant warning flag in calculations, because it is here that most dosage errors occur. As with whole-number equations, simplifying the numbers by eliminating decimal points and reducing the numbers is an optional first step. If you elect to do the entire calculation with a calculator, be sure to enter the decimal points carefully. Double-check all calculator entries and answers.

🔑 Particular care must be taken with calculator entry of decimal numbers to include the decimal point. Each entry and answer must be routinely double-checked.

EXAMPLE 1 **Option 1: Initial Elimination of Decimal Points and Reduction of Fractions**

$$\dfrac{0.3}{1.65} \times \dfrac{2.5}{1}$$

$$\dfrac{30}{165} \times \dfrac{25}{10} \qquad \text{Move the decimal point two places in 0.3 and 1.65 (to become 30 and 165) and one place in 2.5 and 1 (to become 25 and 10).}$$

$$\dfrac{\overset{3}{\cancel{30}}}{\underset{33}{\cancel{165}}} \times \dfrac{\overset{5}{\cancel{25}}}{\underset{1}{\cancel{10}}} \qquad \text{Divide 30 and 10 by 10; then divide 25 and 165 by 5.}$$

$$\dfrac{\overset{1}{\cancel{3}}}{\underset{11}{\cancel{33}}} \times \dfrac{5}{1} \qquad \text{Divide 3 and 33 by 3.}$$

$5 \div 11$ Divide the remaining numerator, 5, by the denominator, 11.

$= 0.454$

Answer: 0.5 (tenth) or 0.45 (hundredth)

Option 2: Calculator Use Throughout

$$\frac{0.3}{1.65} \times \frac{2.5}{1}$$

$0.3 \times 2.5 \div 1.65$ Multiply 0.3 by 2.5; then divide by 1.65.

$= 0.454$

Answer: 0.5 (tenth) or 0.45 (hundredth)

EXAMPLE 2   **Option 1: Initial Elimination of Decimal Points and Reduction of Fractions**

$$\frac{0.3}{1.2} \times \frac{2.1}{0.15}$$

$$\frac{3}{12} \times \frac{210}{15}$$ Eliminate the decimal points by moving them one place in 0.3 and 1.2 (to become 3 and 12) and two places in 2.1 and 0.15 (to become 210 and 15).

$$\frac{\overset{1}{\cancel{3}}}{\underset{4}{\cancel{12}}} \times \frac{\overset{42}{\cancel{210}}}{\underset{3}{\cancel{15}}}$$ Divide 3 and 12 by 3; then divide 210 and 15 by 5.

$$\frac{1}{\underset{2}{\cancel{4}}} \times \frac{\overset{21}{\cancel{42}}}{3}$$ Divide 42 and 4 by 2.

$21 \div 2 \div 3$ Use a calculator to divide the numerator, 21, by 2 and then by 3.

$= 3.5$

Answer: 3.5 (tenth) or 3.5 (hundredth)

Option 2: Calculator Use Throughout

$$\frac{0.3}{1.2} \times \frac{2.1}{0.15}$$

$0.3 \times 2.1 \div 1.2 \div 0.15$ Multiply 0.3 by 2.1; then divide by 1.2 and 0.15.

$= 3.5$

Answer: 3.5 (tenth) or 3.5 (hundredth)

EXAMPLE 3   **Option 1: Initial Elimination of Decimal Points and Reduction of Fractions**

$$\frac{0.15}{0.17} \times \frac{3.1}{2}$$

$$\frac{15}{17} \times \frac{31}{20}$$ Move the decimal point two places in 0.15 and 0.17 and one place in 3.1 and 2 (requires adding a zero to 2).

$$\frac{\overset{3}{\cancel{15}}}{17} \times \frac{31}{\underset{4}{\cancel{20}}} \qquad \text{Divide 15 and 20 by 5.}$$

$3 \times 31 \div 17 \div 4 \qquad$ Complete this with a calculator.

$= 1.367$

Answer: 1.4 (tenth) or 1.37 (hundredth)

Option 2: Calculator Use Throughout

$$\frac{0.15}{0.17} \times \frac{3.1}{2}$$

$0.15 \times 3.1 \div 0.17 \div 2 \qquad$ Multiply 0.15 by 3.1, divide by 0.17, and then divide by 2.

$= 1.367$

Answer: 1.4 (tenth) or 1.37 (hundredth)

EXAMPLE 4 **Option 1: Initial Elimination of Decimal Points and Reduction of Fractions**

$$\frac{2.5}{1.5} \times \frac{1.2}{1.1}$$

$$\frac{25}{15} \times \frac{12}{11}$$

$$\frac{\overset{5}{\cancel{25}}}{\underset{3}{\cancel{15}}} \times \frac{12}{11}$$

$$\frac{5}{\underset{1}{\cancel{3}}} \times \frac{\overset{4}{\cancel{12}}}{11}$$

$5 \times 4 \div 11$

$= 1.818$

Answer: 1.8 (tenth) or 1.82 (hundredth)

Option 2: Calculator Use Throughout

$$\frac{2.5}{1.5} \times \frac{1.2}{1.1}$$

$2.5 \times 1.2 \div 1.5 \div 1.1$

$= 1.818$

Answer: 1.8 (tenth) or 1.82 (hundredth)

PROBLEMS 4-2

Solve the equations. Express answers to the nearest tenth and hundredth. You may use a calculator.

1. $\dfrac{2.1}{1.15} \times \dfrac{0.9}{1.2}$ = _____ _____

2. $\dfrac{3.1}{2.7} \times \dfrac{2.2}{1.4}$ = _____ _____

3. $\dfrac{0.3}{1.2} \times \dfrac{3}{2.1}$ = _____ _____

4. $\dfrac{0.17}{0.3} \times \dfrac{2.5}{1.5}$ = _____ _____

5. $\dfrac{1.75}{0.95} \times \dfrac{1.5}{2}$ = _____ _____

6. $\dfrac{0.75}{1.15} \times \dfrac{3}{1.25}$ = _____ _____

7. $\dfrac{10.2}{1.5} \times \dfrac{2}{5.1}$ = _____ _____

8. $\dfrac{0.125}{0.25} \times \dfrac{2.5}{1.5}$ = _____ _____

9. $\dfrac{0.9}{0.3} \times \dfrac{1.2}{1.4}$ = _____ _____

10. $\dfrac{0.35}{1.7} \times \dfrac{2.5}{0.7}$ = _____ _____

Answers 1. 1.4; 1.37   **2.** 1.8; 1.8   **3.** 0.4; 0.36   **4.** 0.9; 0.94   **5.** 1.4; 1.38   **6.** 1.6; 1.57   **7.** 2.7; 2.67   **8.** 0.8; 0.83   **9.** 2.6; 2.57   **10.** 0.7; 0.74

MULTIPLE-NUMBER EQUATIONS

The calculation steps just practiced are also used for multiple-number equations, which occur frequently in advanced clinical calculations. **Reduction of numbers may be of particular benefit here because calculations of this type sometimes have numbers that cancel and/or reduce dramatically.** Answers are expressed to the nearest whole number in the examples and problems that follow to replicate actual clinical calculations.

EXAMPLE 1   Option 1: Initial Reduction of Fractions

$$\frac{60}{1} \times \frac{1000}{4} \times \frac{1}{1000} \times \frac{6}{1}$$

$$\frac{60}{1} \times \frac{\overset{1}{\cancel{1000}}}{\underset{2}{\cancel{4}}} \times \frac{1}{\underset{1}{\cancel{1000}}} \times \frac{\overset{3}{\cancel{6}}}{1}$$

Eliminate 1000 from the numerator and the denominator; then divide 6 and 4 by 2.

$60 \times 3 \div 2$ Multiply 60 by 3; then divide by 2.

$= 90$

Answer: 90   The answer is obtained by cancellation alone.

Option 2: Calculator Use Throughout

$$\frac{60}{1} \times \frac{1000}{4} \times \frac{1}{1000} \times \frac{6}{1}$$

$60 \times 1000 \times 6 \div 4 \div 1000$ Multiply 60 by 1000, then by 6; divide by 4 and 1000.

$= 90$

Answer: 90

EXAMPLE 2 **Option 1: Initial Reduction of Fractions**

$$\frac{20}{1} \times \frac{75}{1} \times \frac{1}{60}$$

$$\frac{\overset{1}{\cancel{20}}}{1} \times \frac{\overset{25}{\cancel{75}}}{1} \times \frac{1}{\underset{\underset{1}{\cancel{3}}}{\cancel{60}}}$$ Divide 20 and 60 by 20 to become 1 and 3; then divide 75 and 3 by 3 to become 25 and 1.

$= 25$

Answer: 25   The answer is obtained by cancellation alone.

Option 2: Calculator Use Throughout

$$\frac{20}{1} \times \frac{75}{1} \times \frac{1}{60}$$

$20 \times 75 \div 60$ Multiply 20 by 75; then divide by 60.

$= 25$

Answer: 25

EXAMPLE 3 **Option 1: Initial Reduction of Fractions**

$$\frac{2}{0.5} \times \frac{1}{100} \times \frac{275}{1}$$

$$\frac{20}{5} \times \frac{1}{100} \times \frac{275}{1}$$ Eliminate the decimal point by moving it one place in 0.5 and one place in 2, which requires adding a zero to 2 (to become 5 and 20).

$$\frac{\overset{1}{\cancel{20}}}{\underset{1}{\cancel{5}}} \times \frac{1}{\underset{5}{\cancel{100}}} \times \frac{\overset{55}{\cancel{275}}}{1}$$ Divide 20 and 100 by 20; then divide 275 and 5 by 5.

$$\frac{1}{\underset{1}{\cancel{5}}} \times \frac{\overset{11}{\cancel{55}}}{1}$$ Divide 5 and 55 by 5.

$= 11$

Answer: 11   The answer is obtained by cancellation alone.

Option 2: Calculator Use Throughout

$$\frac{2}{0.5} \times \frac{1}{100} \times \frac{275}{1}$$

$2 \times 275 \div 0.5 \div 100$ Multiply 2 by 275; then divide by 0.5 and 100.

$= 11$

Answer: 11

EXAMPLE 4   **Option 1: Initial Reduction of Fractions**

$$\frac{1}{60} \times \frac{1}{12} \times \frac{10}{1} \times \frac{750}{1}$$

$$\frac{1}{\cancel{60}_{6}} \times \frac{1}{\cancel{12}_{6}} \times \frac{\cancel{10}^{1}}{1} \times \frac{\cancel{750}^{375}}{1}$$

$375 \div 6 \div 6$

$= 10.4$

Answer: 10

Option 2: Calculator Use Throughout

$$\frac{1}{60} \times \frac{1}{12} \times \frac{10}{1} \times \frac{750}{1}$$

$10 \times 750 \div 60 \div 12$

$= 10.4$

Answer: 10

PROBLEMS 4-3

Solve the equations. Express answers to the nearest whole number.

1. $\dfrac{15}{1} \times \dfrac{350}{5} \times \dfrac{1}{60}$ = _____

2. $\dfrac{1}{32} \times \dfrac{60}{1} \times \dfrac{7.5}{3.1}$ = _____

3. $\dfrac{10}{1} \times \dfrac{2500}{24} \times \dfrac{1}{60}$ = _____

4. $\dfrac{1.7}{2.3} \times \dfrac{15.3}{12.1} \times \dfrac{6.2}{0.3}$ = _____

5. $\dfrac{20}{1} \times \dfrac{1200}{16} \times \dfrac{1}{60}$ = _____

6. $\dfrac{5}{1} \times \dfrac{320}{1.5} \times \dfrac{1}{60}$ = _____

7. $\dfrac{100}{1} \times \dfrac{1750}{200} \times \dfrac{1}{60}$ = _____

8. $\dfrac{60}{1} \times \dfrac{1150}{200} \times \dfrac{1}{100}$ = _____

9. $\dfrac{25}{4} \times \dfrac{1000}{8} \times \dfrac{1}{60}$ = _____

10. $\dfrac{18}{10} \times \dfrac{120}{7} \times \dfrac{9}{17}$ = _____

Answers **1.** 18 **2.** 5 **3.** 17 **4.** 19 **5.** 25 **6.** 18 **7.** 15 **8.** 3 **9.** 13 **10.** 16

SUMMARY

This concludes the chapter on solving common fraction equations. The important points to remember from this chapter are:

- Most clinical calculations consist of an equation containing one to five common fractions.

- Numbers in an equation may initially be reduced using common denominators/divisors to simplify the final multiplication and division.

- Zeros may be eliminated from the same number of numerators and denominators without altering the value.

- In solving equations, the numerators are multiplied, then divided by the product of the denominators.

- Double-check all calculator entries and answers.

- Answers may be expressed as whole numbers, or to the nearest tenth or hundredth, depending on the calculation being done.

SUMMARY SELF-TEST

Solve the equations. Express answers to the nearest tenth and hundredth. You may use a calculator.

1. $\dfrac{0.8}{0.65} \times \dfrac{1.2}{1}$ = _____ _____

2. $\dfrac{350}{1000} \times \dfrac{4.4}{1}$ = _____ _____

3. $\dfrac{0.35}{1.3} \times \dfrac{4.5}{1}$ = _____ _____

4. $\dfrac{0.4}{1.5} \times \dfrac{2.3}{1}$ = _____ _____

5. $\dfrac{1}{75} \times \dfrac{500}{1}$ = _____ _____

6. $\dfrac{0.15}{0.12} \times \dfrac{1.45}{1}$ = _____ _____

7. $\dfrac{100,000}{80,000} \times \dfrac{1.7}{1}$ = _____ _____

8. $\dfrac{1.45}{2.1} \times \dfrac{1.5}{1}$ = _____ _____

9. $\dfrac{1550}{500} \times \dfrac{0.5}{1}$ = _____ _____

10. $\dfrac{4}{0.375} \times \dfrac{0.25}{1}$ = _____ _____

11. $\dfrac{0.08}{0.1} \times \dfrac{2.1}{1}$ = _____ _____

12. $\dfrac{1.5}{1.25} \times \dfrac{1.45}{1}$ = _____ _____

13. $\dfrac{0.5}{0.15} \times \dfrac{0.35}{1}$ = _____ _____

14. $\dfrac{300,000}{200,000} \times \dfrac{1.7}{1}$ = _____ _____

15. $\dfrac{13.5}{10} \times \dfrac{1.8}{1}$ = _____ _____

16. $\dfrac{1,000,000}{800,000} \times \dfrac{1.4}{1}$ = _____ _____

17. $\dfrac{1.3}{0.2} \times \dfrac{0.25}{1}$ = _____ _____

18. $\dfrac{1.5}{0.1} \times \dfrac{0.25}{1}$ = _____ _____

19. $\dfrac{1.9}{3.5} \times \dfrac{3.2}{1.4}$ = _____ _____

20. $\dfrac{15,000}{7500} \times \dfrac{3.5}{1.2}$ = _____ _____

21. $\dfrac{4.7}{1.3} \times \dfrac{50}{20} \times \dfrac{4}{25} \times \dfrac{8.2}{2.1}$ = _____ _____

22. $\dfrac{40}{24} \times \dfrac{250}{5} \times \dfrac{0.375}{7.5}$ = _____ _____

23. $\dfrac{6.9}{21.6} \times \dfrac{250}{5} \times \dfrac{0.75}{2.1}$ = _____ _____

24. $\dfrac{1}{60} \times \dfrac{1}{25} \times \dfrac{10}{1} \times \dfrac{1000}{1}$

= _____ _____

25. $\dfrac{50.5}{22.75} \times \dfrac{4.7}{6.3} \times \dfrac{31.7}{10.2}$

= _____ _____

Solve the equations. Express answers to the nearest whole number. You may use a calculator.

26. $\dfrac{104}{95} \times \dfrac{20}{15} \times \dfrac{63}{1.6}$

= _____

27. $\dfrac{40,000}{10,000} \times \dfrac{30}{1} \times \dfrac{3.7}{12.5}$

= _____

28. $\dfrac{60}{1} \times \dfrac{500}{50} \times \dfrac{1}{1000} \times \dfrac{116}{1}$

= _____

29. $\dfrac{1.5}{0.6} \times \dfrac{10}{14} \times \dfrac{3.2}{5.3} \times \dfrac{100}{2}$

= _____

30. $\dfrac{60}{1} \times \dfrac{50}{250} \times \dfrac{1}{100} \times \dfrac{455}{1}$

= _____

31. $\dfrac{33.7}{15.9} \times \dfrac{19.2}{2.6} \times \dfrac{2.9}{3.85}$

= _____

32. $\dfrac{20}{4} \times \dfrac{100}{88} \times \dfrac{1200}{250} \times \dfrac{10}{30}$

= _____

33. $\dfrac{14}{7.9} \times \dfrac{88}{8}$

= _____

34. $\dfrac{10}{1} \times \dfrac{325}{1.5} \times \dfrac{1}{60}$

= _____

35. $\dfrac{60}{1} \times \dfrac{300}{400} \times \dfrac{1}{800} \times \dfrac{400}{1}$

= _____

36. $\dfrac{3.7}{1.3} \times \dfrac{12}{8} \times \dfrac{3.1}{7.4} \times \dfrac{5}{1}$

= _____

37. $\dfrac{20}{2} \times \dfrac{125}{25} \times \dfrac{2}{750} \times \dfrac{216}{1}$

= _____

38. $\dfrac{4}{3} \times \dfrac{45}{1} \times \dfrac{22.5}{37.8}$

= _____

39. $\dfrac{7.5}{12.3} \times \dfrac{55}{5} \times \dfrac{23.2}{1.2}$

= _____

40. $\dfrac{1000}{1} \times \dfrac{50}{250} \times \dfrac{20}{1} \times \dfrac{1}{60}$

= _____

41. $\dfrac{15}{1} \times \dfrac{1000}{4000} \times \dfrac{800}{1} \times \dfrac{1}{60}$

= _____

42. $\dfrac{15}{1} \times \dfrac{500}{3} \times \dfrac{1}{60}$

= _____

43. $\dfrac{25}{3} \times \dfrac{750}{8} \times \dfrac{0.1}{1}$ = _____

44. $\dfrac{40}{2} \times \dfrac{250}{50} \times \dfrac{1}{800} \times \dfrac{154}{1}$ = _____

45. $\dfrac{33}{4} \times \dfrac{75}{40} \times \dfrac{2}{150} \times \dfrac{432}{1}$ = _____

46. $\dfrac{22.5}{7} \times \dfrac{100}{5} \times \dfrac{1}{700} \times \dfrac{3}{80} \times \dfrac{3150}{1}$ = _____

47. $\dfrac{100}{250} \times \dfrac{50}{1} \times \dfrac{27.5}{1.375}$ = _____

48. $\dfrac{2.2}{0.25} \times \dfrac{3.6}{1} \times \dfrac{3.7}{7.1}$ = _____

49. $\dfrac{1.3}{0.21} \times \dfrac{0.3}{2} \times \dfrac{10.1}{0.75}$ = _____

50. $\dfrac{27.5}{10} \times \dfrac{40}{7} \times \dfrac{8.5}{1.9}$ = _____

Answers

1. 1.5; 1.48	**14.** 2.6; 2.55	**27.** 36	**40.** 67
2. 1.5; 1.54	**15.** 2.4; 2.43	**28.** 70	**41.** 50
3. 1.2; 1.21	**16.** 1.8; 1.75	**29.** 54	**42.** 42
4. 0.6; 0.61	**17.** 1.6; 1.63	**30.** 55	**43.** 78
5. 6.7; 6.67	**18.** 3.8; 3.75	**31.** 12	**44.** 19
6. 1.8; 1.81	**19.** 1.2; 1.24	**32.** 9	**45.** 89
7. 2.1; 2.13	**20.** 5.8; 5.83	**33.** 19	**46.** 11
8. 1; 1.04	**21.** 5.6; 5.65	**34.** 36	**47.** 400
9. 1.6; 1.55	**22.** 4.2; 4.17	**35.** 23	**48.** 17
10. 2.7; 2.67	**23.** 5.7; 5.7	**36.** 9	**49.** 13
11. 1.7; 1.68	**24.** 6.7; 6.67	**37.** 29	**50.** 70
12. 1.7; 1.74	**25.** 5.1; 5.15	**38.** 36	
13. 1.2; 1.17	**26.** 57	**39.** 130	

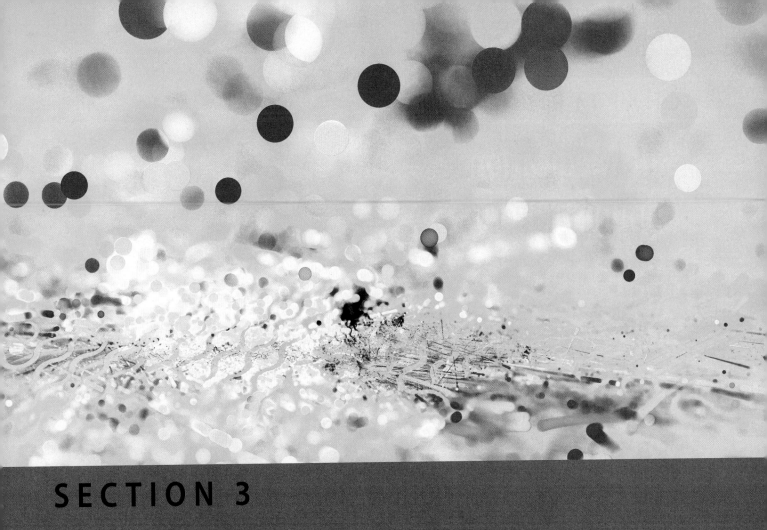

SECTION 3
Safe Medication Administration

CHAPTER 5   Safe Medication Administration

CHAPTER 5

Safe Medication Administration

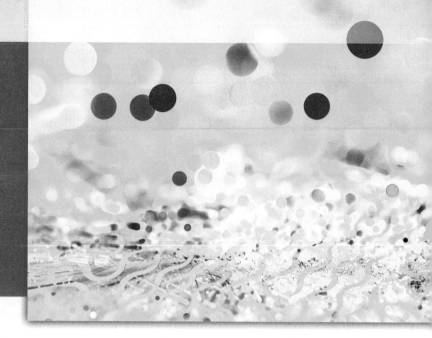

OBJECTIVES

The learner will:

1. Read a medication administration record to identify medications to be administered.

2. Record medications administered.

3. List and discuss the Six Rights of Medication Administration.

4. Explain "partnering with the patient" in medication administration.

5. List common causes of dosage errors.

6. List the five steps to take when a dosage error occurs.

7. List the two major safety concerns addressed by The Joint Commission and the Institute for Safe Medication Practices.

INTRODUCTION

In this chapter you will be introduced to a sample **medication administration record (MAR)** that may be used to prepare, administer, and chart medications. Additional instruction will include the **Six Rights of Medication Administration**, the basic guidelines for all medication administration; information on the most common sources of **medication errors**; and the **actions that you must take when errors occur**. You'll also be introduced to the latest transcription rules for medication dosages and abbreviations that have been addressed by the major watchdog organizations for medication safety: **The Joint Commission** and the **Institute for Safe Medication Practices (ISMP)**.

MEDICATION ADMINISTRATION RECORDS (MAR)

The focus of this section is to familiarize you with a sample MAR so that you will understand the many columns and features it contains. Your instructors will orient you to the actual MARs you will use in your clinical experiences, and you will quickly discover that there is **no one universal form** in use. Each clinical facility using MARs makes its own determination on the particular format that best suits its needs. What you will notice, however, is that **all MARs are more similar than different**. A MAR, simply stated, is **a paper record of all medications a patient is receiving and has received**.

The most prominent MAR feature is a **large column** that lists the medications **given on a continuing basis**. This column will contain a **drug name, dosage, frequency, actual times of administration**, and **precautions related to administration, such as checking blood pressure, pulse, or body weight**. Other columns include an area for the initials of the person who transcribed the dosages; the start date of the medication; an area to record the dosages administered; an area for the initials of the nurse who gives the dosage; and an additional area where all staff initials are identified with a full name. A MAR may consist of a single sheet of paper printed on both sides, or two sheets, to allow separate space for p.r.n. (*pro re nata* or "as needed") medications (available on patient request), for parenteral medications and site identification, and for intravenous (IV) medications and/or fluids.

Refer to the sample MAR in **Figure 5-1**, and locate the following column headings and entries:

- **Column 1:** "Start" and "Stop." The three drugs listed are being given on a continuing basis. They were started on "5–1." None has been discontinued.

- **Column 2:** "Medication and Dose." The first drug listed is Lanoxin®, including its generic name, digoxin. The dosage, "0.25 mg," and frequency, "daily," are next. There is a precautionary designation to "Check pulse" (ck pulse).

- **Column 3:** "Schedule." Gives the actual times of each medication's administration. For Lanoxin, this is 8 am.

- **Column 4:** This column has two designations. The "Route" is oral or "PO" for all three medications. The "Nurse" space, which "HB" has initialed, identifies the transcriber of these medication orders.

- **Column 5:** There are three designations here: "Time," the actual hour the drug is to be given (i.e., "8 am"); "Site" if the drug is parenteral; and "Initials," where the nurse who gave the drug, "JB," verified administration. The pulse, "64," is recorded next to the 8 am dosage.

This particular MAR covers only 4 days of medications, "5–3" through "5–6." However, most MARs provide for longer periods, often up to a month. At the bottom of this MAR is an area for identification of staff initials, where "HB" is clearly identified as "H Baker" and "JB" as "J Brown."

PROBLEMS 5-1

Refer to the MAR provided in Figure 5-1 to answer the following questions.

1. List the second and third listed drugs and dosages on this sample record.

   _____   _____

2. Who administered the 4 pm dosage for the second drug listed?

   _____

3. Drug number 3 is administered twice a day. Identify the hours these dosages are to be given. _____   _____

Answers   1. Hydrodiuril 50 mg, ciprofloxacin 250 mg   **2.** H Baker   **3.** 6 am, 6 pm

MEDICATION ADMINISTRATION RECORD

Start / Stop	Medication and Dose	Schedule	Route / Nurse		Date 5-3	Date 5-4	Date 5-5	Date 5-6
5-1	Lanoxin 0.25 mg (digoxin) daily ck pulse	8 am	PO	Time	8 P6 4			
			HB	Site				
				Initials	JB			
5-1	Hydrodiuril 50 mg twice daily	8 am	PO	Time	8 4			
		4 pm	HB	Site				
				Initials	JB HB			
5-1	Ciprofloxacin 250 mg twice a day	6 am	PO	Time	6 6			
		6 pm	HB	Site				
				Initials	JB HB			
				Time				
				Site				
				Initials				
				Time				
				Site				
				Initials				
				Time				
				Site				
				Initials				
				Time				
				Site				
				Initials				

Initials	Signature	Initials	Signature	Initials	Signature	Initials	Signature
JB	J Brown RN						
HB	H Baker						

Allergies

Physician

Room #   Name

Figure 5-1 Medication administration record.

PROBLEMS 5-2

Use the drug entries on the MAR provided as a guide to enter the next two additional drugs and dosages. Use today's date as the start date.

1. Coumadin® (warfarin) 5 mg PO daily 6 pm.

2. Pronestyl® (procainamide) 1000 mg PO every 6 hours: 6 am, noon, 6 pm, and midnight.

3. Identify your initials as the transcriber of these dosages.

4. Sign for the initial 6 pm dosage administration for each drug.

Answers Verify your answers with your instructor.

Computer-controlled records, usually keyed to drug label bar codes, are becoming more widespread in the healthcare field. The Veterans Administration System in the United States is already completely computerized, and its adoption of such records has resulted in increased safety and lower costs in medication services. It is wise to remember, however, that errors can occur anywhere, and the newer systems of administration will have identified their own safety precautions for error-prone areas.

THE SIX RIGHTS OF MEDICATION ADMINISTRATION

The **Six Rights** of administration consist of the right **drug**, the right **dosage**, the right **route**, the right **time**, to the right **person**, and the right **recording** of a dosage when it is administered. These rights may be covered in more detail in your fundamentals text, but it is appropriate to discuss them briefly here.

RIGHT DRUG

When preparing dosages, the **drug order and drug label are routinely checked against each other three times: when you locate the drug, just before you open or pour it, and immediately before you administer it**. Three specific safety reminders related to reading labels need to be revisited. First, **a drug may be ordered by trade name but available only in a generic form**, so make sure you have the drug that has been ordered. Second, **many drug names, particularly generic names, are very similar**, and must be identified carefully. Third, because it is easy to miss the **special initials that follow a drug name**—a familiar example is CR, for controlled release—look for and identify these if they are present. When doing the three required order and label cross-checks, all of these precautions to locate the correct drug apply.

RIGHT DOSAGE

Dosage is **a particular concern in metric dosages containing a decimal**. Think back to your instruction in conversions between the different units of metric measures containing decimals. You know that in conversions in metric dosages, **the decimal point will always move three places**. If you are **converting from a greater to a lesser unit**—g to mg or mg to mcg—**the number will become larger**; if you are **converting from a lesser to a greater unit**—for example, mcg to mg or mg to g—**the number will become smaller**. If you inadvertently **convert in the wrong direction, the numbers often don't make sense**: 0.25 mg **cannot** be 250 g; and 2 mg **cannot** be 0.002 mcg. Remember that medications are **prepared in average dosages** and usually consist of **one-half to three times the average dose (tablet or capsule) available**. Ask yourself if the conversion makes sense, and recognize when it doesn't.

RIGHT ROUTE

Oral medications are swallowed. This is not always easy for patients to do, and it is why many children's medications are prepared as liquids. This means you must **watch the patient actually take oral medications**. If you have any doubt that the medications have been swallowed, check the patient's mouth.

An additional oral route is the **sublingual—under the tongue**. There has been a considerable increase in the number of sublingual drugs in use in recent years, so this route designation is one to carefully identify. If a sublingual drug is swallowed, it will not have the desired effect, if it has any effect at all, because the acid in the stomach will destroy it.

Drops are another administration route, with eye, nose, and ear drops being quite commonly used. Eye medications are also prepared as **ointments**, and, understandably, they are clearly labeled for their intended **ophthalmic** use. **Locating the ophthalmic designation** is mandatory before the use of any preparation on the eyes.

An increasing number of **topical** drugs, used on the skin, are in use. These are primarily **ointments** or, less commonly, **liquids**. The amount of ointment or liquid to be used is specific, as is the cleansing of a site for repeated ointment applications, and covering or not covering the site after application.

Now in very wide use are **transdermal patches**. The precautions in their use relate to where the patch must be applied, how long it is to stay on, and examination for local skin reaction to the adhesive that secures the patch. Unfortunately, many people are sensitive to transdermal patch adhesives. A rash may appear when a patch is used for the first time, or even after repeated use. Inflamed skin will not absorb the medication well, and inflammation can cause acute discomfort.

A large number of **inhalation** medications are in common use. One of the newest is Exubera®, a form of inhalation insulin. These medications are usually self-administered, and your responsibility will be to ensure that the patient understands how to use the inhalation device, how many activations each dosage requires, how many times a day the medication should be used, and which precautions in use are warranted, such as for temporary dizziness.

The **creams and suppositories** used for the genitorectal systems provide another method of direct medication application. These medications are very clearly labeled and recognizable.

Finally, there are the **parenterals: medications administered under the skin**. The **intravenous (IV)** is the primary parenteral route, with **intramuscular (IM)** and **subcutaneous** coming in second, and **intradermal** a distant third. Most injectable drugs are **site-specific**, and are labeled for either IV, IM, or subcutaneous use. You'll be reading many drug labels that identify specific parenteral site routes in the balance of this text.

RIGHT TIME

The time when each drug is to be given is **often critical**, such as insulin immediately before a meal or, more correctly, a meal as soon as insulin is injected. Drugs may be ordered at **specific hours during the day or only at bedtime**. Some drugs must be given **before or after specific blood tests**. Pain medications are given **p.r.n.**, which means **on request at specified hourly intervals**. Pain medications are extremely **time-sensitive**, and must be given before pain becomes severe in postoperative situations, and at least half an hour before a painful procedure, including postoperative ambulation.

Each clinical facility designates routine administration times; however, "twice a day" may mean 9 am and 5 pm or 9 am and 9 pm, depending on the action of the drug being given. Each MAR identifies two **time-related specifics: frequency**—for example, "twice a day"—and **specific hours**—for example, 9 (am) and 5 (pm) or, in international/military time, 09 and 17, representing 0900 and 1700.

A final consideration, just illustrated, is **standard versus international/military time**. A clinical facility will use **either one time system or the other, but not both**. International/military time uses a 24-hour clock, starting with 0001 for 1 minute after midnight, to 2400 for midnight of the same (next date) day. To convert from standard to international/military time, add 12 hours to each hour beginning with 1 pm standard time. For example, 2 pm plus 12 hours is 1400; 4 pm plus 12 hours is 1600. Using international time, if you are unfamiliar with it, will initially require careful thought. **Table 5-1** compares times in each system.

RIGHT PERSON

Administering medications to the **right person** should be foolproof, but it isn't. All MARs identify patients by the **room number and bed** they occupy. But sometimes patients are moved, so room and bed number cannot be relied on for identification. The current identification procedure is to **ask an individual her or his name**, then check the response against the wrist **Identa-Band®**. Obviously, some people will not be able to state their name. But if they can, they must be asked.

TABLE 5-1 Comparison of Standard and International/Military Time			
Standard am	**International/Military am**	**Standard pm**	**International/Military pm**
1:00	0100	1:00	1300
2:00	0200	2:00	1400
3:00	0300	3:00	1500
4:00	0400	4:00	1600
5:00	0500	5:00	1700
6:00	0600	6:00	1800
7:00	0700	7:00	1900
8:00	0800	8:00	2000
9:00	0900	9:00	2100
10:00	1000	10:00	2200
11:00	1100	11:00	2300
12:00 noon	1200	12:00 midnight	2400

Of considerable concern is the possibility of having two people with the same surname on the same floor or even, though more rarely, in the same room. **Duplicate names** are a source of errors, so **read both the surname and first name** on each Identa-Band. **Do this every time you give a medication— no exceptions. Once a drug is administered, there is no way to get it back**.

RIGHT RECORDING

If an administered drug **is not charted, it can be given again in error**. There is an **absolute rule that a drug given must be recorded immediately**. It is also necessary to **record and report unusual reactions to a medication**, such as nausea or dizziness, or a patient's **refusal to take a medication**. In such an occurrence, **record and report the incident immediately**.

If you give a **parenteral** medication other than by IV, **the injection site used is usually recorded**, so that a different site can be used next time. Patients with diabetes or other conditions who need frequent injections may tell you which site they prefer, which they have a perfect right to do. Or, ask them if they have a preference. In actual practice, **sites are chosen by the condition of the tissues at acceptable sites**, because previous injection sites are generally easy to see and must be avoided.

THE SEVENTH RIGHT: PARTNERING WITH THE PATIENT

Partnering with the patient/recipient is so important a concern that it should be a seventh right. You are only half of a medication administration twosome. **The medication recipient is one of your best assists in preventing errors**. Consider the following, not uncommon, verbal reports:

"I just had my medication."

"My doctor told me he was stopping this drug."

"The doctor said I needed a bigger dose."

"This pill doesn't look the same as the one I had before."

"Where is my . . . pill?"

"This pill made me sick the last time I took it."

Learn to listen very carefully, and **consider the patient correct until proven otherwise**.

You will also be responsible for **helping the patient learn what drugs and dosages he or she is taking, what they are for, what time they must be taken, and how they must be taken**. Most individuals will be discharged with medications, so the sooner they—or, if they are not deemed responsible, their caretaker—can learn what they are taking, the better. They must also learn about common side effects and, if particularly relevant, untoward effects they should watch for. Patients taking medications are essentially under chemical assistance, or assault, and they or their caretakers must be full partners in their medication administration.

> 🔑 An important safety precaution is recognition of the patient/recipient as a full partner in medication administration.

MEDICATION ADMINISTRATION ABBREVIATIONS

We are now moving into the area of drug administration abbreviations. These have been the subject of much review and change in recent years in an effort to cut down on medication errors. This is a good time to learn some of the most common abbreviations you will see. You may already be familiar with some of these because they are often used in regular prescriptions.

Take a good look at **Table 5-2**. Pay particular attention to the use of upper- and lowercase letters and periods in the abbreviations. Then complete the questions that follow.

TABLE 5-2	Drug Administration Abbreviations		
a.c.	before meals	p.c.	after meals
ad lib	as desired	per	by
b.i.d.	two times a day	PO; orally	by mouth
cap	capsule	p.r.n.	when necessary/required
elix.	elixir	soln.	solution
ext	extract	stat.	at once; immediately
IM	intramuscular	subcut.	subcutaneous
IV	intravenous	supp.	suppository
nightly	every night at bedtime	susp.	suspension
NS (N/S)	normal saline	syp.	syrup
OD	right eye	tab.	tablet
OS	left eye	tr. or tinct.	tincture
OU	both eyes	ung	ointment

PROBLEMS 5-3

Identify what the following abbreviations mean.

1. b.i.d. _____

2. IV _____

3. stat   _____

4. OS   _____

5. a.c.   _____

6. p.c.   _____

7. cap   _____

8. OD   _____

9. ad lib   _____

10. tab.   _____

11. NS   _____

12. PO   _____

Answers 1. twice a day **2.** intravenous **3.** at once **4.** left eye **5.** before meal **6.** after meal
7. capsule **8.** right eye **9.** as much as wanted **10.** tablet **11.** normal saline **12.** by mouth (per os)

COMMON MEDICATION ERRORS

Prescription drugs are estimated to kill an estimated 100,000 people each year in the United States, although not all these deaths are hospital-based. Medication errors happen, and they will continue to happen in **all three of the modalities** related to drug orders: **prescribing** (done by a licensed practitioner), **transcribing** (done by a person who specializes in this responsibility, frequently the pharmacy staff), and **administration** (primarily a nursing responsibility). The vast majority of errors occur in the prescribing and transcribing areas, but those attributable to administration still account for a very large number of incidents.

In recent years, there has been a concerted international effort to identify the source of, and take active steps to reduce, the incidence of medication errors caused by the use of administration abbreviations. The primary and an ongoing leader in this project is **The Joint Commission,** formerly known as the **Joint Commission on Accreditation of Healthcare Organizations (JCAHO).**

Most safety recommendations fall into **two major categories**: (1) **abbreviations for administration and drug names** and (2) **metric dosages containing decimals.**

ERRORS IN ABBREVIATIONS AND DRUG NAMES

A number of abbreviations designating **the frequency and routes of medication administration** have been eliminated. Here are some examples: the abbreviations Q.D., QD, q.d., and qd used for a **single daily dose** and Q.O.D., QOD, q.o.d., and qod used for a dosage given **every other day**. These are no longer used, but are now clearly written as **"daily"** or **"every other day."** Similarly, qhs, formerly used for "nightly" and misread as "every hour," is now written "nightly"; SC or sub q, used for "subcutaneous," has been changed to "subcut" or "subcutaneous"; and use of "per os" for "by mouth" has been eliminated in favor of "PO," "by mouth," or "orally." An additional abbreviation, q2h or q2hr (or **any** specific hour) is now clearly written "every 2 hours." Another deletion is the use of a lowercase "u" or uppercase "U" or "IU" for "units." As you have already learned, units is not abbreviated, but written in full as "units." Table 5-2 lists acceptable administration abbreviations, but do keep in mind that there may be future changes in this evolving area of concern.

Common examples of confusing **drug name abbreviations** are MS for morphine sulfate and MSO_4 or $MgSO_4$ for magnesium sulfate. These drugs are now identified using their complete names. **Table 5-3**, the Official "Do Not Use" List, identifies these changes.

TABLE 5-3 Official "Do Not Use" List of Medical Abbreviations[1]		
Do Not Use	**Potential Problem**	**Use Instead**
U (unit)	Mistaken for "0" (zero), the number "4" (four), or "cc"	Write "unit"
IU (international unit)	Mistaken for IV (intravenous) or the number 10 (ten)	Write "international unit"
Q.D., QD, q.d., qd (daily)	Mistaken for each other	Write "daily"
Q.O.D., QOD, q.o.d, qod (every other day)	Period after the Q mistaken for "I" and the "O" mistaken for "I"	Write "every other day"
Trailing zero (X.0 mg)[2]	Decimal point is missed	Write "X mg"
Lack of leading zero (.X mg)		Write "0.X mg"
MS	Can mean morphine sulfate or magnesium sulfate	Write "morphine sulfate"
MSO_4 and $MgSO_4$	Confused for one another	Write "magnesium sulfate"

[1] Applies to all orders and all medication-related documentation that is handwritten (including free-text computer entry) or on preprinted forms.
[2] Exception: A "trailing zero" may be used only where required to demonstrate the level of precision of the value being reported, such as for laboratory results, imaging studies that report size of lesions, or catheter/tube sizes. It may not be used in medication orders or other medication-related documentation.

© The Joint Commission, 2008. Reprinted with permission.

ERRORS IN WRITING METRIC DOSAGES

All the correct rules for writing metric dosages have been covered earlier in this text. Let's revisit the culprit areas, which are also identified in Table 5-3. The first error is in **placing a decimal and a zero (0) following a whole-number dosage** (called a **trailing zero**)—for example, 4.0 g instead of 4 g. The decimal could easily be missed and 10 times the ordered dosage, 40 g, administered. The second error is **failing to place a zero in front of a decimal fraction** (referred to as lack of a **leading zero**)—for example, .5 mg instead of **0**.5 mg. Once again, the decimal could be missed and 5 mg administered. Unfortunately, you may still see an occasional commercial drug label that has not yet been standardized to reflect the new recommended notation rules. But at least on a drug label you will not have the problem of trying to **interpret indecipherable handwriting**, which is often the direct cause of many of the errors just discussed. Commercial drug labels are being redesigned to reflect these new guidelines.

Additional changes have since been recommended by the **Institute for Safe Medication Practices**. Those of you re-entering the healthcare field after a significant absence may want to review the ISMP lists in the Appendix. These tables are for reference only and need not be memorized.

ACTION STEPS WHEN ERRORS OCCUR

You will almost certainly meet with an error in one way or another during your career. So, let's look at the routine steps you must take when one occurs.

> **Step 1: Report error immediately.**
>
> **Step 2: Institute necessary remedial measures.**
>
> **Step 3: Determine the reason for the error.**
>
> **Step 4: Prepare an incident/accident report.**
>
> **Step 5: Institute corrective policies/procedures to prevent recurrence.**

The most important step after ensuring the safety of the patient is reporting the error. If an error isn't reported, no action can be taken. Keep in mind that **an error is an accident, and not necessarily a reflection on competency, nor will reporting an error terminate your career. Distraction and fatigue play a significant role in medication errors**, and when in stressful situations you must be particularly aware and vigilant that you do not become the person making an error.

⚷ The major factors in nursing medication administration errors are distraction and fatigue, and particular vigilance is necessary in these stressful situations.

In time, and with repeat practice, administering medications will become familiar and comfortable. The irony is that when it does, you must **exercise more caution than ever. Routine medication administration must never be routine**.

⚷ Regardless of the source of an error, if you give a wrong drug or dosage, you are legally responsible for it.

SUMMARY

This completes your introduction to safe medication administration. The important points to remember from this chapter are:

- When identifying a drug, pay particular attention to generic names and any initials that identify additional drug components or action.

- When identifying dosages, take special precautions with metric dosages containing a decimal.

- The route of administration is critical to medication safety and effectiveness.

- Parenteral medications are site-specific: IV, IM, subcutaneous, and intradermal.

- Time of administration is especially important for p.r.n. medications for pain, and for drugs with a rapid action such as insulin.

- Identification of the right person begins with asking the patient his or her name, followed by checking the Identa-Band.

- Making the patient or caretaker a full partner in medication administration is a major safety consideration.

- Recent changes in abbreviations for drug names and administration are creating increased safety in the clinical setting.

- Dosage errors must be reported as soon as discovered to set in motion the four additional steps you must take.

- Administering medications must never become routine.

- Fatigue and clinical distractions are major factors in medication errors.

- MARs are the immediate reference for medication administration, and keeping them up-to-the-minute is of prime importance.

SUMMARY SELF-TEST

Answer the questions as succinctly as possible.

1. List the Six Rights of Medication Administration. _____

_____

2. What consideration was stressed regarding reading generic names? _____

_____

3. What might extra initials following a drug name identify? _____

_____

_____

4. List the two major transcribing considerations for metric dosages containing a decimal.

_____

_____

5. What use will you make of the fact that medications are prepared in average dosages?

_____

_____

6. Name and discuss the two time-sensitive medications that were identified in this chapter.

_____

_____

7. Which two patient identification steps follow arrival at the room and bed number indicated on a MAR? _____

_____

8. What will you do if a patient refuses a medication? _____

_____

9. List the steps you must take when a medication error occurs. _____

_____

_____

_____

10. List your medication responsibilities in preparing a patient for discharge.

_____

_____

_____

Answers

1. Drug, dosage, route, person, time, and recording
2. Read carefully; they are often similar.
3. Additional medications in a preparation or special action
4. Use a zero in front of a decimal to draw attention to it; do not include a decimal or zero following a whole-number dosage.
5. An unusual number of oral tablets or capsules or excessively large mL volumes must be questioned.
6. Pain medications—give before pain becomes severe or half an hour before a painful

procedure; insulin—make sure a meal is available shortly after administration
7. Ask the patient for his or her name; check the Identa-Band.
8. Ask why, record it, and report it.
9. Report the error, take remedial measures as necessary, determine the cause, and institute a policy to prevent a repeat.
10. Review all the discharge drugs by asking the patient to explain the dosage, frequency, time, and route of administration for each. Review these again as necessary, including side effects and precautions.

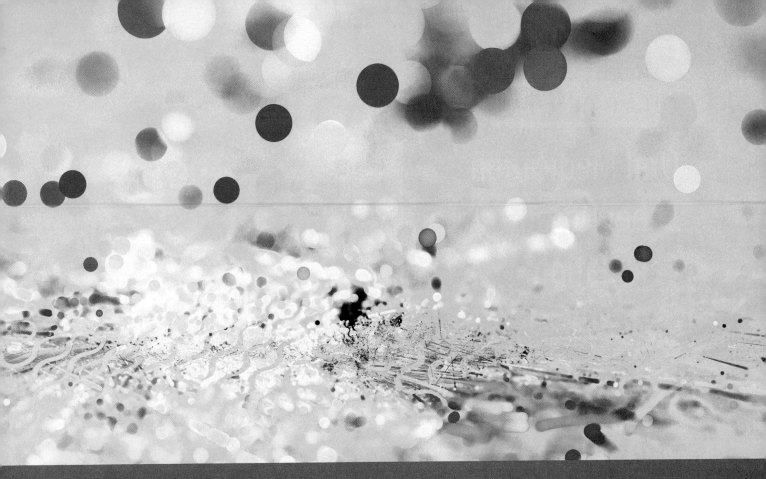

SECTION 4

Introduction to Clinical Calculations

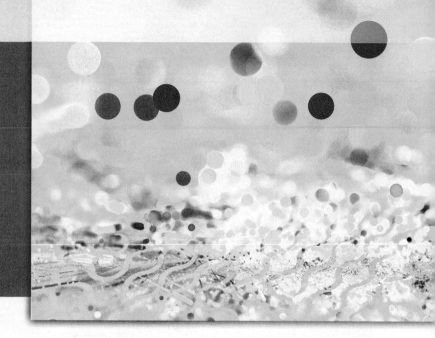

CHAPTER 6

Oral Medication Label Dosage Calculation

OBJECTIVES

The learner will:

1. Identify scored tablets, unscored tablets, and capsules.

2. Read drug labels to identify trade and generic names.

3. Locate dosage strengths and calculate average dosages.

4. Measure oral solutions using a medicine cup.

INTRODUCTION: TYPES OF ORAL MEDICATIONS

This chapter begins your introduction to actual drug dosage labels to demonstrate the simplicity of solving simple dosage calculations. Medication label information includes trade and generic drug names, metric dosage strengths, manufacturer's name, and other details you need to be aware of, primarily so that you can quickly locate the correct dosage strength to calculate ordered dosages. You will then use actual drug labels to calculate a full range of oral medication dosages. **Average dosage calculations require only the information you have already learned on the metric system and in the Refresher Math section on addition and subtraction.** They are routinely done mentally. Advanced calculations are needed primarily in clinical specialty areas, and they will be covered in later chapters.

> 🔑 Most oral dosages consist of one-half to three tablets or capsules, or one-half to double the mL volume of liquid medications, and are done mentally.

We will begin with labels for solid drug preparations (**Figure 6-1**). These include tablets, scored tablets (which contain an indented marking to make breakage for partial dosages possible), enteric-coated tablets (which delay absorption until the drug reaches the small intestine), capsules (which are powdered or oily drugs in a gelatin cover), and sustained- or controlled-release capsules (whose action is spread over a prolonged period of time—for example, 12 hours).

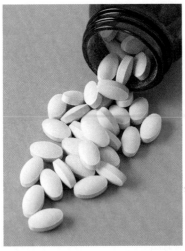

A. Tablets.

© Ramon Espelt Photography/Shutterstock

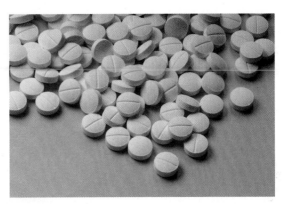

B. Scored tablets.

© MARCELODLT/Shutterstock

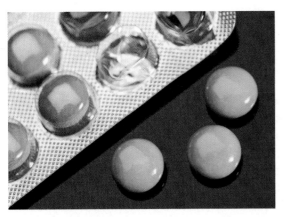

C. Enteric-coated tablets.

© Juanmonino/E+/Getty Images

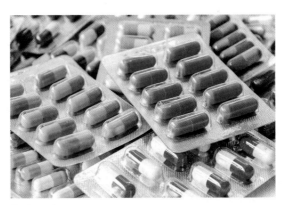

D. Capsules.

© nokwalai/Shutterstock

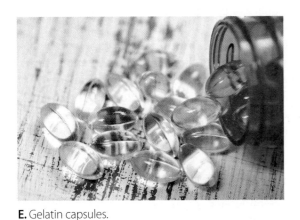

E. Gelatin capsules.

© Alexeysun/Shutterstock

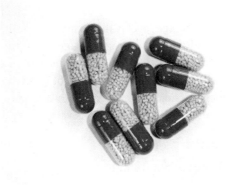

F. Controlled-release capsules.

© Lubov Vis/Shutterstock

Figure 6-1 Solid drug preparations.

TABLET AND CAPSULE LABELS

The most common type of label you will see in the clinical setting is the **unit dosage label**, in which each tablet or capsule is packaged separately. However, the dosage information on both unit and multiple dose labels is identical.

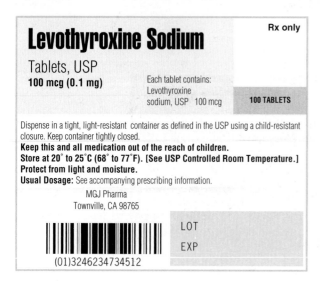

Figure 6-2

Figure 6-3

EXAMPLE 1

Look at the levothyroxine sodium label in **Figure 6-2**. The **name** of the drug is clearly printed at the **top left** of the label. This is the drug's **generic name**, which, in spite of it's capitalization on this label, is normally written using **lowercase letters**. Underneath this is the **drug format, tablets**. Notice the **USP** that follows "Tablets," which refers to **United States Pharmacopeia**, one of several **national listings** of medications. The **generic** is the **official international chemical name** of a drug. Drug labels often contain **trade names**, each for the **exclusive use** of a drug's manufacturer. Levothyroxine sodium, which is the main drug used to treat hypothyroidism, is also marketed under the trade names Synthroid, Levoxyl, Unithroid, and Levothyroid. **Trade names are usually capitalized**, with some form of **trade mark or registration symbol** identifying them. Drugs may be ordered by either name depending on hospital policy or prescriber preference, so recognizing this difference is necessary for accurate identification.

Next on the label is the **dosage strength**, 100 mcg or 0.1 mg. The prepared dosage is often representative of the **average dosage strength: the dosage given to the average patient at one time**.

Notice that **100 TABLETS** is printed near the **top** of the label. This is the **total number** of tablets in the bottle. Be careful not to confuse the quantity of tablets or capsules with the dosage strength. **The dosage strength always has a unit of measure associated with it**—in this case, mcg and mg. Because label designs vary widely, this is an important point to remember.

EXAMPLE 2

The label in **Figure 6-3** is an example of a medication that contains not one but **two drugs**: 5 mg of the narcotic oxycodone and 325 mg of acetaminophen, an analgesic. The dosages in multiple-drug products are routinely written in the same order as the drugs listed in the product. Oxycodone and acetaminophen are generic names. Medications that contain more than one drug are usually **ordered by trade name and number of tablets or capsules** to be given rather than by dosage. Percocet, Endocet, Roxicet, and Tylox are some of the **trade name** medications that contain identical dosages for these pain relieving drugs. Given the country's addictive history of oxycodone, you will already be familiar with this generic name.

 Tablets and capsules that contain more than one drug are usually ordered by trade name and number of tablets or capsules to be given, rather than by dosage.

PROBLEMS 6-1

Refer to the label in **Figure 6-4** and answer the questions about this drug.

1. What is the generic name? _____

2. What is the dosage strength? _____

3. How many tablets are in this container? _____

4. If lisinopril 5 mg is ordered, how many tablets will you give? _____

5. If lisinopril 10 mg is ordered, how many tablets will you give? _____

Lisinopril
Tablets, USP

5 mg

100 Tablets

Rx only

DFE Pharma
Townville, CA 98765

Each uncoated tablet contains:
Lisinopril dihydrate USP equivalent to
Lisinopril anhydrous 10 mg

USUAL DOSAGE: See accompanying
prescribing information.

WARNING: As with all medications,
keep out of the reach of children.
Store at 20˚ to 25˚C (68˚ to 77˚F);
[See USP Controlled Room Temperature].
Protect from moisture, freezing and
excessive heat.
Dispense in a tight container.

ONCE-DAILY

**Change in
tablet description**

LOT   EXP

Figure 6-4

Answers 1. lisinopril   **2.** 5 mg   **3.** 100 tablets   **4.** 1 tab   **5.** 2 tab

Refer to the label in **Figure 6-5**, which is another example of a combined drug tablet. The **generic** names of these drugs are **carbidopa** and **levodopa**, major drugs used in the treatment of Parkinson's disease. Two other labels for these combined drugs are included to show different dosage preparations. The label in Figure 6-5 identified a 25 mg/100 mg carbidopa-levodopa preparation. Contrast this with the labels in **Figures 6-6** and **6-7**.

In Figure 6-6, the dosage strengths are different. The strengths of carbidopa and levodopa are **10 mg** and **100 mg**, respectively, which are actually lower dosages. And, finally, Figure 6-7 is a label for a controlled-release or sustained-release tablet with yet another dosage strength of 50–200: **carbidopa 50 mg** and **levodopa 200 mg**. Unlike the previous combined drug tablet discussed, an order for Sinemet **must** include the dosage because it is available in several strengths.

⚷ Extra numbers after a drug name may be used to identify the dosage strengths of more than one drug in a preparation, and extra initials may be used to identify a special drug action.

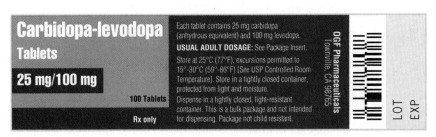

Carbidopa-levodopa
Tablets

25 mg/100 mg

100 Tablets

Rx only

Each tablet contains 25 mg carbidopa
(anhydrous equivalent) and 100 mg levodopa.
USUAL ADULT DOSAGE: See Package Insert.
Store at 25°C (77°F), excursions permitted to
15°-30°C (59°-86°F) [See USP Controlled Room
Temperature]. Store in a tightly closed container,
protected from light and moisture.
Dispense in a tightly closed, light-resistant
container. This is a bulk package and not intended
for dispensing. Package not child resistant.

OGF Pharmaceuticals
Townville, CA 98765

LOT   EXP

Figure 6-5

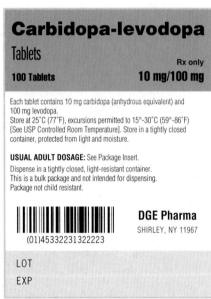

Figure 6-6

Figure 6-7

Refer to the labels in Figures 6-5 through 6-7 to answer these questions.

1. What is the dosage of carbidopa-levodopa in Figure 6-6? _____

2. What is the dosage in Figure 6-7? _____

3. What form are these medications prepared as? _____

4. The tablets in Figure 6-7 have a different action. Identify this. _____

Answers 1. 10 mg/100 mg   **2.** 50 mg/ 200 mg   **3.** tablets   **4.** Extended-Release

TABLET AND CAPSULE DOSAGE CALCULATION

When the time comes for you to administer medications, you will have to read a medication administration record (MAR) to prepare the dosage. The MAR will tell you the name and amount of drug to be given, but it will not tell you how many tablets or capsules contain this dosage. This you must calculate yourself. However, remember that most tablets/capsules are prepared in average dosage strengths, and most orders will involve giving one-half to three tablets (or one to three capsules, since capsules cannot be broken in half). **Learn to question orders for more than three tablets or capsules.**

🔑 An unusual number of tablets or capsules could be a warning of an error in prescribing, transcribing, or calculation.

Let's now look at some sample orders and do some actual dosage calculations. **Assume that tablets are scored and can be broken in half**.

PROBLEMS 6-3

Refer to the label in Figure 6-8 to answer these questions.

1. What is the dosage strength?   _____

2. If you have an order for 120 mg, give   _____

3. If you have an order for 60 mg, give   _____

4. What is the generic name of this drug?   _____

5. What is the total number of capsules in this package?   _____

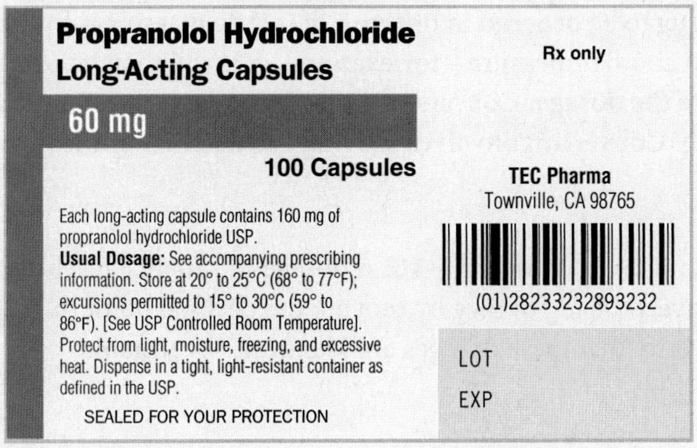

**Propranolol Hydrochloride
Long-Acting Capsules**

Rx only

60 mg

100 Capsules

TEC Pharma
Townville, CA 98765

Each long-acting capsule contains 160 mg of propranolol hydrochloride USP.
Usual Dosage: See accompanying prescribing information. Store at 20° to 25°C (68° to 77°F); excursions permitted to 15° to 30°C (59° to 86°F). [See USP Controlled Room Temperature]. Protect from light, moisture, freezing, and excessive heat. Dispense in a tight, light-resistant container as defined in the USP.

SEALED FOR YOUR PROTECTION

(01)28233232893232

LOT

EXP

Figure 6-8

Answers **1.** 60 mg   **2.** 2 cap   **3.** 1 cap   **4.** propranolol hydrochloride   **5.** 100 capsules

---

PROBLEMS 6-4

Refer to the label in Figure 6-9 to answer these questions.

1. What is the dosage strength?   _____

2. If 10 mg is ordered, give   _____

3. If 2.5 mg is ordered, give   _____

4. If 5 mg is ordered, give   _____

5. What is the generic name of this drug?   _____

6. What is the total number of tablets in this package?   _____

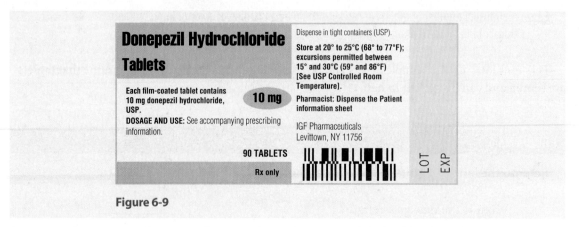

Figure 6-9

Answers 1. 10 mg **2.** 1 tab **3.** 2½ tab **4.** ½ tab **5.** donepezil HCl (hydrochloride is often reduced to chemical HCl) **6.** 90 tablets

In reading this label, you were asked to calculate a dosage that required a half tablet, which is not common. However, in a number of problems you will be asked to calculate these, just so you will be familiar with them.

It is common for a drug to be **ordered** in one unit of metric measure—**for example, mg**—and discover that it is **labeled** in another measure—**for example, g**. It will then be necessary to **convert the metric units to calculate the dosage.** Conversions will always be between touching units of measure: g and mg or mg and mcg. **Converting involves moving the decimal point three places.**

EXAMPLE 1

Refer to the triazolam label in **Figure 6-10**. A dosage of 250 mcg has been ordered. The label reads 0.25 mg. Convert the mg to mcg by moving the decimal point three places to the right, and you can mentally verify that these dosages are identical. Give 1 tablet.

EXAMPLE 2

Refer to the clonazepam label in **Figure 6-11**. A dosage of 1000 mcg is ordered. The label reads 0.5 mg, so you must give 2 tablets (1 tab = 500 mcg, so 1000 mcg requires 2 tab). The decimal moves three places to the right in this conversion from mg to mcg.

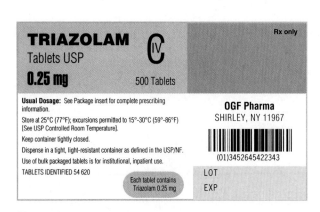

Figure 6-10

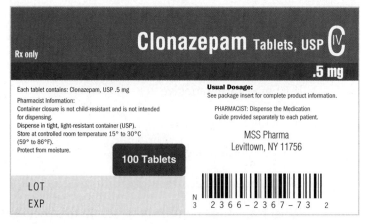

Figure 6-11

PROBLEMS 6-5

Locate the appropriate labels for the following dosages, and indicate how many tablets or capsules are needed to give them. Assume all tablets are scored and can be broken in half. Labels may be used in more than one problem.

1. verapamil HCl 0.12 g _____ cap

2. loxapine succinate 10 mg _____ cap

3. loxapine succinate 5000 mcg _____ cap

4. methylphenidate HCl 5000 mcg _____ tab

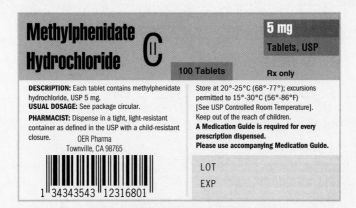

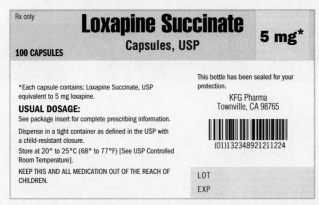

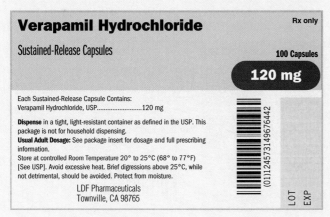

Answers **1.** 1 cap **2.** 2 cap **3.** 1 cap **4.** 1 tab

PROBLEMS 6-6

Locate the appropriate labels for the following drug orders, and indicate the number of tablets/capsules that will be required to administer the dosages ordered. Assume that all tablets are scored and can be broken in half. A label may be used in more than one problem.

1. isosorbide dinitrate 60 mg   _____ tab

2. sulfasalazine 0.5 g   _____ tab

3. sulfasalazine 1 g   _____ tab

4. terbutaline sulfate 2500 mcg   _____ tab

5. chlordiazepoxide HCl 50 mg   _____ cap

6. chlordiazepoxide HCl 25 mg   _____ cap

7. isosorbide dinitrate 80 mg   _____ tab

8. levothyroxine 0.2 mg   _____ tab

9. levothyroxine Na 0.2 mg   _____ tab

10. terbutaline sulfate 2500 mcg   _____ tab

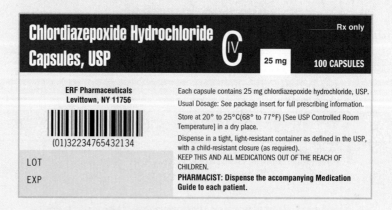

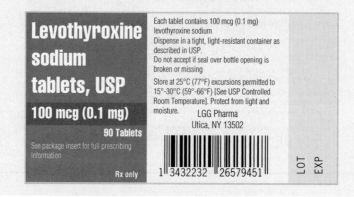

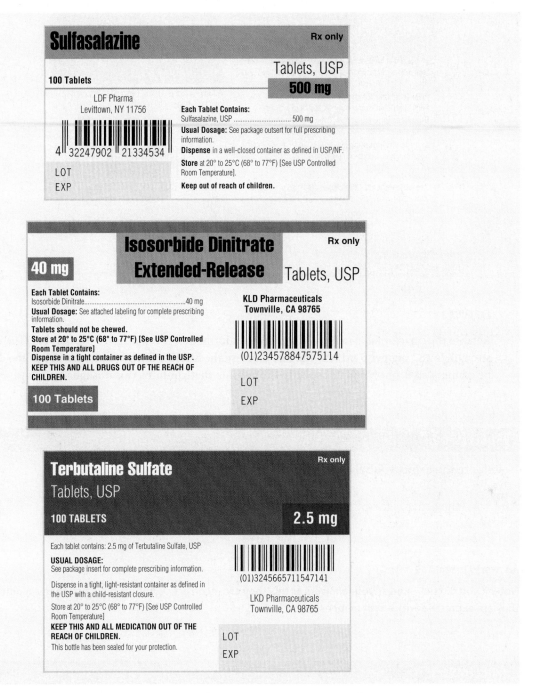

Answers **1.** 1½ tab **2.** 1 tab **3.** 2 tab **4.** 1 tab **5.** 2 cap **6.** 1 cap **7.** 2 tab **8.** 2 tab
9. 2 tab **10.** 1 tab

ORAL SOLUTION LABELS

In liquid drug preparations, the dosage is contained in a certain mL **volume of solution**. Let's review
dosages in some solid and liquid drug preparations to illustrate the difference.

EXAMPLE 1	**Solid:** 250 mg in **1 tablet**	**Liquid:** 250 mg in **5 mL**
EXAMPLE 2	**Solid:** 100 mg in **1 capsule**	**Liquid:** 100 mg in **10 mL**

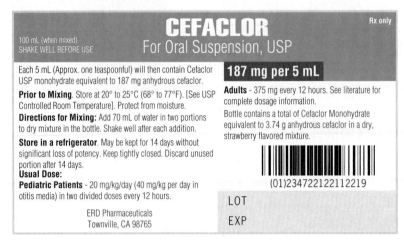

Figure 6-12

EXAMPLE 3

Refer to the cefaclor label in **Figure 6-12**. The information it contains will be familiar. The dosage strength is **187 mg per 5 mL**. As with solid drugs, the MAR will tell you the **dosage of the drug** to be administered, but it **will not specify the volume that contains this dosage**.

PROBLEMS 6-7

Refer to the cefaclor label in Figure 6-12 to calculate these dosages.

1. The order is for cefaclor 187 mg. Give   _____

2. The order is for cefaclor 374 mg. Give   _____

Answers   1. 5 mL   **2.** 10 mL

Note: If you did not express your answers as mL, they are incorrect. Numbers have no meaning unless they are expressed with a unit of measure.

PROBLEMS 6-8

Refer to the solution labels in **Figures 6-13** and **6-14** to calculate these dosages.

1. fluoxetine soln. 10 mg   _____

2. cefaclor susp. 187 mg   _____

3. cefaclor susp. 374 mg   _____

4. fluoxetine HCl soln. 30 mg   _____

5. fluoxetine soln. 40 mg   _____

6. fluoxetine HCl soln. 20 mg   _____

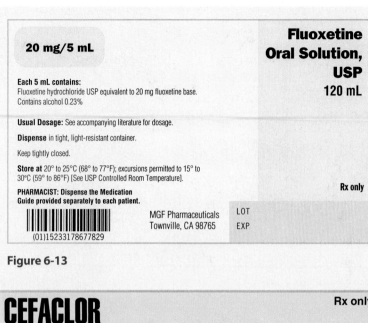

Figure 6-13

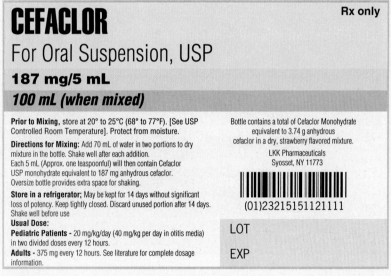

Figure 6-14

Answers 1. 2.5 mL   **2.** 5 mL   **3.** 10 mL   **4.** 7.5 mL   **5.** 10 mL   **6.** 5 mL

MEASUREMENT OF ORAL SOLUTIONS

Oral solutions are most commonly measured using a disposable **calibrated medication cup**. Take a close look at the schematic drawing of the medication cup calibrations in **Figure 6-15**. Many disposable medication cups, like this one, still contain the TSP (teaspoon), TBS (tablespoon), and OZ (ounce) calibrations of the household system and the obsolete DR (for dram) calibration of the apothecary system. Some also contain the increasingly disused cc (cubic centimeter) calibration, which is identical to a mL. Oral solutions are **most safely poured at eye level**. Because of the number of units of measure on these cups, **always read calibrations very carefully**.

Small-volume solution dosages can also be measured using specially calibrated **oral syringes**, such as those illustrated in **Figure 6-16**. Oral syringes have safety features built into their design to prevent them from being mistaken for hypodermic syringes. The main safety feature of oral syringes is the syringe tip, which is larger and a different shape. Other oral syringe features you may see are an off-center tip, termed **eccentric**, or an **amber color**. Hypodermic syringes are not colored, although their packaging and needle covers are colored to aid in identification. Hypodermic syringes **without a needle** can also be used to measure and administer oral dosages.

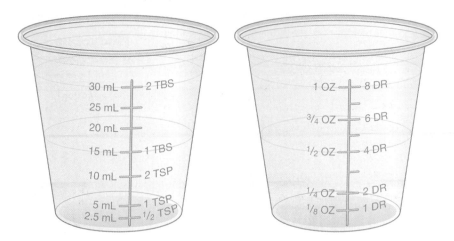

Figure 6-15

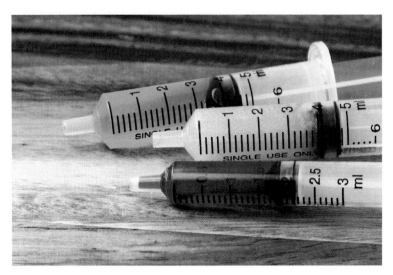

Figure 6-16
© mangpor_2004/iStock/Getty Images

The main concern with **correct oral syringe identification** is that they **are not sterile**, and they must not be confused and used for **hypodermic medications, which are sterile**. This mistake **has** actually been made, despite the fact that hypodermic needles do not fit correctly on oral syringes. Therefore, this precaution does need to be stressed.

Oral solutions may also be ordered as drops (gtt), and when this is the case, the dropper is attached to the bottle stopper. Medicine droppers are often calibrated in mL or by actual dosage, such as 125 mg, and so forth. (Refer to the *Pediatric IV Medications* chapter for more information on droppers.)

SUMMARY

This concludes the chapter on reading oral medication labels. The important points to remember from this chapter are:

- Most labels contain both generic and trade names.

- Dosages are clearly printed on the label, including preparations containing multiple drugs.

- Combined-dosage tablets and capsules may be ordered by trade name and number of tablets/capsules to be given and may include dosages.

- Additional letters that follow a drug name are used to identify additional drugs in the preparation or a special action of the drug.

- Most dosages of tablets or capsules consist of one-half to three tablets (or one to three capsules, which cannot be broken in half). An unusual number of tablets or capsules may indicate an error.

- For accurate measurement, pour solutions at eye level when a medicine cup is used.

- Liquid oral medications may be measured and administered using an oral medication syringe or a hypodermic syringe without a needle.

- Care must be taken not to use oral syringes for hypodermic medication preparation because these are not sterile.

SUMMARY SELF-TEST

Answer the following questions.

1. What guideline were you given on the number of tablets/capsules in an average dosage? _____

2. Which type of oral medication can provide a half-dosage order? _____

3. Which type of oral medications cannot be crushed? _____

4. How are generic names written and identified on labels? _____

5. What is the key to distinguishing between total tablets and dosage on a label? _____

Answers

1. 1–3
2. scored tab
3. enteric coated tab
4. printed lower case
5. dosage contains a quantity

CHAPTER 7

Hypodermic Syringe Management

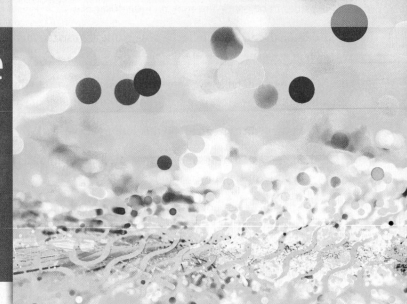

OBJECTIVES

The learner will measure parenteral solutions using:

1. A standard 3 mL syringe.

2. A tuberculin syringe.

3. 5 and 10 mL syringes.

4. A 20 mL syringe.

INTRODUCTION

A variety of hypodermic syringes are in clinical use. This chapter focuses most heavily on the frequently used 3 mL syringe. However, larger-volume syringes are used on occasion, so it is necessary that you learn the **differences** as well as the **similarities** of all syringes in use.

Regardless of a syringe's volume or capacity—0.5, 1, 3, 5, 10, or 20 mL—all except specialized insulin syringes **are calibrated in mL**. Because some syringe manufacturers have not yet replaced the labeling on their syringes with the official mL volume measurement, you may still see cc on syringes. Keep in mind, however, that these two measures, mL and cc, are essentially identical. They will be correctly referred to throughout this text as mL. The various capacity syringes contain **calibrations that differ from each other**. Recognizing the difference in syringe calibrations is the chief safety concern of this chapter.

> ⚷ The calibrations on different volume syringes differ from each other, requiring
> particular care in dosage measurement.

STANDARD 3 mL SYRINGE

The most commonly used hypodermic syringe is the 3 mL size illustrated in **Figure 7-1**. Notice the calibrations for the metric mL scale, and that **longer calibrations** identify zero (0) and each ½ and full mL measure. These longer calibrations are numbered: ½, 1, 1½, 2, 2½, and 3.

Next, notice the **number of calibrations in each mL**, which is **10**, indicating that on this syringe, each mL is **calibrated in tenths**. Tenths of a mL are written as **decimal fractions**—for example 1.2 mL, 2.5 mL, or 0.4 mL. Also, notice the arrow on this syringe, which identifies a 0.8 mL dosage.

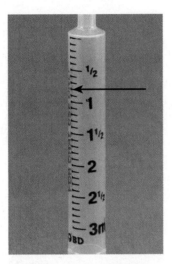

Figure 7-1 A 3 mL syringe.

PROBLEMS 7-1

Use decimal numbers—for example, 2.2 mL—to identify the measurements indicated by the arrows on the standard 3 mL syringes that follow.

1. _____   2. _____   3. _____

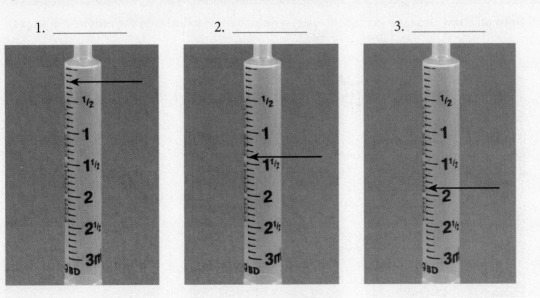

Answers 1. 0.2 mL   **2.** 1.4 mL   **3.** 1.9 mL

Did you have difficulty with the 0.2 mL calibration in Problem 1? Remember that **the first long calibration on all syringes is zero**. It is slightly longer than the 0.1 mL and subsequent one-tenth calibrations. Be careful not to mistakenly count it as 0.1 mL.

You have just been looking at photos of syringe barrels only. In assembled syringes, the colored suction tip of the plunger has two widened areas in contact with the barrel that look like two distinct rings. **Calibrations are read from the front, or top, ring**. Do not become confused by the second, or bottom, ring or by the raised middle section of the suction tip.

PROBLEMS 7-2

What dosages are measured by the following three assembled syringes?

1. _____   2. _____   3. _____

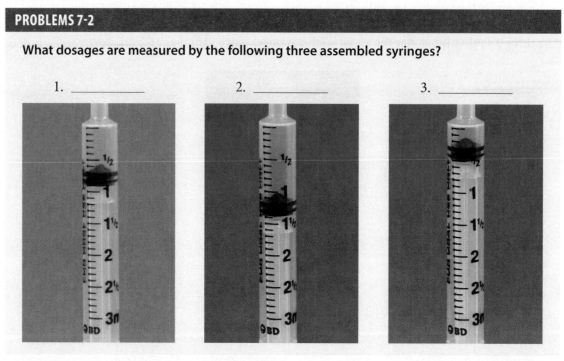

Answers **1.** 0.7 mL   **2.** 1.2 mL   **3.** 0.3 mL

PROBLEMS 7-3

Draw an arrow or shade in the following syringe barrels to indicate the required dosages.

1. 1.3 mL   2. 2.4 mL   3. 0.9 mL

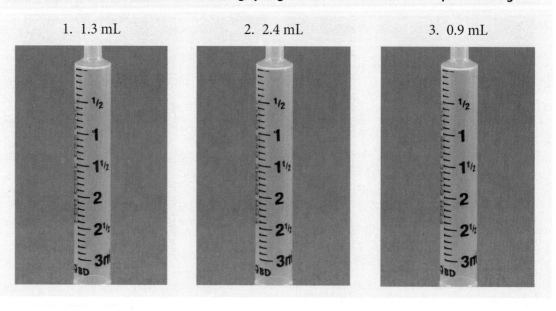

4. 2.5 mL   5. 1.7 mL   6. 2.1 mL

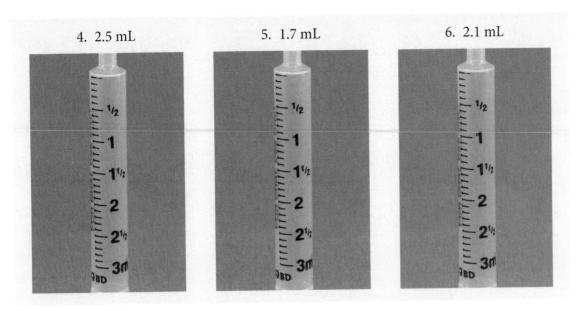

Answers Verify your answers with your instructor.

PROBLEMS 7-4

Identify the dosages measured on the following 3 mL syringes.

1. _____   2. _____   3. _____

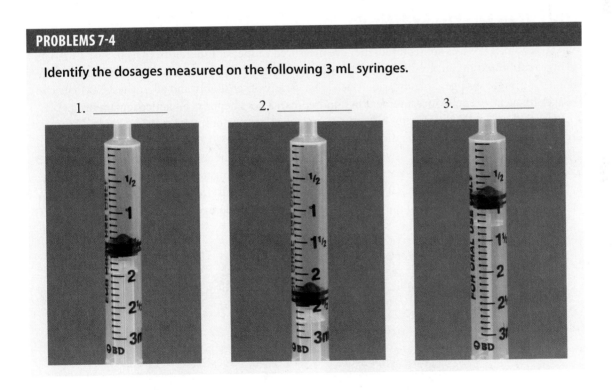

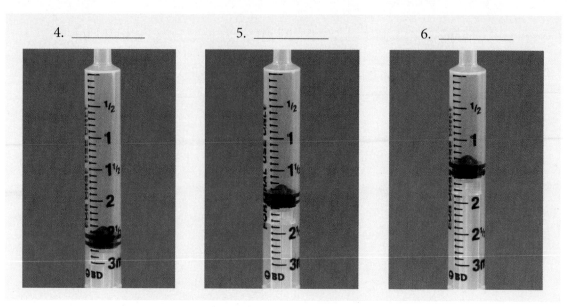

4. _____   5. _____   6. _____

Answers 1. 1.5 mL   **2.** 2.3 mL   **3.** 0.8 mL   **4.** 2.6 mL   **5.** 1.9 mL   **6.** 1.4 mL

TUBERCULIN (TB) SYRINGE

When very small dosages are required, they are measured in special **tuberculin (TB) 0. 5 or 1 mL syringes calibrated in hundredths**. Originally designed for the small dosages required for tuberculin skin testing, these syringes are now widely used in a variety of sensitivity and allergy tests. Pediatric dosages frequently require measurement in hundredths, as does heparin, an anticoagulant drug.

Refer to the 0.5 mL TB syringe in **Figure 7-2**, and take a careful look at its metric calibrated hundredths scale. Slightly longer calibrations identify zero, 0.05, 0.1, 0.15, 0.2, and so on through the 0.5 mL measure. Shorter calibrations lie between these to measure the hundredths. Each tenth mL—0.1, 0.2, 0.3, 0.4, and 0.5—is numbered on this particular TB syringe. Take a moment to study the dosage measured by the arrow in Figure 7-2, which is 0.43 mL. The closeness and small size of the TB syringe calibrations mandate particular care and an unhurried approach in TB syringe dosage measurement.

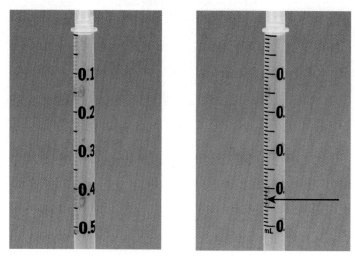

Figure 7-2 A tuberculin (TB) syringe.

PROBLEMS 7-5

Identify the measurements on the six TB syringes provided.

1. _____

2. _____

3. _____

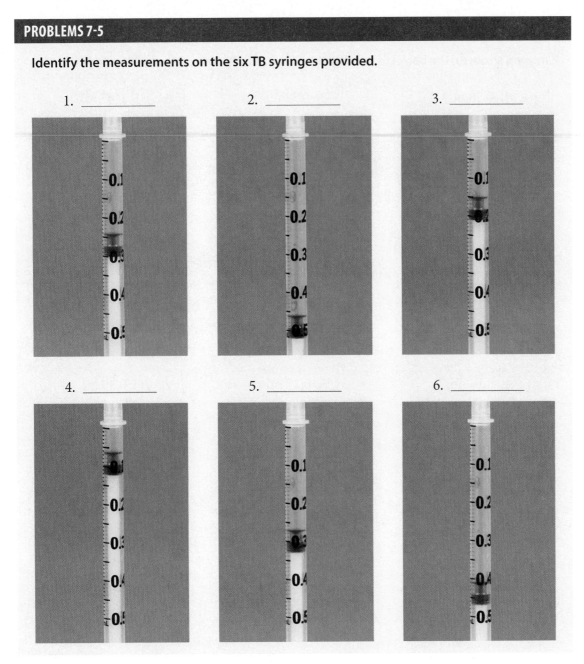

4. _____

5. _____

6. _____

Answers **1.** 0.24 mL   **2.** 0.46 mL   **3.** 0.15 mL   **4.** 0.06 mL   **5.** 0.27 mL   **6.** 0.41 mL

PROBLEMS 7-6

Draw an arrow on the barrel to identify the dosages indicated on these TB syringes.

1. 0.28 mL   2. 0.32 mL   3. 0.45 mL

4. 0.12 mL   5. 0.27 mL   6. 0.35 mL

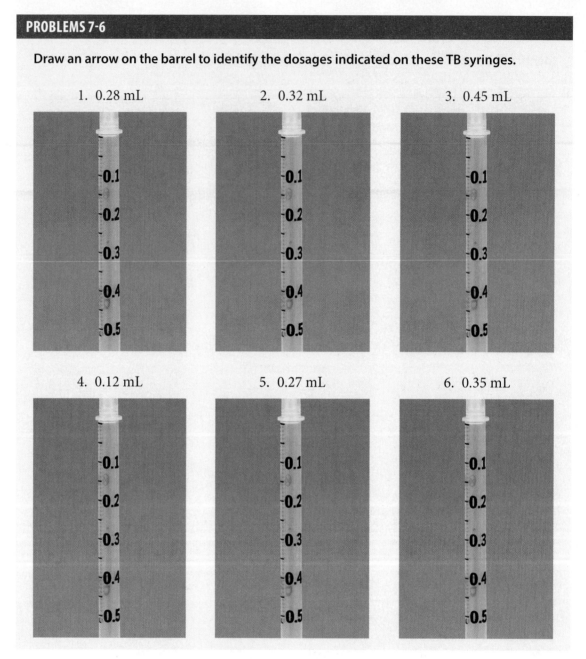

Answers Verify your answers with your instructor.

5 AND 10 mL SYRINGES

When volumes larger than 3 mL are required, a 5 or 10 mL syringe is typically used. Refer to **Figure 7-3**, and examine the calibrations between the numbered mLs to determine how these syringes are calibrated.

As you may have discovered, the calibrations divide each mL of these syringes into **five sections**, so that **each shorter calibration actually measures 0.2 mL**. The 5 mL syringe in Figure 7-3A measures 4.6 mL, and the 10 mL syringe in Figure 7-3B measures 7.6 mL. These syringes are most often used to measure whole rather than fractional dosages, but in your practice readings, we will include a full range of measurements.

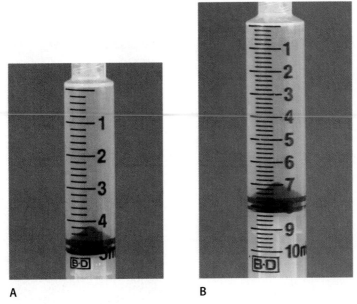

Figure 7-3   A. A 5 mL syringe; **B.** A 10 mL syringe.

PROBLEMS 7-7

What dosages are measured on the following syringes?

1. _____   2. _____   3. _____

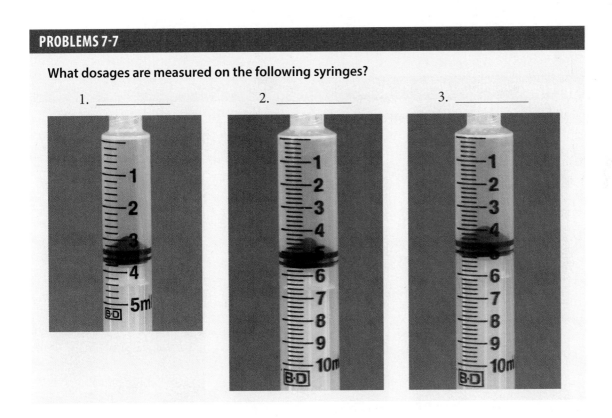

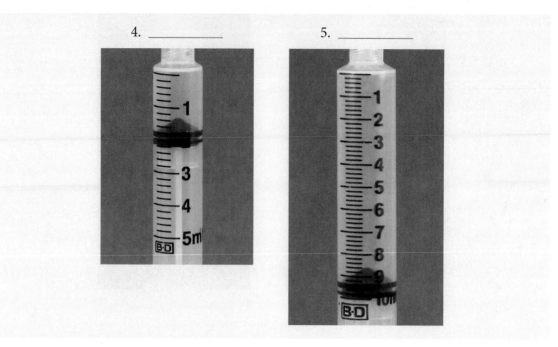

4. _____   5. _____

Answers **1.** 3.4 mL   **2.** 5 mL   **3.** 4.6 mL   **4.** 1.8 mL   **5.** 9.4 mL

PROBLEMS 7-8

Measure the dosages indicated on the syringes provided.

1. 1.4 mL   2. 3.2 mL   3. 6.8 mL

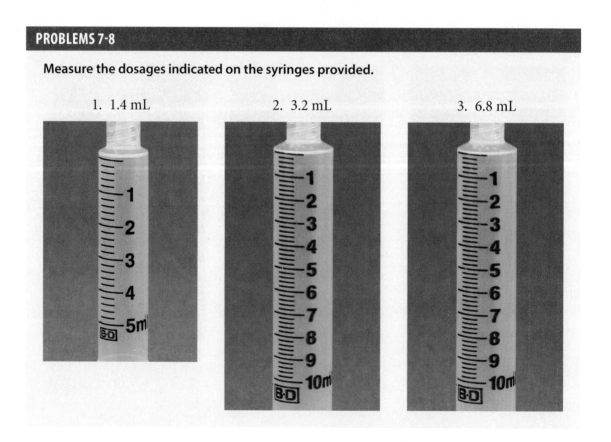

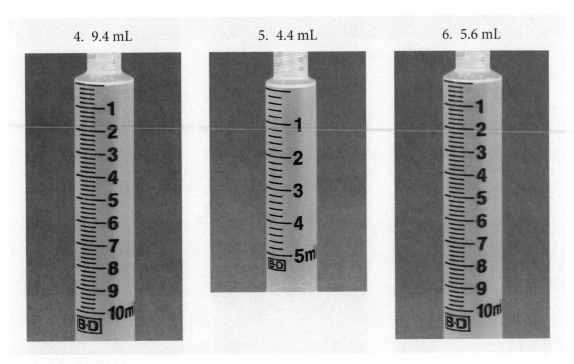

4. 9.4 mL   5. 4.4 mL   6. 5.6 mL

Answers Verify your answers with your instructor.

20 mL AND LARGER SYRINGES

Examine the 20 mL syringe in **Figure 7-4**. As you can see, this syringe is calibrated in **1 mL increments**, with longer calibrations identifying the 0, 5, 10, 15, and 20 mL volumes. Syringes with a capacity larger than 20 mL are also calibrated in full mL measures. These syringes are used only for measurement of very large volumes.

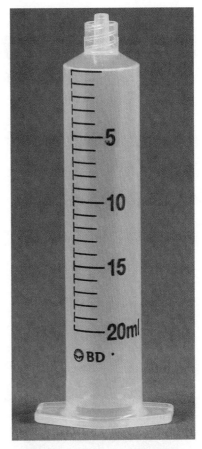

Figure 7-4 A 20 mL syringe.

PROBLEMS 7-9

What dosages are measured on these syringes?

1. _____   2. _____   3. _____

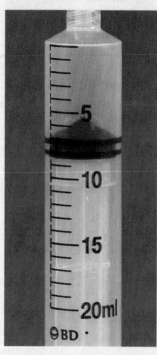   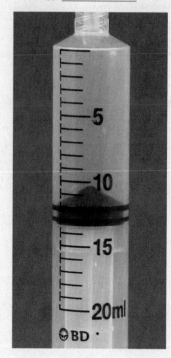   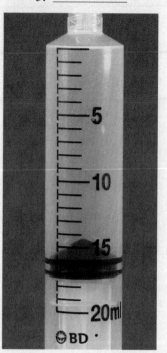

Answers 1. 7 mL   **2.** 12 mL   **3.** 16 mL

PROBLEMS 7-10

Draw an arrow or shade in the following syringe barrels provided to identify the volumes listed.

1. 11 mL   2. 17 mL   3. 9 mL

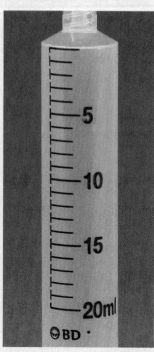   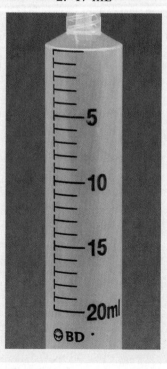   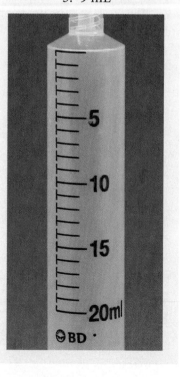

Answers Verify your answers with your instructor.

SUMMARY

This concludes your introduction to syringe calibrations. The important points to remember from this chapter are:

- 3 mL syringes are calibrated in tenths.

- TB syringes are calibrated in hundredths.

- 5 and 10 mL syringes are calibrated in fifths (two-tenths).

- Syringes larger than 10 mL are calibrated in full mL measures.

- The first long calibration on all syringes indicates zero.

- All syringe calibrations must be read from the top, or front, ring of the plunger's suction tip.

SUMMARY SELF-TEST

Identify the dosages measured on the following syringes.

1. _____   2. _____   3. _____

4. _____   5. _____   6. _____

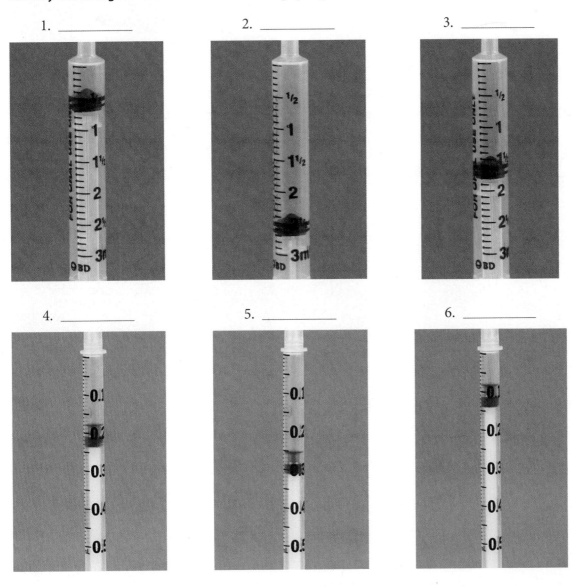

7. _____

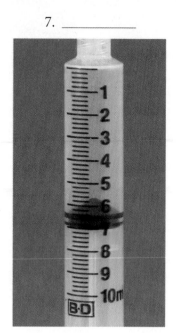

8. _____

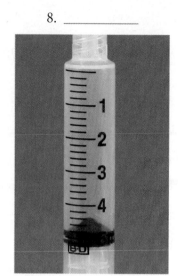

9. _____

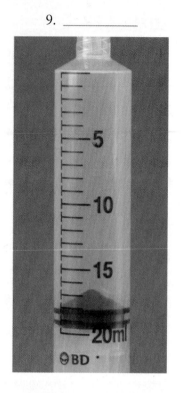

Draw an arrow or shade in the following syringes/cartridges to measure the indicated dosages.

10. 0.42 mL

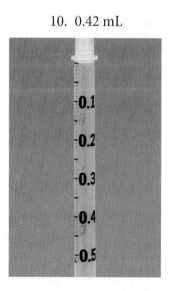

11. 0.31 mL

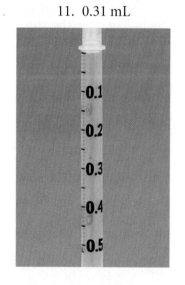

12. 0.44 mL

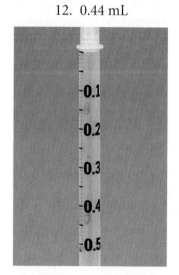

13. 13 mL

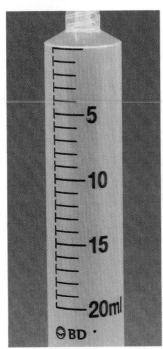

14. 1.2 mL

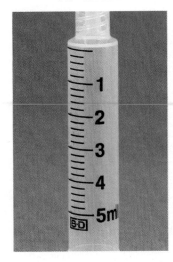

15. 7.6 mL

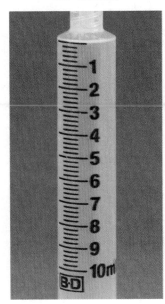

16. 1.7 mL

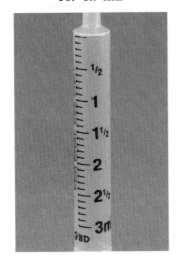

17. 2.2 mL

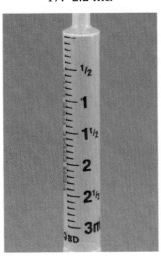

18. 0.9 mL

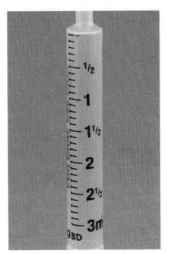

Answers

1. 0.5 mL
2. 2.5 mL
3. 1.6 mL

4. 0.18 mL
5. 0.25 mL
6. 0.08 mL

7. 6.4 mL
8. 4.8 mL
9. 18 mL

Verify your answers for **10–18** with your instructor.

CHAPTER 8

Parenteral Medication Label Dosage Calculation

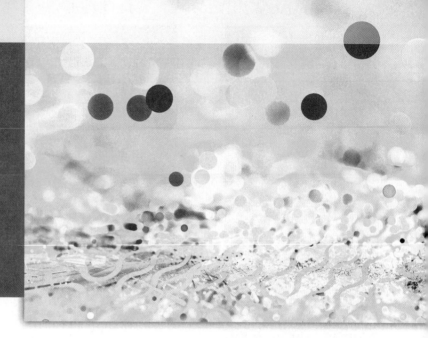

OBJECTIVES

The learner will:

1. Read parenteral solution labels and identify dosage strengths.

2. Calculate average parenteral dosages from the labels provided.

3. Measure parenteral dosages in metric, milliequivalent, unit, percentage, and ratio strengths using 3 mL, TB, 5 mL, 10 mL, and 20 mL syringes.

INTRODUCTION

Parenteral medications are administered by injection, with the intravenous (IV), intramuscular (IM), and subcutaneous (subcut) routes being the most frequently used. The labels of oral and parenteral solutions are very similar, but the size of the average parenteral dosage label is much smaller. Intramuscular solutions are manufactured so that the **average adult dosage will be contained in a volume of between 0.5 mL and 3 mL**, with subcutaneous injections being smaller, and seldom exceeding 1 mL. Excessively larger or smaller volumes would need to be questioned, or calculations rechecked.

> 🔑 Volumes larger than 3 mL are difficult for a single IM injection site to absorb, and the 0.5 to 3 mL volume can be used as a guideline for accuracy of calculations in IM and subcutaneous dosages.

Intravenous medication administration is usually a two-step procedure. The dosage is prepared first, then may be further diluted in IV fluids before administration. In this chapter, we will be concerned only with the **first step of IV drug preparation, which is accurate measurement of the prescribed dosage**.

Parenteral medications are packaged in a variety of single-use glass ampules, single- and multiple-use rubber-stoppered vials, and premeasured syringes and cartridges (**Figure 8-1**).

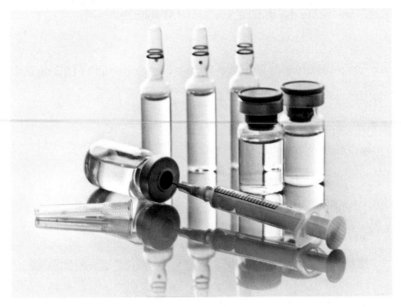

Figure 8-1 Ampules, vials, and a prefilled cartridge.
© Alexander Raths/Shutterstock

READING METRIC SOLUTION LABELS

Let's begin by looking at parenteral solution labels on which the dosages are expressed in metric units of measure.

EXAMPLE 1

Refer to the hydroxyzine HCl label in **Figure 8-2**. The immediate difference you will notice between this label and oral solution labels is the **size**. Ampules and vials are small and their labels are small, which requires that they be **read with particular care**. The information, however, is similar to oral labels. Hydroxyzine hydrochloride is the generic name, and an example of trade name of this drug is Vistaril®. The dosage strength is 50 mg per mL (in the rectangular area). Locate the total volume of this vial, which is 10 mL (in black, center). Keep in mind that average intramuscular and subcutaneous dosages usually consist of one-half to double the average dosage strength, which for this IM Vistaril is 50 mg per mL.

For 50 mg, you would give 1 mL.

For 25 mg, you would give 0.5 mL.

For 100 mg, you would give 2 mL.

For 75 mg, you would give 1.5 mL.

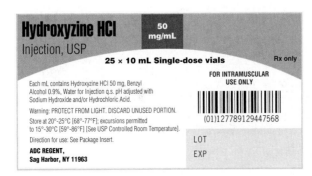

Figure 8-2

These average dosages are within the usual 0.5 to 3 mL IM volume.

EXAMPLE 2

The glycopyrrolate medication in **Figure 8-3** has a dosage strength of 0.2 mg/mL.

For a 0.2 mg dosage, you would give 1 mL.

For a 0.1 mg dosage, you would give 0.5 mL.

For a 200 mcg dosage, you would give 1 mL.

For a 100 mcg dosage, you would give 0.5 mL.

For a 0.4 mg dosage, you would give 2 mL.

For a 400 mcg dosage, you would give 2 mL.

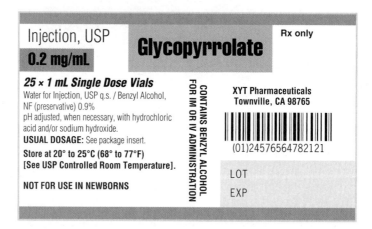

Figure 8-3

PROBLEMS 8-1

Refer to the betamethasone sodium phosphate and betamethasone acetate label in **Figure 8-4** to answer the following questions.

1. What is the dosage strength of this solution?   _____

2. How many mL are required for a dosage of 3 mg?   _____

3. How many mL for a 6 mg dosage?   _____

4. How many mL for a 9 mg dosage?   _____

5. How many mL for a 12 mg dosage?   _____

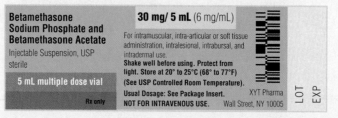

Figure 8-4

Answers **1.** 30 mg/5 mL (6 mg/mL)   **2.** 0.5 mL   **3.** 1 mL   **4.** 1.5 mL   **5.** 2 mL

PROBLEMS 8-2

Refer to the gentamicin label in **Figure 8-5** to answer the following questions.

1. What is the dosage strength? _____

2. If 80 mg were ordered, how many mL would this be? _____

3. If 60 mg were ordered, how many mL would this be? _____

4. How many mL would you need to prepare a
   20 mg IV dosage? _____

Gentamicin
Injection, USP
80 mg per 2 mL
(40 mg per mL*)
Multiple Dose Vials

Each mL contains: Gentamicin sulfate equivalent to 40 mg gentamicin;
1.8 mg methylparaben and 0.2 mg propylparaben as preservatives: 3.2 mg
sodium metabisulfite; 0.1 mg disodium edetate; water for injection, q.s.;
sodium hydroxide and/or sulfuric acid may have been added for pH
adjustment.
Usual Dosage: See package insert.
Warning: Patients treated with gentamicin sulfate and other
aminoglycosides should be under close clinical observation because of the
potential toxicity. See WARNINGS and PRECAUTIONS in the insert.
STORE AT: 20° to 25°C (68° to 77°F) [See USP Controlled Room
Temperature]. The container closure is not made with natural rubber latex.

Rx only

*****Gentamicin equivalent**
For intramuscular or intravenous use.
MUST BE DILUTED FOR IV USE.

AFT Pharma
Townville, CA 98765

(01)12314342368016

LOT

EXP

Figure 8-5

Reprinted with permission of APP Pharmaceuticals, LLC.

Answers 1. 80 mg/2 mL (40 mg/mL) **2.** 2 mL **3.** 1.5 mL **4.** 0.5 mL

PERCENTAGE (%) AND RATIO SOLUTION LABELS

Drugs labeled as **percentage solutions** often express the dosage strength in **metric measures in addition to percentage strength**. The lidocaine label in **Figure 8-6**, a 2% solution, is an example.

However, notice that sideways near the percentage strength is a "20 mg/mL" designation. Lidocaine HCl is most often ordered in mg, but it is also used as a local anesthetic, and when it is, a physician may ask you to prepare a larger volume specifying % dosage strength.

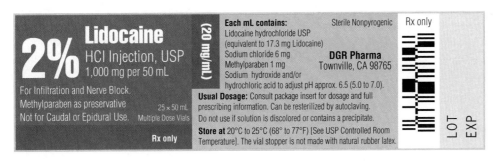

2% Lidocaine
HCl Injection, USP
1,000 mg per 50 mL
(20 mg/mL)
For Infiltration and Nerve Block.
Methylparaben as preservative
Not for Caudal or Epidural Use.
25 × 50 mL
Multiple Dose Vials
Rx only

Each mL contains:
Lidocaine hydrochloride USP
(equivalent to 17.3 mg Lidocaine)
Sodium chloride 6 mg
Methylparaben 1 mg
Sodium hydroxide and/or
hydrochloric acid to adjust pH approx. 6.5 (5.0 to 7.0).
Usual Dosage: Consult package insert for dosage and full
prescribing information. Can be resterilized by autoclaving.
Do not use if solution is discolored or contains a precipitate.
Store at 20°C to 25°C (68° to 77°F) [See USP Controlled Room
Temperature]. The vial stopper is not made with natural rubber latex.

Sterile Nonpyrogenic   Rx only

DGR Pharma
Townville, CA 98765

LOT EXP

Figure 8-6

PROBLEMS 8-3

Refer to the lidocaine label in Figure 8-6 to answer the following questions.

1. How many mL are needed for a 10 mg dosage? _____

2. How many mL for a 20 mg dosage? _____

3. If you are asked to prepare 5 mL of a 2% solution? _____

4. If you are asked to prepare 15 mg? _____

Answers 1. 0.5 mL **2.** 1 mL **3.** 5 mL **4.** 0.75 mL

PROBLEMS 8-4

Refer to the lidocaine label in **Figure 8-7** to answer the following questions.

1. What is the percentage strength of this lidocaine solution? _____

2. How many mL does the vial contain? _____

3. If you are asked to prepare 20 mL of a 1% lidocaine solution, how many mL will you draw up in the syringe? _____

4. If you are asked to prepare 25 mg from this vial, what volume will you draw up? _____

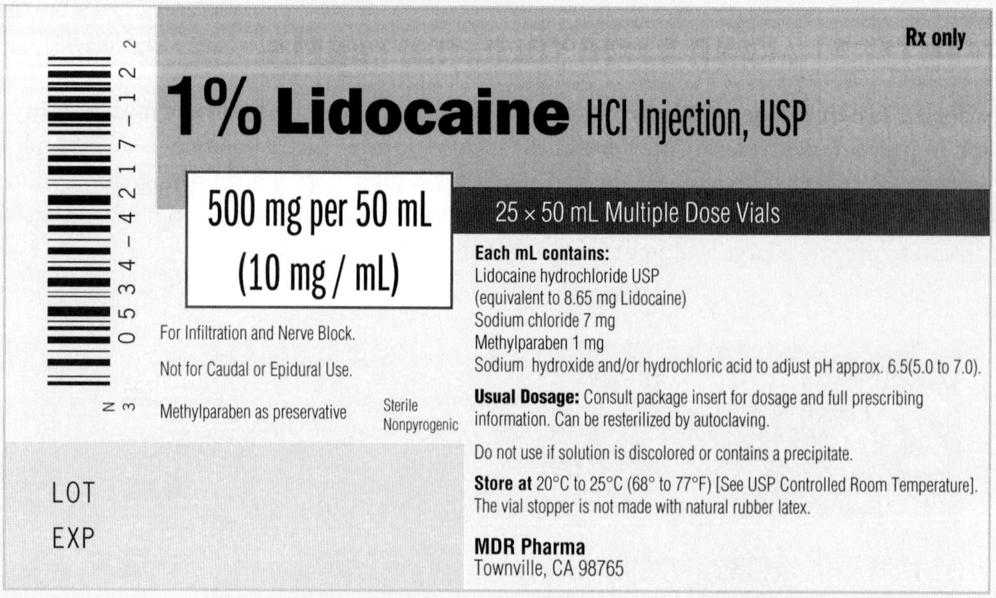

Rx only

N 3 0534-4217-122

1% Lidocaine HCl Injection, USP

500 mg per 50 mL (10 mg / mL)

25 × 50 mL Multiple Dose Vials

For Infiltration and Nerve Block.

Not for Caudal or Epidural Use.

Methylparaben as preservative

Sterile Nonpyrogenic

Each mL contains:
Lidocaine hydrochloride USP
(equivalent to 8.65 mg Lidocaine)
Sodium chloride 7 mg
Methylparaben 1 mg
Sodium hydroxide and/or hydrochloric acid to adjust pH approx. 6.5(5.0 to 7.0).

Usual Dosage: Consult package insert for dosage and full prescribing information. Can be resterilized by autoclaving.

Do not use if solution is discolored or contains a precipitate.

Store at 20°C to 25°C (68° to 77°F) [See USP Controlled Room Temperature]. The vial stopper is not made with natural rubber latex.

MDR Pharma
Townville, CA 98765

LOT

EXP

Figure 8-7

Refer to the calcium gluconate label in Figure 8-8 to answer the following questions.

5. What is the strength of this solution? _____

6. How many mL does this preparation contain? _____

7. What is the mEq dosage strength of this solution? _____

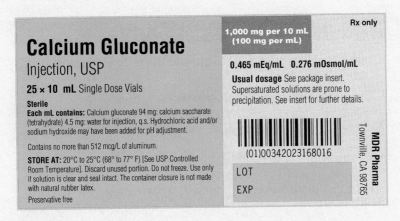

Figure 8-8

Answers 1. 1% **2.** 50 mL **3.** 20 mL **4.** 2.5 mL **5.** 1000 mg/10 mL (100 mg/mL) **6.** 10 mL
7. 0.465 mEq/mL

Parenteral medications expressed in **ratio strengths** are not common, but **when they are ordered, it will be by number of mL**. Ratio labels may also contain dosages in metric weights.

PROBLEMS 8-5

Refer to the epinephrine label in Figure 8-9 to answer the following questions.

1. What is the ratio strength of this solution? _____

2. What volume is this contained in? _____

3. What is the metric dosage strength of this solution? _____

Epinephrine
Injection, USP

1 mg/mL
(1 mg/mL) 1:1000

Rx only

XBD Pharmaceuticals
Levittown, NY 11756

Dosage: See prescribing information.

Store between 20°C to 25°C (68° to 77° F).
Protect from moisture and freezing.

(01)00342023168016

LOT

EXP

**For Intramuscular, Subcutaneous,
and Intraocular Use**
Dilute Before Intraocular Use

Figure 8-9

Answers 1. 1:1000 **2.** 1 mL **3.** 1 mg/mL

SOLUTIONS MEASURED IN UNITS

A number of drugs are measured in **international units**, measured in international units; antibiotics, heparin, and insulin are common examples.

🔑 While "UNITS" is frequently capitalized on commercial drug labels, in clinical dosage orders it is correctly written in lowercase as "units."

PROBLEMS 8-6

Refer to the heparin label in **Figure 8-10** to answer the following questions.

1. What is the dosage strength of this heparin solution? _____

2. If a volume of 1.5 mL is prepared, how many units will this be? _____

3. How many mL will you need for a dosage of 5500 units for an IV? _____

4. If 0.25 mL of this medication is prepared, what dosage will this be? _____

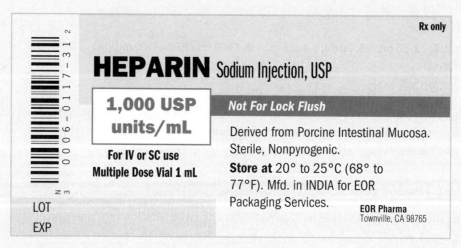

Figure 8-10

Refer to the penicillin G benzathine and procaine label in **Figure 8-11** to answer the following questions.

5. What is the dosage strength of this medication? _____

6. If 600,000 units is ordered, how many mL would this require? _____

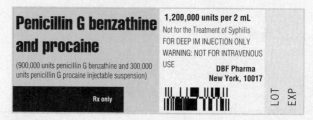

Figure 8-11

Answers **1.** 1000 units/mL   **2.** 1500 units   **3.** 5.5 mL   **4.** 250 units   **5.** 1,200,000 units/2 mL   **6.** 1 mL

SOLUTIONS MEASURED AS MILLIEQUIVALENTS (mEq)

The next four labels will introduce you to milliequivalent (mEq) dosages. Refer to the calcium gluconate label in **Figure 8-12** and notice that this vial has a dosage of 0.465 mEq/mL. If a dosage of 0.465 mEq were ordered, you would draw up 1 mL in the syringe.

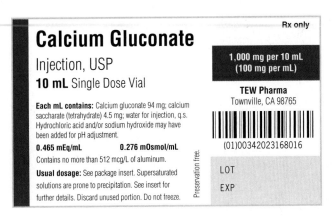

Figure 8-12

PROBLEMS 8-7

Refer to the potassium chloride label in Figure 8-13 to answer the following questions.

1. What are the total dosage and volume of this vial? _____

2. What is the dosage in mEq per mL? _____

3. If you were asked to prepare 15 mEq for addition to an IV, what volume would you draw up? _____

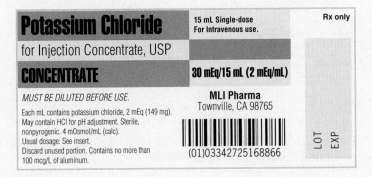

Figure 8-13

Refer to the potassium acetate label in Figure 8-14 to answer the following dosage questions.

4. What is the strength of this solution in mEq per mL? _____

5. If you were asked to prepare 40 mEq for addition to an IV solution, what volume would you draw up in the syringe? _____

6. What volume would you need for a dosage of 20 mEq? _____

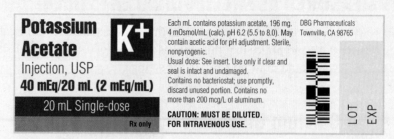

Figure 8-14

Refer to the sodium bicarbonate label in Figure 8-15. Notice that this solution lists the drug strength in mEq and percentage. Read the label very carefully to answer the following questions.

7. What is the dosage strength expressed in mEq/mL?   _____

8. What is the total volume of the vial, and how many mEq does this volume contain?   _____

9. If you were asked to prepare 10 mL of an 8.4% sodium bicarbonate solution, what volume would you draw up in a syringe?   _____

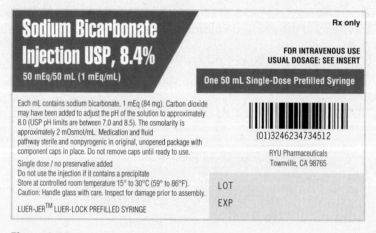

Figure 8-15

Answers 1. 15 mL   **2.** 2 mEq/mL   **3.** 7.5 mL   **4.** 40 mEq/20 mL (2 mEq/mL)   **5.** 20 mL   **6.** 10 mL
7. 1 mEq/mL   **8.** 50 mL/50 mEq; 1 mEq/mL   **9.** 10 mL

SUMMARY

This concludes the introduction to parenteral solution labels. The important points to remember from this chapter are:

■ The most commonly used parenteral administration routes are IV, IM, and subcutaneous.

■ The labels of most parenteral solutions are quite small and must be read with particular care.

■ The average IM dosage will be contained in a volume of between 0.5 mL and 3 mL.

- These 0.5 to 3 mL volumes can be used as a guideline to accuracy of IM calculations.

- The average subcutaneous dosage volume is between 0.5 and 1 mL.

- IV medication preparation is usually a two-step procedure: measurement of the dosage, then dilution according to manufacturer's recommendations or a physician's or prescriber's order.

- Parenteral drugs may be measured in metric, ratio, percentage, unit, or mEq dosages.

- If dosages are ordered by percentage or ratio strength, they are usually specified in mL to be administered.

- Most IM dosages are prepared using a 3 mL syringe.

- Most subcutaneous dosages are prepared using a 3 mL or tuberculin syringe.

SUMMARY SELF-TEST

Read the parenteral drug labels provided to measure the following dosages. Then, indicate on the syringe provided exactly how much solution you will draw up to obtain these dosages. Have your instructor check your answers to be sure you have measured the dosages correctly.

Dosage Ordered   **mL Needed**

1. terbutaline sulfate 500 mcg   _____

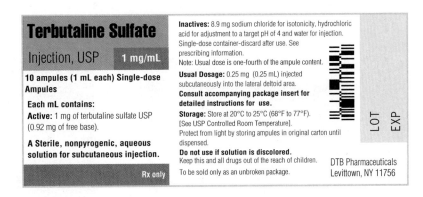

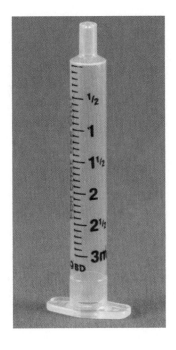

Dosage Ordered

mL Needed

2. furosemide 10 mg

_____

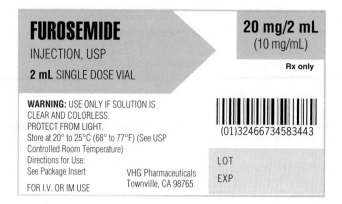

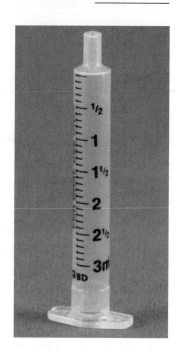

3. heparin 2500 units

_____

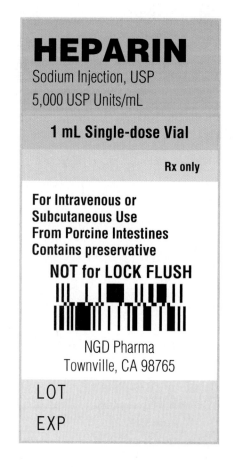

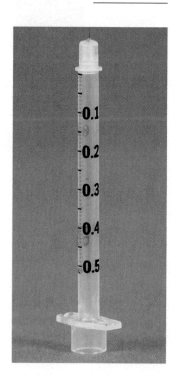

Dosage Ordered

mL Needed

4. acyclovir Na 100 mg

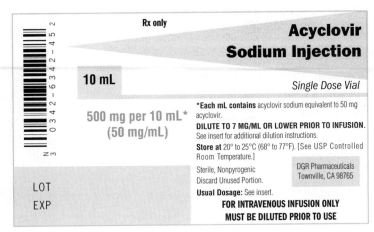

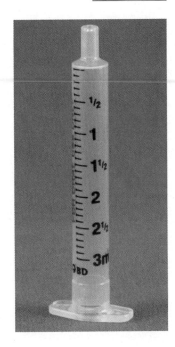

5. atropine 0.2 mg

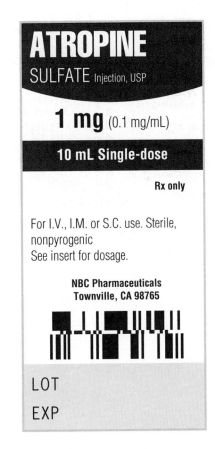

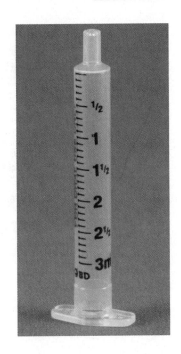

Dosage Ordered

mL Needed

6. hydroxyzine HCl 25 mg

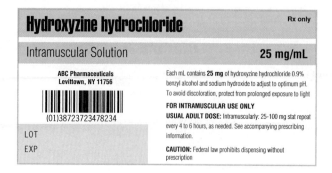

Hydroxyzine hydrochloride

Rx only

Intramuscular Solution

25 mg/mL

ABC Pharmaceuticals
Levittown, NY 11756

(01)38723723478234

LOT

EXP

Each mL contains **25 mg** of hydroxyzine hydrochloride 0.9% benzyl alcohol and sodium hydroxide to adjust to optimum pH. To avoid discoloration, protect from prolonged exposure to light

FOR INTRAMUSCULAR USE ONLY
USUAL ADULT DOSE: Intramuscularly: 25-100 mg stat repeat every 4 to 6 hours, as needed. See accompanying prescribing information.

CAUTION: Federal law prohibits dispensing without prescription

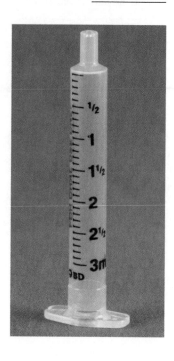

_____

7. glycopyrrolate 100 mcg

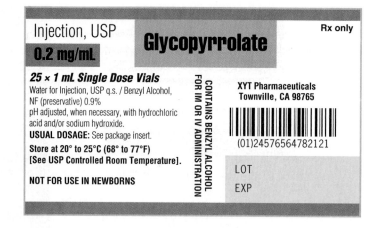

Injection, USP   **Glycopyrrolate**

Rx only

0.2 mg/mL

25 × 1 mL Single Dose Vials
Water for Injection, USP q.s. / Benzyl Alcohol, NF (preservative) 0.9%
pH adjusted, when necessary, with hydrochloric acid and/or sodium hydroxide.
USUAL DOSAGE: See package insert.
Store at 20° to 25°C (68° to 77°F)
[See USP Controlled Room Temperature].

NOT FOR USE IN NEWBORNS

CONTAINS BENZYL ALCOHOL
FOR IM OR IV ADMINISTRATION

XYT Pharmaceuticals
Townville, CA 98765

(01)24576564782121

LOT

EXP

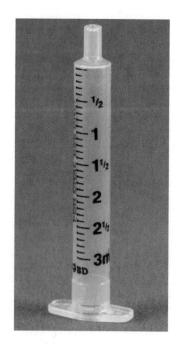

_____

Dosage Ordered

mL Needed

8. nitroglycerine 25 mg

_____

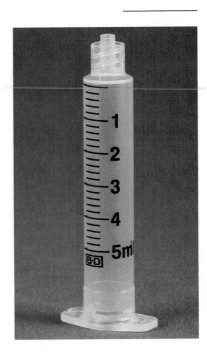

NITROGLYCERIN

INJECTION, USP

50 mg/10 mL (5 mg/mL)

Rx only

25 × 10 mL
SINGLE DOSE VIALS

Each mL contains: Nitroglycerin 5 mg, Alcohol 30% (v/v), Propylene Glycol 30%, Water for Injection q.s. pH (range 3.0 - 6.5) adjusted with Sodium Hydroxide and/or Hydrochloric Acid.

Sterile. PROTECT FROM LIGHT. RETAIN IN CARTON UNTIL TIME OF USE.

Store at 20°-25°C (68°-77°F); excursions permitted to 15°-30°C (59°-86°F) (See USP Controlled Room Temperature).
DISCARD UNUSED PORTION.
Directions for Use: See Package Insert.

MUST BE DILUTED BEFORE USE. ONLY GLASS INTRAVENOUS BOTTLES SHOULD BE USED IN PREPARING THE INTRAVENOUS ADMIXTURE (SEE INSERT).

NOT FOR DIRECT INTRAVENOUS INJECTION.
FOR INTRAVENOUS INFUSION ONLY.

FGS Pharma
SHIRLEY, NY 11967

(01)3452645422343

LOT

EXP

9. methotrexate 0.25 g

_____

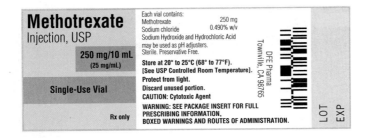

Methotrexate
Injection, USP

250 mg/10 mL
(25 mg/mL)

Single-Use Vial

Rx only

Each vial contains:
Methotrexate   250 mg
Sodium chloride   0.490% w/v
Sodium Hydroxide and Hydrochloric Acid
may be used as pH adjusters.
Sterile. Preservative Free.

Store at 20° to 25°C (68° to 77°F).
[See USP Controlled Room Temperature].
Protect from light.
Discard unused portion.
CAUTION: Cytotoxic Agent
WARNING: SEE PACKAGE INSERT FOR FULL
PRESCRIBING INFORMATION,
BOXED WARNINGS AND ROUTES OF ADMINISTRATION.

DFE Pharma
Townville, CA 98765

LOT
EXP

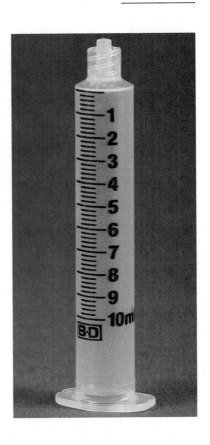

Dosage Ordered

mL Needed

10. cyanocobalamin 1 mg

_____

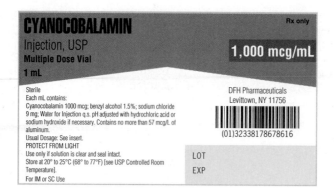

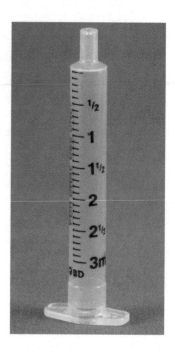

11. hydralazine hydrochloride 10 mg

_____

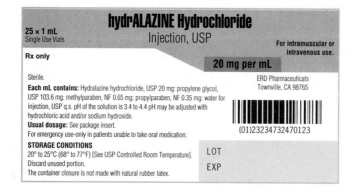

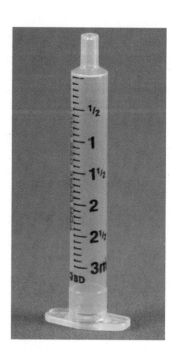

Dosage Ordered

mL Needed

12. epinephrine 2 mg

_____

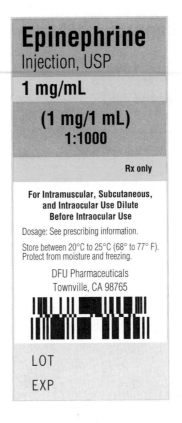

Epinephrine
Injection, USP

1 mg/mL

(1 mg/1 mL)
1:1000

Rx only

For Intramuscular, Subcutaneous,
and Intraocular Use Dilute
Before Intraocular Use

Dosage: See prescribing information.

Store between 20°C to 25°C (68° to 77° F).
Protect from moisture and freezing.

DFU Pharmaceuticals
Townville, CA 98765

LOT

EXP

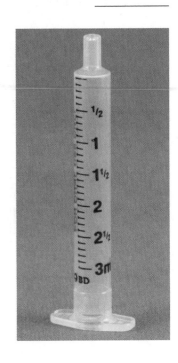

13. fentanyl 125 mcg

_____

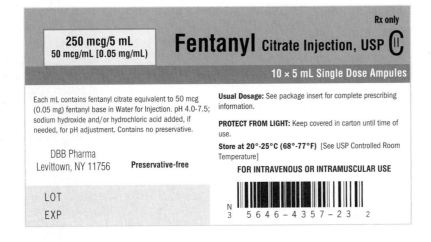

250 mcg/5 mL
50 mcg/mL [0.05 mg/mL]

Rx only

Fentanyl Citrate Injection, USP Ⓒ

10 × 5 mL Single Dose Ampules

Each mL contains fentanyl citrate equivalent to 50 mcg
(0.05 mg) fentanyl base in Water for Injection. pH 4.0-7.5;
sodium hydroxide and/or hydrochloric acid added, if
needed, for pH adjustment. Contains no preservative.

DBB Pharma
Levittown, NY 11756   **Preservative-free**

LOT

EXP

Usual Dosage: See package insert for complete prescribing
information.

PROTECT FROM LIGHT: Keep covered in carton until time of
use.

Store at 20°-25°C (68°-77°F) [See USP Controlled Room
Temperature]

FOR INTRAVENOUS OR INTRAMUSCULAR USE

N
3   5 6 4 6 – 4 3 5 7 – 2 3   2

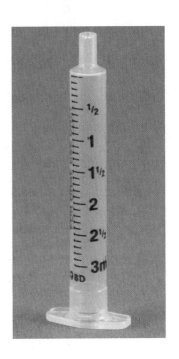

Dosage Ordered

mL Needed

14. calcium gluconate 0.93 mEq

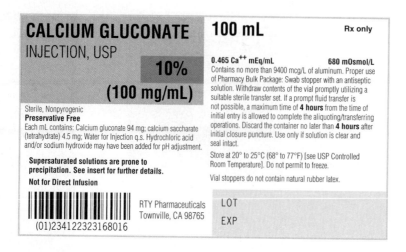

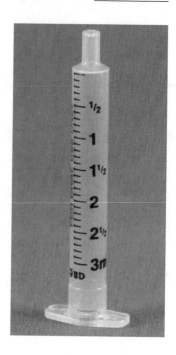

_____

15. ceftriaxone 0.5 g

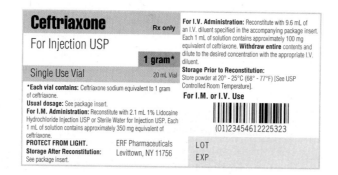

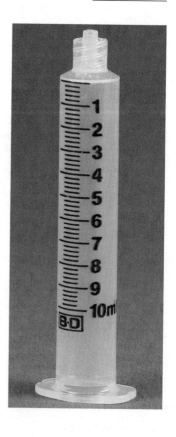

_____

Dosage Ordered

mL Needed

16. heparin 500 units

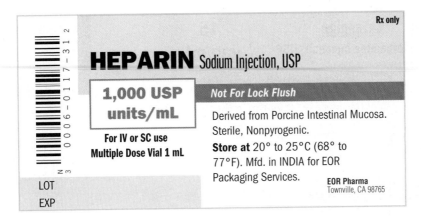

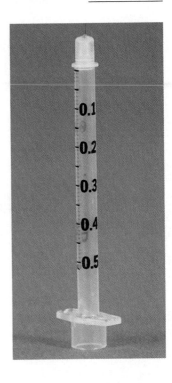

17. epinephrine 0.5 mg

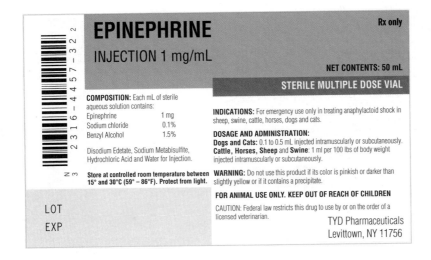

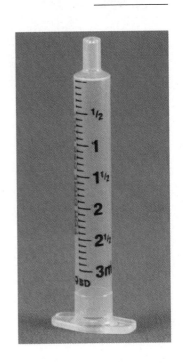

Dosage Ordered

mL Needed

18. ketorolac tromethamine 30 mg
_____

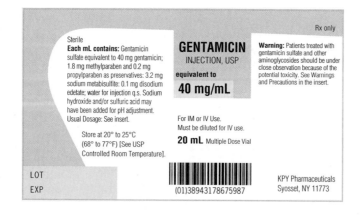

| **Ketorolac** | **15** |
| Tromethamine Injection, USP | **mg/mL** |

Rx only   25 × 1 mL Single Dose Vials   EPS Pharmaceuticals
Valley Stream, NY 11581

Each vial contains 15 mg ketorolac tromethamine, USP, 10% (w/v) alcohol, USP. 6.68 mg sodium chloride, 1 mg citric acid, anhydrous, sterile water for injection. pH adjusted to approximately 7.4 with sodium hydroxide or hydrochloric acid. Sealed under nitrogen. Discard unused portion.

Usual Dosage: For dosage recommendations and other important prescribing information, read accompanying insert.
Store at 20°-25°C [68°-77°F] [See USP Controlled Room Temperature].
PROTECT FROM LIGHT. Retain in carton until time of use.

FOR INTRAVENOUS OR INTRAMUSCULAR USE
Sterile
(01)1325578677829

LOT
EXP

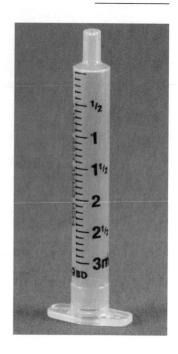

19. gentamicin 60 mg
_____

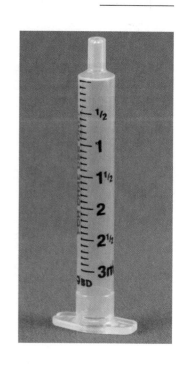

Rx only

Sterile
Each mL contains: Gentamicin sulfate equivalent to 40 mg gentamicin; 1.8 mg methylparaben and 0.2 mg propylparaben as preservatives: 3.2 mg sodium metabisulfite: 0.1 mg disodium edetate; water for injection q.s. Sodium hydroxide and/or sulfuric acid may have been added for pH adjustment. Usual Dosage: See insert.

Store at 20° to 25°C (68° to 77°F) [See USP Controlled Room Temperature].

GENTAMICIN
INJECTION, USP
equivalent to
40 mg/mL

For IM or IV Use.
Must be diluted for IV use.
20 mL Multiple Dose Vial

Warning: Patients treated with gentamicin sulfate and other aminoglycosides should be under close observation because of the potential toxicity. See Warnings and Precautions in the insert.

LOT
EXP

(01)38943178675987

KPY Pharmaceuticals
Syosset, NY 11773

Dosage Ordered

20. lidocaine HCl 50 mg

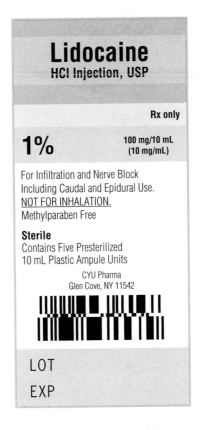

Lidocaine
HCl Injection, USP

Rx only

1%   100 mg/10 mL
(10 mg/mL)

For Infiltration and Nerve Block
Including Caudal and Epidural Use.
<u>NOT FOR INHALATION.</u>
Methylparaben Free

Sterile
Contains Five Presterilized
10 mL Plastic Ampule Units

CYU Pharma
Glen Cove, NY 11542

LOT

EXP

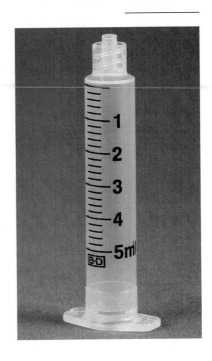

_____

21. sodium chloride 40 mEq

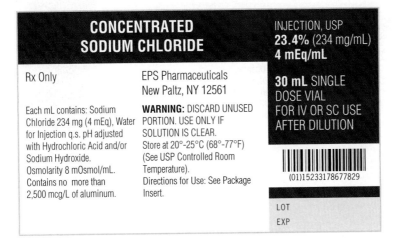

**CONCENTRATED
SODIUM CHLORIDE**

INJECTION, USP
23.4% (234 mg/mL)
4 mEq/mL

Rx Only

EPS Pharmaceuticals
New Paltz, NY 12561

Each mL contains: Sodium
Chloride 234 mg (4 mEq), Water
for Injection q.s. pH adjusted
with Hydrochloric Acid and/or
Sodium Hydroxide.
Osmolarity 8 mOsmol/mL.
Contains no more than
2,500 mcg/L of aluminum.

WARNING: DISCARD UNUSED
PORTION. USE ONLY IF
SOLUTION IS CLEAR.
Store at 20°-25°C (68°-77°F)
(See USP Controlled Room
Temperature).
Directions for Use: See Package
Insert.

30 mL SINGLE
DOSE VIAL
FOR IV OR SC USE
AFTER DILUTION

(01)15233178677829

LOT
EXP

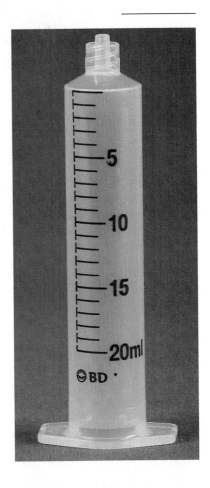

_____

Dosage Ordered

22. atropine 200 mcg

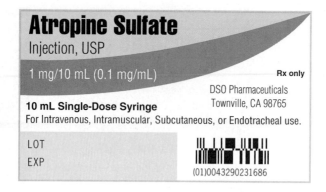

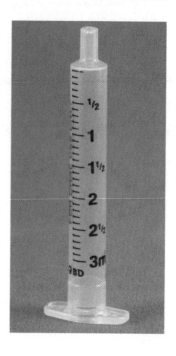

mL Needed

_____

23. meperidine 50 mg

_____

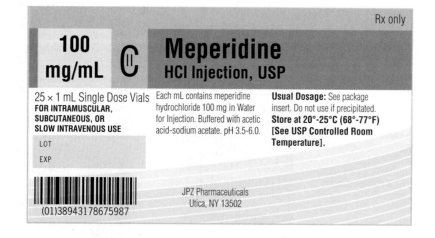

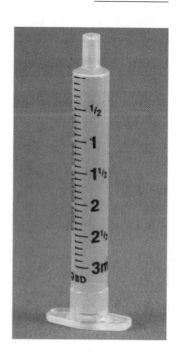

Dosage Ordered

mL Needed

24. clindamycin 0.3 g

_____

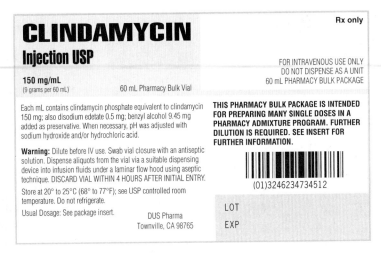

CLINDAMYCIN

Injection USP

Rx only

150 mg/mL
(9 grams per 60 mL)

60 mL Pharmacy Bulk Vial

FOR INTRAVENOUS USE ONLY
DO NOT DISPENSE AS A UNIT
60 mL PHARMACY BULK PACKAGE

Each mL contains clindamycin phosphate equivalent to clindamycin 150 mg; also disodium edetate 0.5 mg; benzyl alcohol 9.45 mg added as preservative. When necessary, pH was adjusted with sodium hydroxide and/or hydrochloric acid.

THIS PHARMACY BULK PACKAGE IS INTENDED FOR PREPARING MANY SINGLE DOSES IN A PHARMACY ADMIXTURE PROGRAM. FURTHER DILUTION IS REQUIRED. SEE INSERT FOR FURTHER INFORMATION.

Warning: Dilute before IV use. Swab vial closure with an antiseptic solution. Dispense aliquots from the vial via a suitable dispensing device into infusion fluids under a laminar flow hood using aseptic technique. DISCARD VIAL WITHIN 4 HOURS AFTER INITIAL ENTRY.

Store at 20° to 25°C (68° to 77°F); see USP controlled room temperature. Do not refrigerate.

Usual Dosage: See package insert.

DUS Pharma
Townville, CA 98765

(01)3246234734512

LOT

EXP

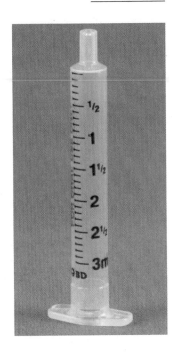

25. morphine sulfate 15 mg

_____

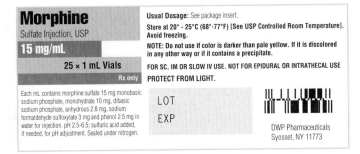

Morphine

Sulfate Injection, USP

15 mg/mL

25 × 1 mL Vials

Rx only

Each mL contains morphine sulfate 15 mg monobasic sodium phosphate, monohydrate 10 mg, dibasic sodium phosphate, anhydrous 2.8 mg, sodium formaldehyde sulfoxylate 3 mg and phenol 2.5 mg in water for injection. pH 2.5-6.5; sulfuric acid added, if needed, for pH adjustment. Sealed under nitrogen.

Usual Dosage: See package insert.

Store at 20° - 25°C (68°-77°F) [See USP Controlled Room Temperature]. Avoid freezing.

NOTE: Do not use if color is darker than pale yellow. If it is discolored in any other way or if it contains a precipitate.

FOR SC, IM OR SLOW IV USE. NOT FOR EPIDURAL OR INTRATHECAL USE

PROTECT FROM LIGHT.

LOT

EXP

DWP Pharmaceuticals
Syosset, NY 11773

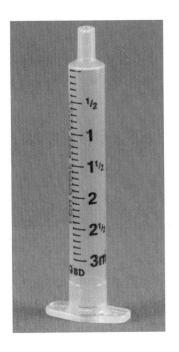

Dosage Ordered   **mL Needed**

26. acyclovir Na 150 mg   _____

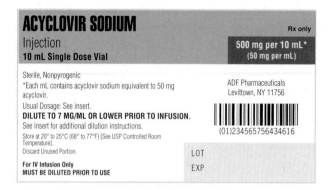

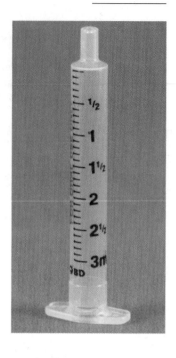

27. cisplatin 20 mg   _____

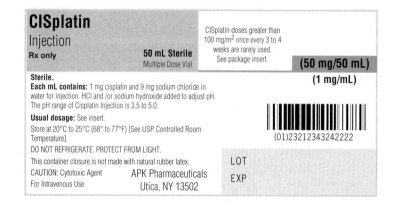

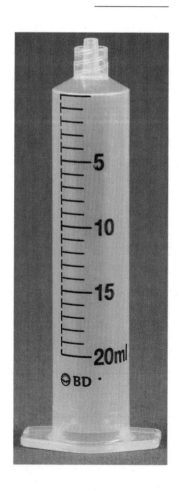

Dosage Ordered

mL Needed

28. sodium chloride 20 mEq

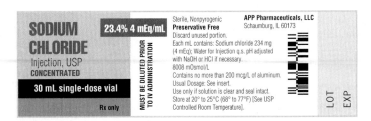

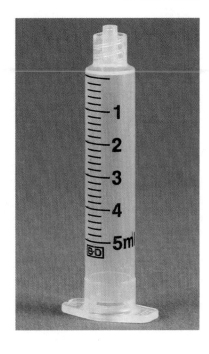

29. meperidine 50 mg

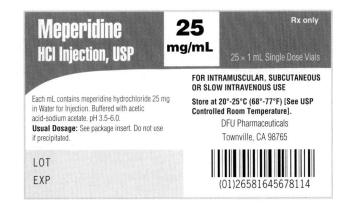

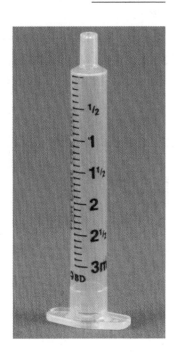

Dosage Ordered

mL Needed

30. furosemide 30 mg

_____

FUROSEMIDE
Injection, USP

40 mg/4 mL
(10 mg/mL)

4 mL Single Dose Vial
For IM or IV use only

Each mL contains 10 mg Furosemide USP,
Water for Injection, q.s., Sodium Chloride
for isotonicity, Sodium Hydroxide and,
if necessary, Hydrochloric acid to adjust
pH between 8.0 and 9.3.

Rx only

WARNING: DISCARD UNUSED PORTION.
USE ONLY IF SOLUTION IS CLEAR AND COLORLESS.
PROTECT FROM LIGHT.
Store at controlled room temperature 20° - 25°C
(68° - 77°F) (See USP)
Direction for Use: See Package Insert.

LOT
EXP

DGH Pharma
Great Neck, NY 11021

(01)9985202316324

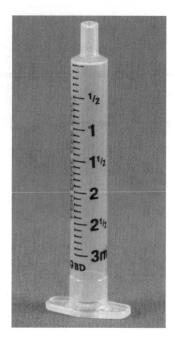

31. gentamicin 60 mg

_____

Each mL contains: Gentamicin sulfate
equivalent to 40 mg gentamicin: 1.8 mg
methylparaben and 0.2 mg propylparaben as
preservatives; 3.2 mg sodium metabisulfite;
0.1 mg disodium edetate; Water for Injection,
q.s.; sodium hydroxide and/or sulfuric acid
may have been added for a pH adjustment.

STORE AT: 20° TO 25°C (68° to 77°F)
[See USP Controlled Room Temperature]. The
container closure is not made with natural
rubber latex.

25 × 2 mL
Multiple Dose Vials

Rx only

Gentamicin
Injection, USP

80 mg per 2 mL
(40 mg per mL*)

Warning: Patients treated with gentamicin
sulfate and other aminoglycosides should
be under close clinical observation because
of the potential toxicity.
See WARNINGS and PRECAUTIONS in the
insert.
Usual dosage: See package insert.

*Gentamicin equivalent
For intramuscular or intravenous use.
MUST BE DILUTED FOR IV USE.

LOT
EXP

(01)54798244225323

PMA Pharmaceuticals
Cortland, NY 13045

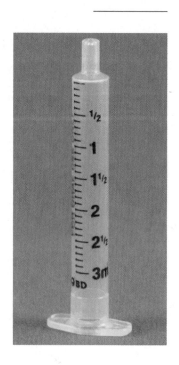

Dosage Ordered

mL Needed

32. meperidine 50 mg _____

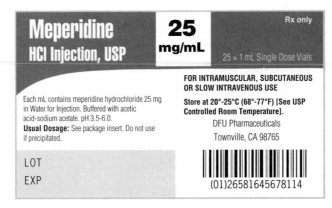

Meperidine
HCl Injection, USP

25 mg/mL

Rx only

25 × 1 mL Single Dose Vials

FOR INTRAMUSCULAR, SUBCUTANEOUS
OR SLOW INTRAVENOUS USE

Each mL contains meperidine hydrochloride 25 mg
in Water for Injection. Buffered with acetic
acid-sodium acetate. pH 3.5-6.0.
Usual Dosage: See package insert. Do not use
if precipitated.

Store at 20°-25°C (68°-77°F) [See USP
Controlled Room Temperature].

DFU Pharmaceuticals
Townville, CA 98765

LOT

EXP

(01)26581645678114

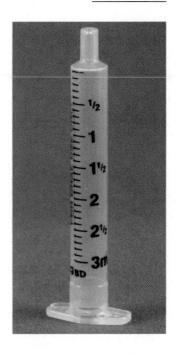

33. dexamethasone 2 mg _____

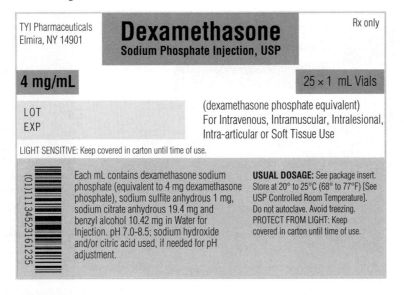

TYI Pharmaceuticals
Elmira, NY 14901

Dexamethasone
Sodium Phosphate Injection, USP

Rx only

4 mg/mL

25 × 1 mL Vials

LOT
EXP

(dexamethasone phosphate equivalent)
For Intravenous, Intramuscular, Intralesional,
Intra-articular or Soft Tissue Use

LIGHT SENSITIVE: Keep covered in carton until time of use.

Each mL contains dexamethasone sodium
phosphate (equivalent to 4 mg dexamethasone
phosphate), sodium sulfite anhydrous 1 mg,
sodium citrate anhydrous 19.4 mg and
benzyl alcohol 10.42 mg in Water for
Injection. pH 7.0-8.5; sodium hydroxide
and/or citric acid used, if needed for pH
adjustment.

USUAL DOSAGE: See package insert.
Store at 20° to 25°C (68° to 77°F) [See
USP Controlled Room Temperature].
Do not autoclave. Avoid freezing.
PROTECT FROM LIGHT: Keep
covered in carton until time of use.

(01)11134523161235

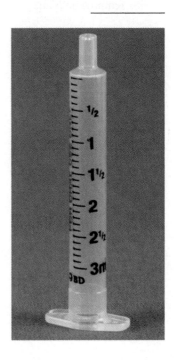

Dosage Ordered

mL Needed

34. hydroxyzine hydrochloride 50 mg

_____

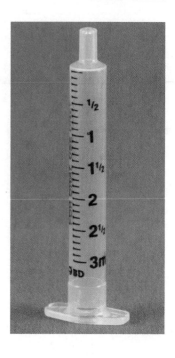

Rx only

Hydroxyzine hydrochloride

25 mg/mL

FOR INTRAMUSCULAR USE ONLY
USUAL ADULT DOSE: Intramuscularly:
25-100 mg stat repeat every 4 to 6 hours,
as needed, see accompanying prescribing
information.
CAUTION: Federal law prohibits dispensing
without prescription

Each ml contains **25 mg** of hydroxyzine hydrochloride
0.9% benzyl alcohol and sodium hydroxide to adjust to
optimum pH.
To avoid discoloration, protect from prolonged exposure
to light

RMZ Pharmaceuticals
Yonkers, NY 10703

10 mL (01)212548963168147 **Intramuscular Solution** LOT EXP

35. fentanyl 0.05 mg

_____

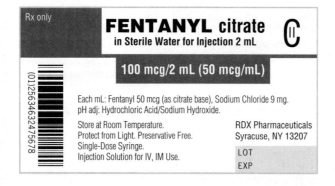

Rx only

FENTANYL citrate C
in Sterile Water for Injection 2 mL

100 mcg/2 mL (50 mcg/mL)

Each mL: Fentanyl 50 mcg (as citrate base), Sodium Chloride 9 mg.
pH adj: Hydrochloric Acid/Sodium Hydroxide.

Store at Room Temperature.
Protect from Light. Preservative Free.
Single-Dose Syringe.
Injection Solution for IV, IM Use.

RDX Pharmaceuticals
Syracuse, NY 13207
LOT
EXP

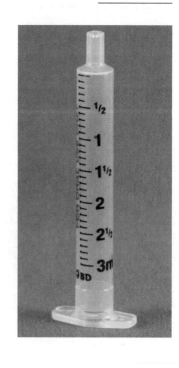

Dosage Ordered   **mL Needed**

36. morphine 15 mg   _____

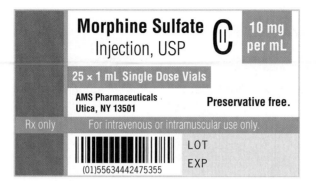

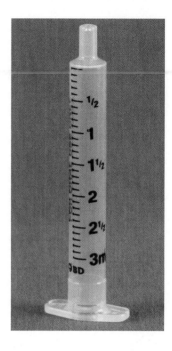

37. cyanocobalamin 1 mg   _____

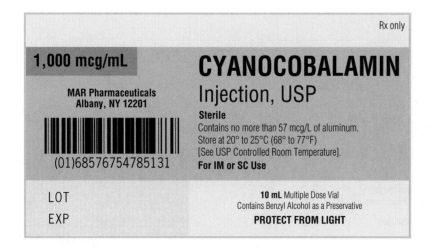

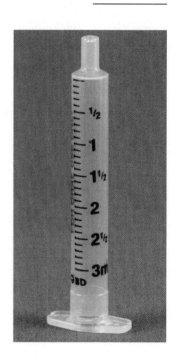

Dosage Ordered

mL Needed

38. ketorolac tromethamine 15 mg

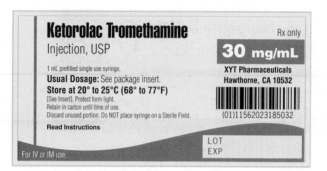

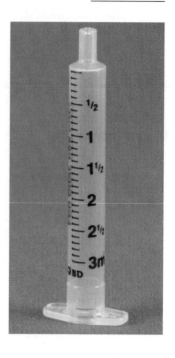

39. glycopyrrolate 200 mcg

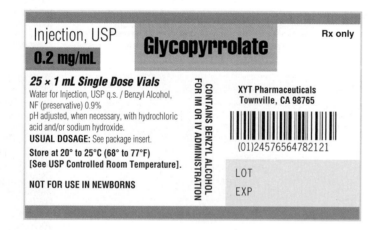

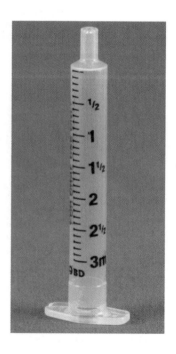

Answers

1. 0.5 mL
2. 1 mL
3. 0.5 mL
4. 2 mL
5. 2 mL
6. 1 mL
7. 0.5 mL
8. 5 mL
9. 10 mL
10. 1 mL

11. 0.5 mL
12. 2 mL
13. 2.5 mL
14. 2 mL
15. 10 mL
16. 0.5 mL
17. 0.5 mL
18. 2 mL
19. 1.5 mL
20. 5 mL

21. 10 mL
22. 2 mL
23. 0.5 mL
24. 2 mL
25. 1 mL
26. 3 mL
27. 20 mL
28. 5 mL
29. 2 mL
30. 3 mL

31. 1.5 mL
32. 2 mL
33. 0.5 mL
34. 2 mL
35. 1 mL
36. 1.5 mL
37. 1 mL
38. 0.5 mL
39. 1 mL

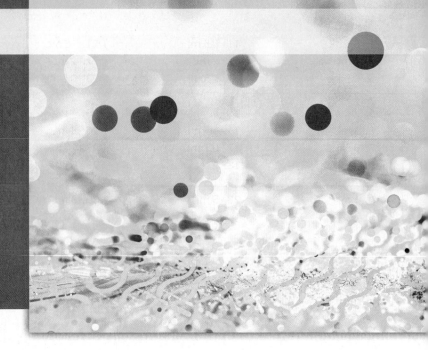

CHAPTER 9

Measuring Insulin Dosages

OBJECTIVES

The learner will:

1. Read insulin labels to identify type.

2. Read calibrations on 100 units/mL insulin syringes.

3. Measure single insulin dosages.

4. Measure combined insulin dosages.

5. Recognize that rapid-acting insulin injection requires that the patient eat immediately.

INTRODUCTION

Diabetes is one of the fastest-growing health problems in both the United States and Canada, and since the advent of technology to manipulate DNA in the 1980s, the number of insulin products has almost quadrupled in an effort to keep pace with treatment needs.

Type 2/adult-onset diabetes can often be **reversed** if an individual **dedicates herself or himself to weight loss, exercise, and dramatic changes in diet**. Unfortunately, many people will not or cannot do this, and they may initially require injectable insulin for treatment of their disease. However, numerous oral and several inhalation insulin medications are widely and effectively used to treat symptoms of type 2 diabetes.

Type 1 diabetes is an autoimmune disease, in which the body destroys its insulin-producing cells. Since insulin is vital to convert food into energy, these patients **require ongoing insulin administration by injection or pump to sustain life**.

This chapter introduces the current insulin preparations available; provides simulated vial labels to familiarize you with the different insulins; describes the physical appearance of insulins; explains insulin action times in relation to dietary intake; instructs you in the use of specialized insulin syringes; and provides a step-by-step procedure for the combination of Regular and N (NPH) insulin in a single syringe, a skill you may use on an ongoing basis throughout your career.

TYPES OF INSULIN

Prior to the 1980s, all insulin was produced from animal sources. Today, **all insulins are products of DNA**. The two earliest DNA-based insulins, **R (Regular)** and **N (NPH)**, are made from **recombinant DNA** (cut and spliced DNA fragments). Both of these insulins incorporate the "**lin**" of the word insu**lin** in their trade names: Humu**lin**® R and Humu**lin**® N, manufactured by Eli Lilly Co., and Novo**lin**® R and Novo**lin**® N, from Novo Nordisk.

   Regular insulin is a **clear** solution, and it is **fast acting**, while **N** insulin is **cloudy**, classified as **intermediate acting**, and has a **slower start but longer action**. Regular and N insulin can safely be (and often are) **combined in a single syringe** to reduce the number of injections an individual must have. They may be combined at first to determine an individual's R and NPH insulin requirements, then ordered in **actual combined insulin preparations**, such as the Humulin and Novolin **70/30** and **50/50** mixes, to provide both fast and more prolonged action.

   Another type of DNA preparation is the **analogs**, which are **chemically altered DNA**. Depending on their structure, the analogs may offer an extremely rapid action, or they may provide for longer and more balanced control of blood glucose levels. Once again, some of the trade names of these products reflect their origin: The "**log**" of ana**log** is incorporated in two of the frequently used trade-named insulins, Huma**log**® and Novo**log**®. Among the analogs whose trade names do not identify their analog structure are Apidra® (glulisine), Lantis® (glargine), and Levemir® (detemir).

> 🗝 Most clinical multi-use insulin vial solution labels look very much alike, and special precaution must be taken in their identification.

INSULIN LABEL IDENTIFICATION

Like other medications, insulin preparations have both trade and generic names. Eli Lilly and Novo Nordisk are the major insulin manufacturers; however, there are now other manufacturers producing and marketing insulin. In the insulin label identification problems that follow, you will be asked to identify insulin manufacturers, as well as insulin types and dosages. Some of the labels included are from **insulin pen** preparations: **prefilled, self-injection syringes** that contain **multiple doses** of insulin.

PROBLEMS 9-1

Refer to the insulin labels provided to answer the specific questions pertaining to each.

1. What kind of insulin does the label in **Figure 9-1** identify? _____

2. What is the dosage strength of this insulin? _____

3. How must this insulin be stored when opened? _____

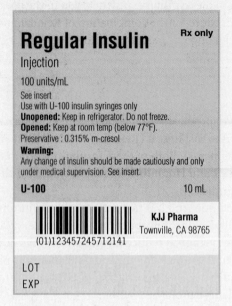

Figure 9-1

4. What kind of insulin is in **Figure 9-2**?   _____

5. What dosage strength does this insulin have?   _____

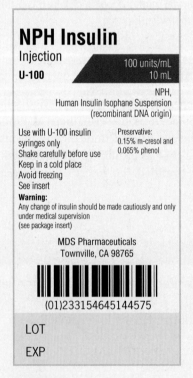

Figure 9-2

6. What does the 70/30 on the label in **Figure 9-3** represent? _____

7. What is the dosage strength of this insulin? _____

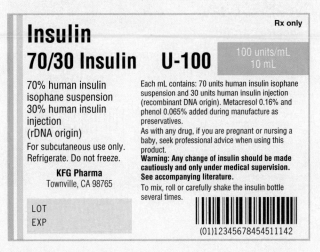

Figure 9-3

8. What is the dosage strength in **Figure 9-4**? _____

9. What does the 50/50 designation mean? _____

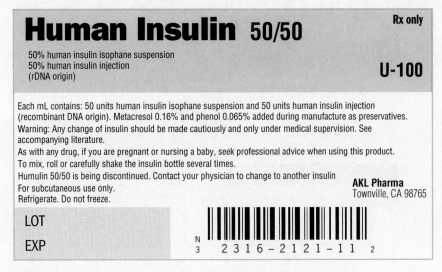

Figure 9-4

10. What is the total volume of the insulin vial in **Figure 9-5**? _____

11. What is the dosage strength of this insulin? _____

12. What is the generic name of this preparation?   _____

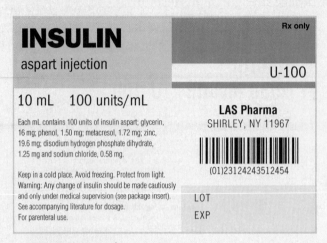

Figure 9-5

13. What is the generic name of the insulin preparation in **Figure 9-6**?   _____

14. What is the dosage strength?   _____

15. What volume of insulin does each cartridge contain?   _____

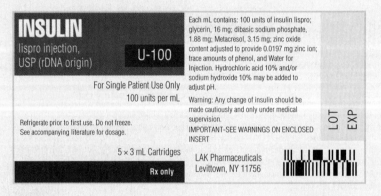

Figure 9-6

16. What is the generic name of the insulin in **Figure 9-7**? _____

17. What is the dosage strength of this preparation? _____

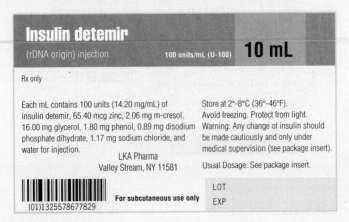

Insulin detemir

(rDNA origin) injection   100 units/mL (U-100)   **10 mL**

Rx only

Each mL contains 100 units (14.20 mg/mL) of insulin detemir, 65.40 mcg zinc, 2.06 mg m-cresol, 16.00 mg glycerol, 1.80 mg phenol, 0.89 mg disodium phosphate dihydrate, 1.17 mg sodium chloride, and water for injection.
LKA Pharma
Valley Stream, NY 11581

Store at 2°-8°C (36°-46°F). Avoid freezing. Protect from light. Warning: Any change of insulin should be made cautiously and only under medical supervision (see package insert).

Usual Dosage: See package insert.

(01)1325578677829   **For subcutaneous use only**   LOT   EXP

Figure 9-7

18. What is the generic name of the insulin in **Figure 9-8**? _____

19. What is the total volume of this vial? _____

20. What is the insulin dosage strength? _____

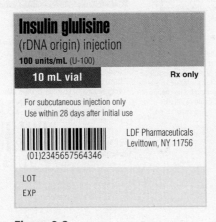

Insulin glulisine
(rDNA origin) injection
100 units/mL (U-100)

10 mL vial   Rx only

For subcutaneous injection only
Use within 28 days after initial use

(01)2345657564346   LDF Pharmaceuticals
Levittown, NY 11756

LOT
EXP

Figure 9-8

21. What does the R on the label in **Figure 9-9** identify? _____

22. Is this a short-acting or long-acting insulin? _____

23. What is the total volume of this vial? _____

24. What is the dosage strength of this insulin? _____

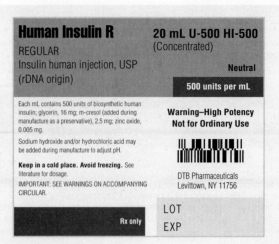

Figure 9-9

25. What is the generic name of the insulin label in **Figure 9-10**? _____

26. What is the total volume of this vial? _____

27. What is its dosage strength? _____

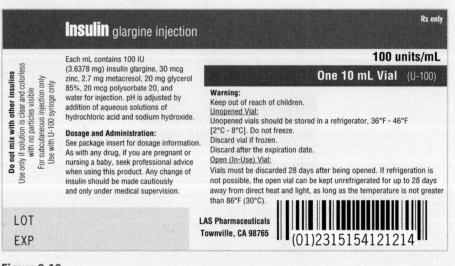

Figure 9-10

Answers 1. regular   **2.** 100 units/mL   **3.** room temperature   **4.** NPH   **5.** 100 units/mL   **6.** combined R and NPH   **7.** 100 units/mL   **8.** 100 units/mL   **9.** combined R and NPH   **10.** 10 mL   **11.** 100 units/mL   **12.** aspart   **13.** lispro   **14.** 100 units/mL   **15.** 3 mL   **16.** detemir   **17.** 100 units/mL   **18.** glulisine   **19.** 10 mL   **20.** 100 units/mL   **21.** regular   **22.** short   **23.** 20 mL   **24.** 500 units/mL   **25.** glargine   **26.** 10 mL   **27.** 100 units/mL

INSULIN ACTION TIMES

As equally important as insulin type and dosage is **the timing of insulin administration**, based on **onset of action, peak and duration, and relationship to dietary intake**. Insulin is classified by action as **rapid, short, intermediate, or long acting**. Refer to the **Medical Criteria** charts on the **Pharmacokinetics of Insulin Preparations** in **Figure 9-11** and **Table 9-1**, which illustrate the onset, peak, and duration of the insulins in current clinical use.

The **rapid-acting** insulins aspart, glulisine, and lispro, whose onset of action varies from 10 to 30 minutes, **must be followed immediately by a meal**. Failure to immediately ingest food would result

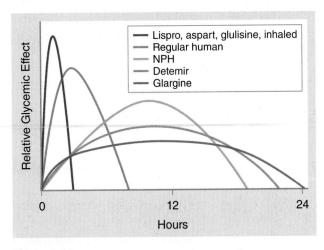

Figure 9-11

Reproduced from Firman, G. (2009). Pharmacokinetics of insulin preparations. *MedicalCriteria*. Retrieved from http://
medicalcriteria.com/web/dbtinsulin.

TABLE 9-1	Medical Criteria Chart on the Pharmacokinetics of Insulin Preparations		
	Time of Action		
Preparation	**Onset, h**	**Peak, h**	**Effective Duration, h**
Short-Acting, Subcutaneous			
Lispro	< 0.25	0.5–1.5	3–4
Aspart	< 0.25	0.5–1.5	3–4
Glulisine	< 0.25	0.5–1.5	3–4
Regular	0.5–1.0	2–3	4–6
Short-Acting, Inhaled			
Inhaled regular insulin	< 0.25	0.5–1.5	4–6
Long-Acting			
NPH	1–4	6–10	10–16
Detemir	1–4	—[1]	12–20
Glargine	1–4	—[1]	24
Degludec	1–4	—	> 40
Insulin Combinations			
75/25–75% protamine lispro, 25% lispro	< 0.25	1.5 h[2]	Up to 10–16
70/30–70% protamine aspart, 30% aspart	< 0.25	1.5 h[2]	Up to 10–16
50/50–50% protamine lispro, 50% lispro	< 0.25	1.5 h[2]	Up to 10–16
70/30–70% NPH, 30% regular insulin	0.5–1	Dual	10–16
50/50–50% NPH, 50% regular insulin	0.5–1	Dual	10–16

[1]Glargine has minimal peak activity; detemir has some peak activity at 6–14 h.

[2]Dual: two peaks; one at 2–3 h; the second several hours later.

Reproduced from Firman, G. (2009). Pharmacokinetics of insulin preparations. *MedicalCriteria*. Retrieved from http://medicalcriteria.com/web/dbtinsulin.

in a rapidly lowered blood glucose level and **insulin reaction from hypoglycemia**. Also note that these rapid-acting insulins have a peak and duration of action from 0.5 to 5 hours. Their action is considered relatively short.

🔑 Rapid- and short-acting insulins must be followed immediately by a meal.

The **intermediate-acting** NPH, detemir, and glargine insulins have a slower onset of 1 to 4 hours, and a sustained peak up to 24 hours.

🔑 Long-acting insulins are not administered in relation to immediate food ingestion.

The number of diabetes-treatment products will continue to increase because of the rapidly rising incidence of type 2 diabetes. Inhalation insulins are now in use, and new drugs are in development that will act to change the body's response to food, either by promoting insulin secretion, delaying gastric emptying, and/or altering glucose metabolism.

INSULIN SYRINGES

Insulin is administered using special **insulin syringes calibrated in units**. In diameter, these are quite like the smaller TB syringes, but the calibrations are totally different. Insulin syringes are used **only for insulin administration**, and they are available in **100 unit, 50 unit, and 30 unit sizes (Figure 9-12)**. The 30 and 50 unit syringe calibrations are larger than the calibrations on the 100 unit syringes, and they provide an added degree of safety in measurement of small dosages.

Because of their small diameter, insulin syringe calibrations and numbering wrap around the small syringe barrel. Refer to the insulin syringes in Figure 9-12 again, and notice the calibrations on them.

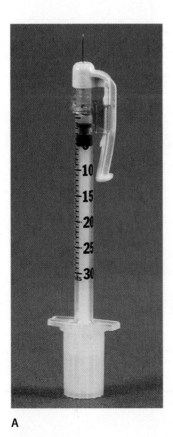
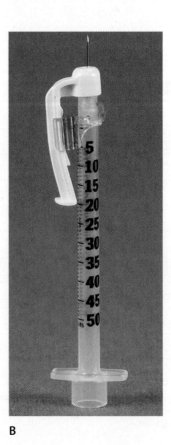
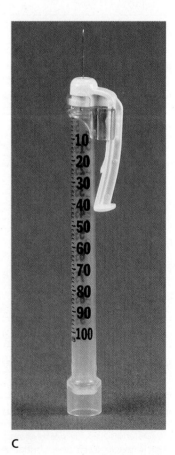

A   B   C

Figure 9-12 Insulin syringes. **A.** 30 unit. **B.** 50 unit. **C.** 100 unit.

For accurate measurement, you will learn **to rotate insulin syringes from side to side to locate the calibration you need and to draw up the insulin dosage ordered**. To make your instruction in measuring insulin dosages easier, the syringe manufacturers have provided the actual art (the calibrations) they use on their insulin syringes. You will be using these "flattened out" calibrations next for your initial instruction in preparing insulin dosages.

The calibrations for the 50 unit dosage syringes are used in the first problems that follow. Notice that the **first long calibration**, as on all other syringes, identifies **zero**, and that **each subsequent calibration measures 1 unit. Each 5 unit calibration is numbered: 5, 10, 15, 20, and so forth**.

PROBLEMS 9-2

Refer to the syringe calibrations for the 50 unit calibrated syringes provided to identify the dosages indicated by the shaded areas and arrows.

1. _____ 2. _____ 3. _____

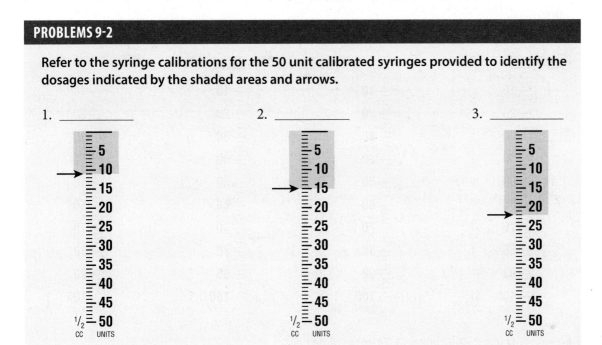

Answers 1. 11 units   **2.** 15 units   **3.** 22 units

PROBLEMS 9-3

Use the 50 unit calibrations provided to shade in the following dosages.

1. 33 units 2. 38 units 3. 18 units

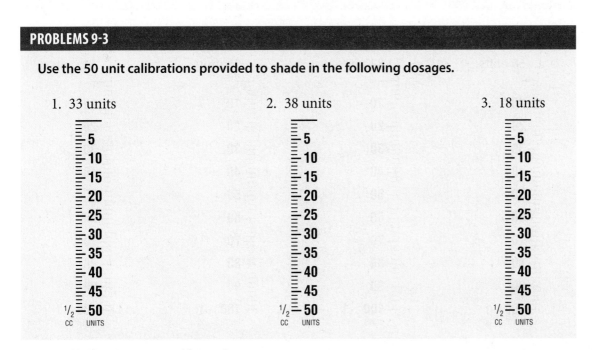

Answers Verify your answers with your instructor.

There are two 100 unit insulin syringes in common use. The first of these syringe calibrations is shown in Problems 9-4. First, notice the 100 unit capacity and observe that, in contrast to the smaller-dose syringes, only **each 10 unit increment is numbered: 10, 20, 30, and so forth**. Next, notice the number of calibrations in each 10 unit increment, which is 5, indicating that **this syringe is calibrated in 2 unit increments. Odd-numbered units cannot be measured accurately using this syringe.**

PROBLEMS 9-4

Identify the dosages indicated by the shading and arrows on the 100 unit syringes provided.

1. _____   2. _____   3. _____   4. _____

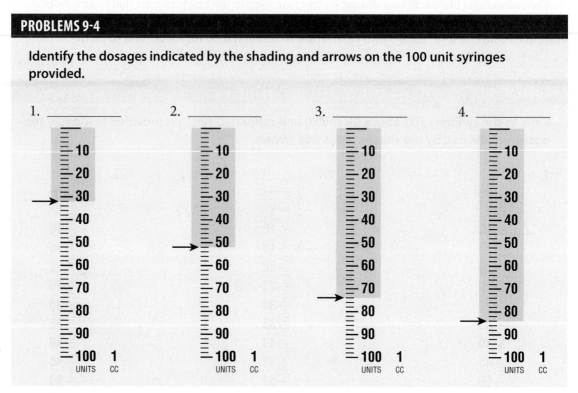

Answers   1. 32 units   **2.** 52 units   **3.** 74 units   **4.** 84 units

PROBLEMS 9-5

Shade in the syringe calibrations provided to measure the dosages indicated.

1. 66 units   2. 84 units   3. 28 units   4. 44 units

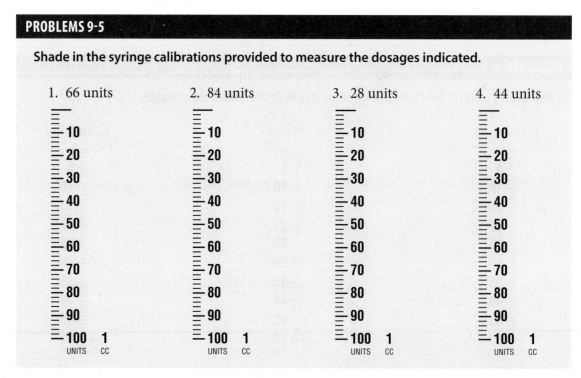

Answers Verify your answers with your instructor.

The second type of 100 unit syringe calibration is illustrated in **Figure 9-13**. Notice that this syringe has a **double scale: The odd numbers are on the left, and the even numbers are on the right**. Each 5 unit increment is numbered, but on **opposite sides** of the syringe. This syringe does have a calibration for each 1 unit increment, but to count every calibration to measure a dosage, the syringe would have to be rotated back and forth. This could cause confusion.

There is a safer way to read the calibrations. **To measure uneven numbered dosages**—for example, 7, 13, 27, and so forth—**use the uneven (left) scale only; for even-numbered dosages**—such as 6, 10, 56, and so forth—**use the even (right) scale only. Count each calibration (on one side only) as 2 units, because that is what each calibration is measuring.**

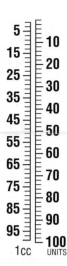

Figure 9-13

EXAMPLE 1

To prepare an 89 unit dosage, start at 85 units on the uneven left scale. Count the first calibration above this mark as 87 units and the next as 89 units. **Each calibration on the same side measures 2 units.**

EXAMPLE 2

To measure a 26 unit dosage, use the even-numbered right-side calibrations. Start at 20 units, move up one calibration to 22 units, another to 24 units, and one more to 26 units. **Each calibration is 2 units.**

PROBLEMS 9-6

Identify the dosages measured on the 100 unit syringe calibrations provided.

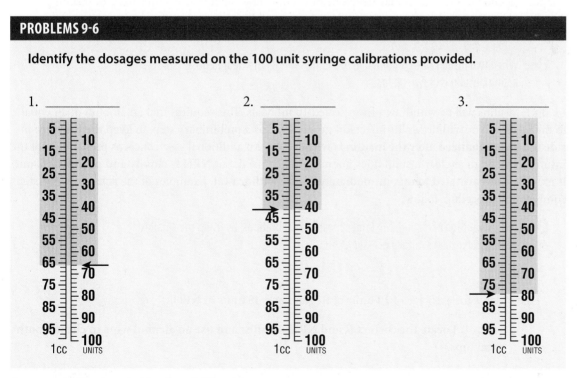

1. _____   2. _____   3. _____

Answers 1. 66 units   **2.** 41 units   **3.** 79 units

PROBLEMS 9-7

Shade in the syringe calibrations provided to identify the following dosages.

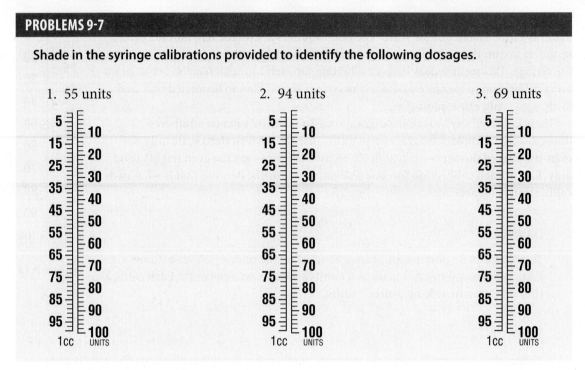

1. 55 units   2. 94 units   3. 69 units

Answers Verify your answers with your instructor.

COMBINING INSULIN DOSAGES

Insulin-dependent individuals may need one or even several subcutaneous injections of insulin per day. To reduce the number of injections as much as possible, it is common to combine two insulins in a single syringe: a short-acting Regular with an intermediate-acting NPH.

> When two insulins are combined in the same syringe, the clear Regular (shortest-acting) insulin is drawn up first.

Both insulins will be withdrawn from sealed 10 mL vials. This requires that an amount of air equal to the insulin to be withdrawn be injected into each vial as a preliminary step, to **keep the pressure inside the vials equalized after the insulin is withdrawn**. An additional step concerns preparation of the insulin itself. Regular clear insulin does not need to be mixed, but **NPH is cloudy and precipitates out**. It must be **gently rotated to mix immediately before withdrawal**. Examples of the actual step-by-step combination procedure follow.

> Take advantage of reading the largest possible calibrations, by using the smallest capacity of insulin syringe necessary.

EXAMPLE 1

The order is for a dosage of 10 units of Regular and 48 units of NPH.

> **Step 1: Locate the correct R and NPH insulins and use an alcohol wipe to cleanse both vial tops.**
>
> **Step 2: The combined dosage, 10 units of Regular and 48 of NPH, is 58 units. This requires the use of a 100 unit syringe.**

Step 3: Draw up 48 units of replacement air for the NPH in the syringe, and insert the needle tip into the NPH vial. Keep the needle tip above the insulin level so as to not inject air into the insulin and possibly distort the dosage. Inject the air and remove the needle.

Step 4: Draw up 10 units of replacement air for the Regular insulin vial. Insert the needle into the vial, again above the insulin level, and inject the air. Draw up the 10 units of Regular.

Step 5: Pick up and gently rotate the NPH vial until the insulin is mixed. Insert the needle back into the vial and draw up the 48 units of NPH.

Step 6: Administer the insulin dosage at once so that the NPH has no chance to precipitate out. Chart the administration.

EXAMPLE 2

A dosage of 16 units Regular and 22 units of NPH has been ordered.

Step 1: Locate the correct Regular and NPH insulins and use an alcohol wipe to cleanse both vial tops.

Step 2: The combined dosage, 16 units of Regular and 22 of NPH, totals 38 units. For this administration, you can use a 50 unit volume syringe.

Step 3: Draw up 22 units of replacement air for the NPH in the syringe. Insert the needle tip into the NPH vial. Keep the needle tip above the insulin level so as to not inject air into the insulin and possibly distort the dosage. Inject the air and remove the needle.

Step 4: Draw up 16 units of replacement air for the Regular insulin vial. Insert the needle into the vial, again above the insulin level, and inject the air. Draw up the 16 units of Regular insulin.

Step 5: Pick up and gently rotate the NPH vial until the insulin is mixed. Insert the needle and draw up the 22 units of NPH.

Step 6: Administer the insulin at once so that the NPH has no chance to precipitate out. Chart the administration.

INSULIN INJECTION SITES AND TECHNIQUES

Insulin is injected subcutaneously. As with other parenteral medications, the **injection sites must be rotated**, keeping the latest injection **at least an inch away from each previously used site**. The abdomen has the most rapid absorption, followed by the upper arm. The outer thigh, a full hand's breadth above the knee and below the hip, may be used, but absorption is somewhat slower at this site. Your responsibility is, and will continue to be, to give the correct insulin and dosage at the correct time, taking special care to assure that a meal immediately follows rapid- and short-acting insulin injection.

For each of the following combined Regular and NPH insulin dosages, indicate the total volume of the combined dosage and the smallest capacity syringe you can use to prepare it; 30, 50, and 100 unit capacity syringes are available.

	Total Volume	Syringe Size
1. 28 units Regular, 64 units NPH	_____	_____
2. 16 units NPH, 6 units Regular	_____	_____
3. 33 units Regular, 41 units NPH	_____	_____
4. 21 units Regular, 52 units NPH	_____	_____
5. 13 units Regular, 27 units NPH	_____	_____

Answers 1. 92 units; 100 unit **2.** 22 units; 30 unit **3.** 74 units; 100 unit **4.** 73 units; 100 unit **5.** 40 units; 50 unit

SUMMARY

This concludes the chapter on insulin dosages. The important points to remember from this chapter are:

- Insulin labels must be read with extreme care because they look very similar.

- Insulin is measured using specially calibrated insulin syringes.

- Insulin syringes are available in 100, 50, and 30 unit capacities.

- The smaller 30 or 50 unit capacity syringes provide a greater degree of safety because of their larger calibrations.

- Each calibration on the 30 and 50 unit volume syringes measures 1 unit.

- Calibrations on 100 unit capacity insulin syringes may measure 1 or 2 unit increments, depending on their design.

- Regular (R) and N (NPH) insulins can be mixed in a single syringe.

- Regular insulin is drawn up first in combination R and NPH dosages.

- N insulins are cloudy because they contain insoluble particles.

- Because N insulins precipitate out, they must be gently and thoroughly mixed before withdrawal from the vial and injected immediately after preparation.

- Insulin is administered subcutaneously.

- The abdomen and upper arm provide the most rapid subcutaneous absorption sites.

- Insulin injection sites are routinely rotated.

SUMMARY SELF-TEST

Use the syringe calibrations provided to measure the following dosages. For combined insulin dosages, use arrows to indicate the exact calibration to be used for each insulin ordered.

1. 37 units Regular

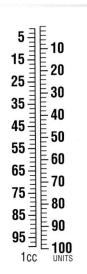

2. 17 units Regular;
   12 units NPH

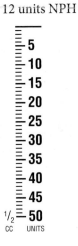

3. 48 units NPH

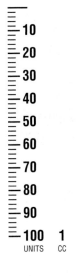

4. 14 units Regular;
   58 units NPH

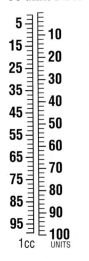

5. 12 units NPH

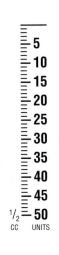

6. 18 units Regular;
   8 units NPH

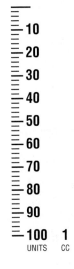

7. 23 units Regular;
   14 units NPH

8. 8 units Regular;
   20 units NPH

9. 24 units Regular

10. 57 units NPH

11. 22 units Regular

12. 14 units Regular;
    44 units NPH

13. 24 units Regular;
    27 units NPH

14. 33 units Regular;
    10 units NPH

15. 56 units Regular

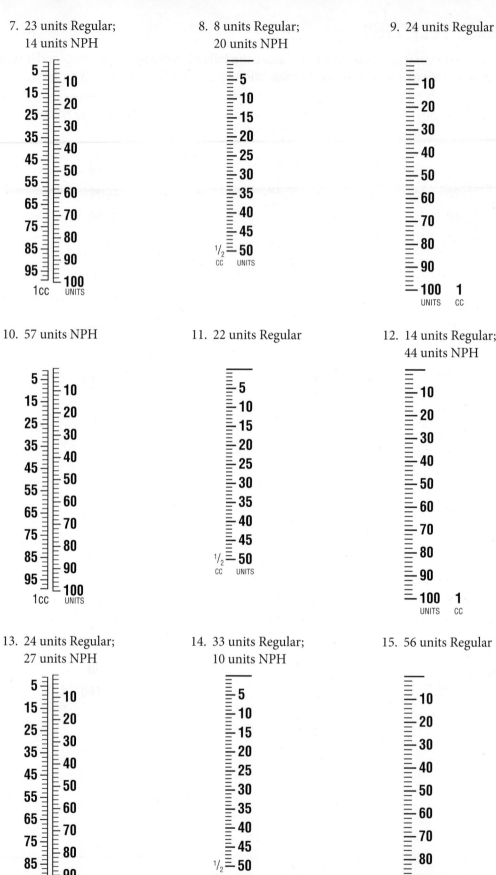
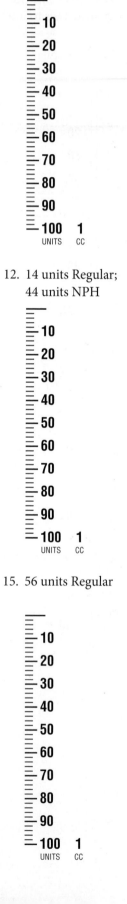

Identify the dosages measured on the following syringes.

16. _____

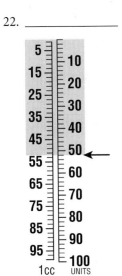

17. _____

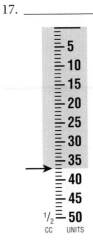

18. _____

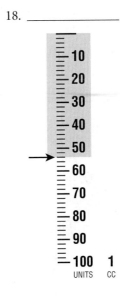

19. _____

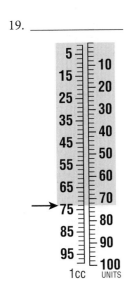

20. _____

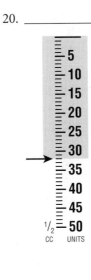

21. _____

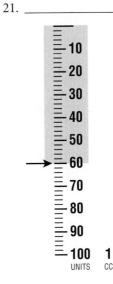

22. _____

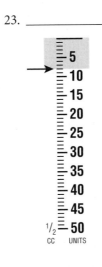

23. _____

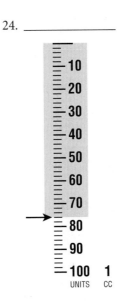

24. _____

25. _____

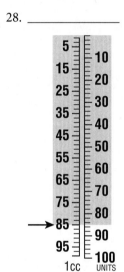

26. _____

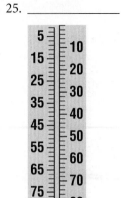

27. _____

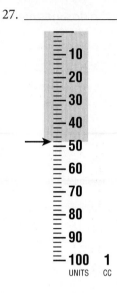

28. _____

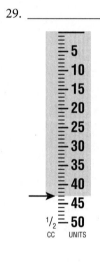

29. _____

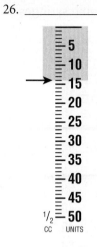

30. _____

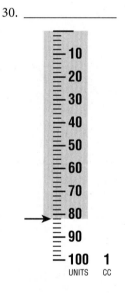

Answers

Verify your answers for **1–15** with your instructor.

16. 67 units	**20.** 32 units	**24.** 76 units	**28.** 85 units
17. 37 units	**21.** 60 units	**25.** 92 units	**29.** 43 units
18. 54 units	**22.** 52 units	**26.** 14 units	**30.** 82 units
19. 73 units	**23.** 8 units	**27.** 48 units	

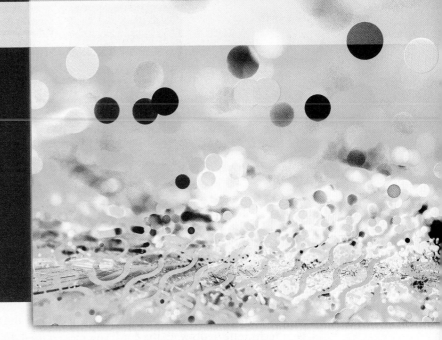

CHAPTER 10

Reconstitution of Powdered Drugs

INTRODUCTION

Many drugs are shipped in powdered form because they **retain their potency for only a short time in solution**. Reconstitution of these drugs is often the responsibility of clinical pharmacies, but you will need to know how to read and follow reconstitution directions and how to label drugs with an expiration date and time once they have been reconstituted. The drug label, or instructional package insert, will give specific directions for reconstitution of the drug. Reading these requires care, and this chapter will take you step by step through the entire process.

RECONSTITUTION OF A SINGLE-STRENGTH SOLUTION

Let's start with the simplest type of reconstitution instructions, for a single-strength solution. Examine the label for the methylprednisolone 500 mg vial in **Figure 10-1**.

> ⚿ Reconstitution directions on vial labels may be small and difficult to read, and extreme care in reading them is essential.

The first step in reconstitution is to locate the directions. They are on the left side of this label. Locate the **Reconstitute with 8 mL Bacteriostatic Water for Injection with Benzyl Alcohol** instructions. Water, or any other solution specified for reconstitution, is called the **diluent**. The **type**

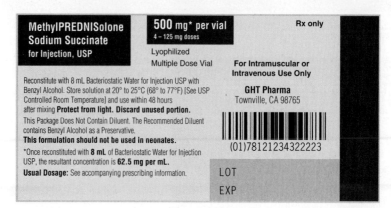

Figure 10-1

of diluent specified will be **different for different drugs**. The **volume of diluent will also vary**. Therefore, reading the label carefully to identify both the type and the volume of diluent to be used is mandatory.

Once you have identified the type of diluent, the next step is to use a **sterile syringe and aseptic technique** to draw up the 8 mL volume required. Inject it slowly into the vial **above the medication level, because air bubbles can distort drug dosages**. If the diluent volume is large, as in this case, be aware that **the syringe plunger will be forced out to expel air to re-equalize the internal vial pressure as you inject the diluent**. Very large volumes of diluent will have to be injected in divided amounts to keep the internal vial pressure equalized. When all the diluent has been injected, rotate and upend the vial until all the medication has been dissolved. **Do not shake the vial** unless directed to do so, because this can add air bubbles to some medications and distort dosages.

> Inject the diluent ABOVE the precipitated medication, then rotate the vial briskly rather than shake it to thoroughly mix the solution.

After reconstitution of the medication, locate the information that relates to the **length of time the reconstituted solution may be stored** and **how it must be stored**. Look again at the methylpredniso-lone directions and locate this information. You will find that this solution can be stored at room temperature and that it must be used within 48 hours of reconstitution.

> If all of the solution is not used immediately, the medication will precipitate out, and require brisk rotation to thoroughly remix the solution prior for reuse.

The next step is to **print your initials on the label as the person who reconstituted the drug**, in case any questions subsequently arise concerning the preparation. Next, **add the expiration date and time to the label**. Let's assume you reconstituted this methylprednisolone solution at **2 pm on January 3**. Which expiration (EXP) date and time will you print on the label? The reconstituted drug lasts only 48 hours at room temperature, so you would print **Exp. Jan. 5, 2 pm**, which is 48 hours (2 days) from the time you reconstituted it.

> The person who reconstitutes a drug is responsible for labeling it with the date and time of expiration, and with his or her initials.

Next, identify the total dosage strength of this vial, which is **500 mg**. Near the top of the label, you can locate the individual dosage strength: **4–125 mg** doses. Because you have injected 8 mL of diluent, this will be approximately **2 mL for each 125 mg** dose, but if you read the small print on the label, you will see that the individual dosage is clearly identified as **62.5 mg per mL**.

Reconstituted volumes do not always exactly equal the amount of diluent added—in fact, most do not. This is because the medication itself has a volume, and it usually makes the total volume somewhat larger than the amount of diluent injected. Our next examples of a single-strength reconstitution will illustrate this increased volume concept.

If a 62.5 mg dosage is ordered, you will need 1 mL.

If a 125 mg dosage is needed, you will need 2 mL (125 mg = 62.5 mg × 2).

If a 250 mg dosage is needed, you will need 4 mL; and if 500 mg is ordered, the total is 8 mL.

🔑 Reconstituted volumes may exceed the volume of the diluent added, because the drug itself has a volume.

PROBLEMS 10-1

Other drugs shipped in powdered form are antibiotics. Read the label in **Figure 10-2** to answer the following questions about reconstituting this drug.

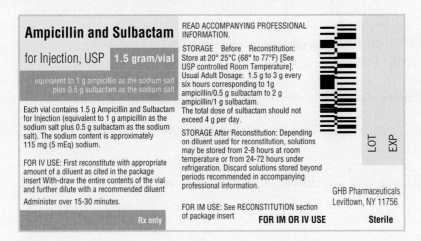

Ampicillin and Sulbactam
for Injection, USP   **1.5 gram/vial**

equivalent to 1 g ampicillin as the sodium salt
plus 0.5 g sulbactam as the sodium salt

Each vial contains 1.5 g Ampicillin and Sulbactam for Injection (equivalent to 1 g ampicillin as the sodium salt plus 0.5 g sulbactam as the sodium salt). The sodium content is approximately 115 mg (5 mEq) sodium.

FOR IV USE: First reconstitute with appropriate amount of a diluent as cited in the package insert With-draw the entire contents of the vial and further dilute with a recommended diluent Administer over 15-30 minutes.

Rx only

READ ACCOMPANYING PROFESSIONAL INFORMATION.

STORAGE Before Reconstitution: Store at 20° 25°C (68° to 77°F) [See USP controlled Room Temperature]. Usual Adult Dosage: 1.5 g to 3 g every six hours corresponding to 1g ampicillin/0.5 g sulbactam to 2 g ampicillin/1 g sulbactam. The total dose of sulbactam should not exceed 4 g per day.

STORAGE After Reconstitution: Depending on diluent used for reconstitution, solutions may be stored from 2-8 hours at room temperature or from 24-72 hours under refrigeration. Discard solutions stored beyond periods recommended in accompanying professional information.

FOR IM USE: See RECONSTITUTION section of package insert   **FOR IM OR IV USE**

LOT   EXP

GHB Pharmaceuticals
Levittown, NY 11756

Sterile

Figure 10-2

1. How is this drug administered?   _____

2. How long will this solution retain its potency at room temperature after reconstitution?   _____

3. How long if refrigerated?   _____

4. If you reconstitute this drug at 10:10 am on October 3 and it is refrigerated, what expiration time will you print on the label?   _____

5. What else will you print on the label?   _____

6. What is the total dosage of this reconstituted IV solution?   _____

Answers 1. IM or IV **2.** 2–8 hours **3.** 24–72 hours **4.** Exp. Oct. 4 10:10 am to Oct. 6 10:10 am (your answer must include "Exp." to be correct) **5.** your initials **6.** 1.5 g

PROBLEMS 10-2

Refer to the penicillin V potassium oral suspension label in **Figure 10-3** to answer the following questions.

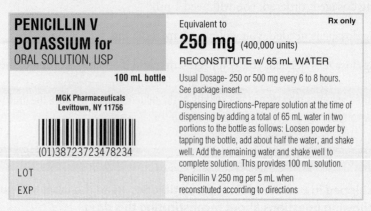

PENICILLIN V POTASSIUM for ORAL SOLUTION, USP

100 mL bottle

MGK Pharmaceuticals
Levittown, NY 11756

(01)38723723478234

LOT

EXP

Rx only

Equivalent to

250 mg (400,000 units)

RECONSTITUTE w/ 65 mL WATER

Usual Dosage- 250 or 500 mg every 6 to 8 hours. See package insert.

Dispensing Directions-Prepare solution at the time of dispensing by adding a total of 65 mL water in two portions to the bottle as follows: Loosen powder by tapping the bottle, add about half the water, and shake well. Add the remaining water and shake well to complete solution. This provides 100 mL solution.

Penicillin V 250 mg per 5 mL when reconstituted according to directions

Figure 10-3

1. How much diluent is needed to reconstitute this large-volume oral suspension preparation?   _____

2. What kind of diluent will you use?   _____

3. The label is specific about how to add this diluent. What does it tell you?   _____

4. This is an oral suspension. Does the diluent need to be sterile?   _____

5. What is the mg dosage strength of the prepared solution?   _____

6. If the dosage ordered is 125 mg, how many mL are needed?   _____

7. For a 500 mg dosage, how many mL are needed?   _____

8. How many units of medication will there be in a 5 mL dose?   _____

9. What should you do to this medication before administering it?   _____

10. What must the person who reconstitutes the medication print on the label?   _____

Answers 1. 65 mL   **2.** water   **3.** tap to loosen powder, add half of water, shake well, add rest of water and shake again   **4.** No, this is an oral medication   **5.** 250 mg or 400,000 units per 5 mL   **6.** 2.5 mL   **7.** 10 mL   **8.** 400,000 units   **9.** shake well to thoroughly mix   **10.** expiration date & time, initials

PROBLEMS 10-3

Refer to the ceftriaxone label in **Figure 10-4** to answer the following questions.

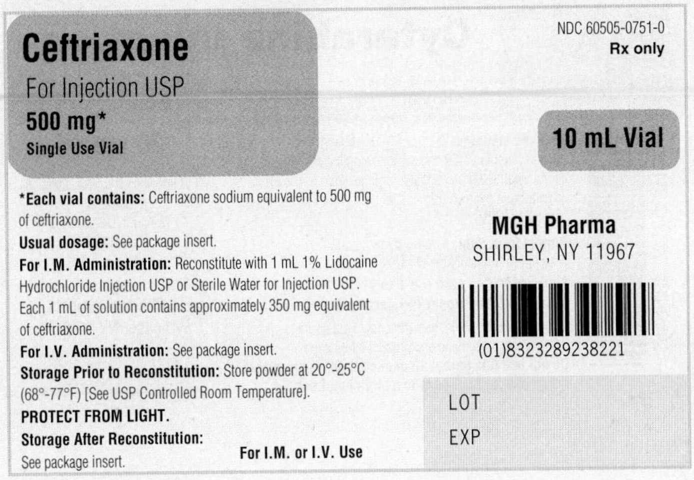

Ceftriaxone
For Injection USP
500 mg*
Single Use Vial

NDC 60505-0751-0
Rx only

10 mL Vial

*****Each vial contains:** Ceftriaxone sodium equivalent to 500 mg of ceftriaxone.
Usual dosage: See package insert.
For I.M. Administration: Reconstitute with 1 mL 1% Lidocaine Hydrochloride Injection USP or Sterile Water for Injection USP. Each 1 mL of solution contains approximately 350 mg equivalent of ceftriaxone.
For I.V. Administration: See package insert.
Storage Prior to Reconstitution: Store powder at 20°-25°C (68°-77°F) [See USP Controlled Room Temperature].
PROTECT FROM LIGHT.
Storage After Reconstitution:
See package insert. **For I.M. or I.V. Use**

MGH Pharma
SHIRLEY, NY 11967

(01)8323289238221

LOT
EXP

Figure 10-4

1. What is the total dosage of this vial? _____

2. How much diluent is used for IM reconstitution? _____

3. What kind of diluent is specified for IM reconstitution? _____

4. What dosage will 1 mL of IM reconstituted solution contain? _____

5. Where does it tell you to look for information on the kind of diluent to use for IV reconstitution? _____

6. Where will you find storage and expiration details? _____

7. What will you print on the label in addition to the expiration date? _____

Answers 1. 500 mg **2.** 1 mL **3.** 1% lidocaine hydrochloride injection or sterile water for injection
4. 350 mg **5.** package insert **6.** package insert **7.** your initials

PROBLEMS 10-4

Refer to the cytarabine label in **Figure 10-5** to answer the following questions.

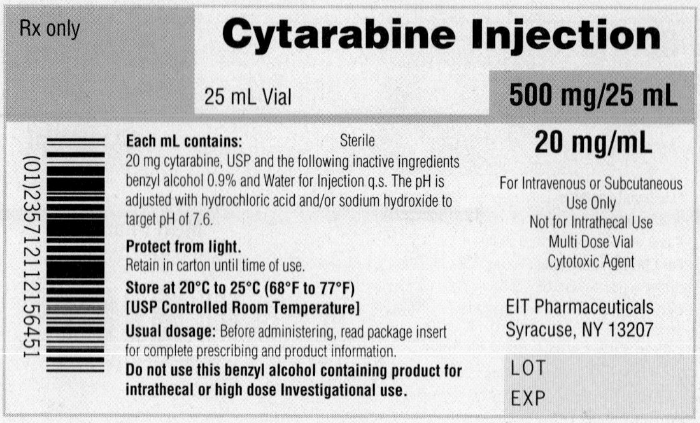

Rx only

Cytarabine Injection

25 mL Vial

500 mg/25 mL

20 mg/mL

Each mL contains: Sterile
20 mg cytarabine, USP and the following inactive ingredients
benzyl alcohol 0.9% and Water for Injection q.s. The pH is
adjusted with hydrochloric acid and/or sodium hydroxide to
target pH of 7.6.

Protect from light.
Retain in carton until time of use.

Store at 20°C to 25°C (68°F to 77°F)
[USP Controlled Room Temperature]

Usual dosage: Before administering, read package insert
for complete prescribing and product information.

Do not use this benzyl alcohol containing product for
intrathecal or high dose Investigational use.

For Intravenous or Subcutaneous
Use Only
Not for Intrathecal Use
Multi Dose Vial
Cytotoxic Agent

EIT Pharmaceuticals
Syracuse, NY 13207

LOT
EXP

(01)2357121121156451

Figure 10-5

1. What is the total dosage strength of this vial? _____

2. By what routes may this drug be administered? _____

3. How is this medication stored? _____

4. Calculate a 30 mg dosage. _____

5. Calculate a 50 mg dosage. _____

Answers 1. 500 mg **2.** IV or subcutaneous **3.** room temperature **4.** 1.5 mL **5.** 2.5 mL

RECONSTITUTION FROM PACKAGE INSERT DIRECTIONS

The reconstitution directions provided in the package insert represent just a small portion of the information that the insert contains. Additional information includes specific use of the drug for diagnosed conditions, such as bacterial meningitis, infections of the gastrointestinal or genitourinary tracts, and so forth; dosage recommendations if the vial label does not contain them; and untoward or adverse reactions, to name just a sample of the topics covered.

Refer to the selected package insert information in **Figure 10-6** to answer the following questions.

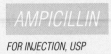

FOR INJECTION, USP

Directions For Use

Use only freshly prepared solutions. Intramuscular and intravenous injections should be administered within one hour after preparation since the potency may decrease significantly after this period.

For Intramuscular Use

Dissolve contents of a vial with the amount of Sterile Water for Injection, USP, or Bacteriostatic Water for Injection, USP, listed in the table below:

Vial Amount	Recommended Amount of Diluent	Approximate Available Volume	Approximate Concentration (in mg/mL)
250 mg	1 mL	1 mL	250 mg
500 mg	1.8 mL	2 mL	250 mg
1 gram	3.5 mL	4 mL	250 mg
2 grams	6.8 mL	8 mL	250 mg

While Ampicillin for Injection, USP, 1 gram and 2 grams, are primarily for intravenous use, they may be administered intramuscularly when the 250 mg or 500 mg vials are unavailable. In such instances, dissolve in 3.5 or 6.8 mL Sterile Water for Injection, USP, or Bacteriostatic Water for Injection, USP, respectively. The resulting solution will provide a concentration of 250 mg per mL.
Ampicillin for Injection, USP 125 mg, is intended primarily for pediatric use. It also serves as a convenient dosage form when small parenteral doses of the antibiotic are required.

For Direct Intravenous Use

Add 5 mL Sterile Water for Injection, USP, or Bacteriostatic Water for Injection, USP to the 250, and 500 mg vials and administer slowly over a 3- to 5- minute period. Ampicillin for Injection, USP, 1 gram or 2 grams, may also be given by direct Intravenous administration. Dissolve in 7.4 or 14.8 mL Sterile Water for Injection, USP, or Bacteriostatic Water for Injection, USP, respectively, and administer slowly over at least 10 to 15 minutes.

CAUTION: More rapid administration may result in convulsive seizures.

Figure 10-6

Information from DailyMed; National Institutes of Health.

1. Identify the types of diluent that may be used for reconstitution under the section labeled **For Intramuscular Use**. _____

2. Look next at the four-column table for reconstitution, and notice that information is provided for the four different strengths of vials available: 250 mg, 500 mg, 1 g, and 2 g. What volume of diluent is specified for a 250 mg vial? _____

3. How much diluent is required for a 500 mg vial? _____

4. How much diluent is required for a 1 g vial? _____

5. How much diluent is required for a 2 g vial? _____

6. The mL dosage strength of all four reconstituted solutions is the same. What is it? _____

7. Refer to the information under **For Direct Intravenous Use**. How much diluent must be added to the 250 mg or 500 mg vials? _____

Answers 1. Sterile Water for Injection or Bacteriostatic Water for Injection   **2.** 1 mL   **3.** 1.8 mL   **4.** 3.5 mL   **5.** 6.8 mL   **6.** 250 mg per 1 mL   **7.** 5 mL

In this section, you were concentrating specifically on locating vial label and package insert directions for reconstitution of a single-strength solution. As you quickly discovered, there is no standard way that this information is presented. Nevertheless, all of the information is there somewhere; you must persist until you locate it.

The next section will introduce you to labels and package inserts that contain directions for preparation of multiple-strength solutions.

RECONSTITUTION OF MULTIPLE-STRENGTH SOLUTIONS

Some powdered drugs offer a choice of dosage strengths. When this is the case, you must choose the strength most appropriate for the dosage ordered. For example, in the penicillin label in **Figure 10-7**, the dosage strengths that can be obtained are listed in the middle.

Notice that three dosage strengths are listed: 250,000 units, 500,000 units, and 1,000,000 units/mL. If the dosage ordered is 500,000 units, the most appropriate strength to mix would be 500,000 units/mL. Read across from this strength, and determine how much diluent must be added to obtain it. The answer is 33 mL. If the dosage ordered is 1,000,000 units, what would be the most appropriate strength to prepare, and how much diluent would this require? The answers are 1,000,000 units/mL and 11.5 mL.

    A multiple-strength solution requires that you add one additional piece of information to the label after reconstitution: the dosage strength just mixed.

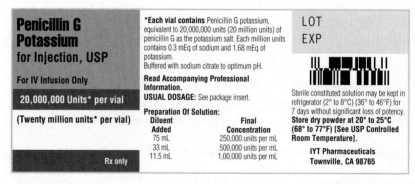

Figure 10-7

PROBLEMS 10-6

Refer to the penicillin G label in Figure 10-7 to answer these additional questions.

1. If you add 75 mL of diluent to prepare a solution of penicillin, what dosage strength will you print on the label?   _____

2. Does this prepared solution require refrigeration?   _____

3. If you reconstitute it on June 1 at 2 pm, what expiration time and date will you print on the label?   _____

4. What is the total dosage strength of this vial?   _____

5. What else do you print on the label besides the dosage strength just reconstituted?   _____

6. Where will you locate information on the diluent to be used?   _____

Answers 1. 250,000 units per mL   **2.** yes   **3.** Exp. June 8 2 pm   **4.** 20 million units   **5.** expiration date and time; your initials   **6.** package insert

The next problems focus on a simulated vial label with a solution strength of 500 mg and a package insert that gives the reconstitution directions.

PROBLEMS 10-7

Refer to the vancomycin HCl label in Figure 10-8 and answer the following questions.

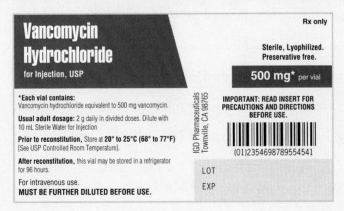

Figure 10-8

1. What is the dosage of this vial? _____

2. What type of diluent must be used for dilution? _____

3. How much diluent must be used? _____

4. What storage directions are listed? _____

5. How long will the medication last after reconstitution? _____

6. Calculate a 30 mg dosage. _____

7. Calculate a 70 mg dosage. _____

Use the 500 mg antibiotic insert in Figure 10-9 to answer the following questions.

ANTIBIOTIC

FOR INJECTION, USP

Preparation and Stability

At the time of use, reconstitute by adding either 10 mL of Sterile Water for Injection to the 500-mg vial or 20 mL of Sterile Water for Injection to the 1-g vial of dry, sterile powder. Vials reconstituted in this manner will give a solution of 50 mg/mL. FURTHER DILUTION IS REQUIRED.

After reconstitution, the vials may be stored in a refrigerator for 14 days without significant loss of potency. Reconstituted solutions containing 500 mg must be diluted with at least 100 mL of diluent. Reconstituted solutions containing 1g must be diluted with at least 200 mL of diluent. The desired dose, diluted in this manner, should be administered by intermittent intravenous infusion over a period of at least 60 minutes.

Figure 10-9

Information from DailyMed; National Institutes of Health.

8. How much diluent must be used to reconstitute a 500 mg vial? _____

9. How much diluent would be needed for a 1 g vial? _____

10. What kind of diluent is specified? _____

11. What is the reconstituted dosage per mL of these dosage strengths? _____

12. How long can the solution be used if it is stored in a refrigerator? _____

13. If the drug is reconstituted on May 4 at 1350, what expiration date and time will you print on the label? _____

14. What else must you print on the label? _____

Answers 1. 500 mg   **2.** Sterile Water   **3.** 10 mL   **4.** refrigerate   **5.** 96 hours   **6.** 0.06 mL   **7.** 0.14 mL
8. 10 mL   **9.** 20 mL   **10.** Sterile Water for Injection   **11.** 50 mg per mL   **12.** 14 days   **13.** Exp. May 18
1350   **14.** your initials

SUMMARY

This concludes the chapter on the reconstitution of powdered drugs. The important points to remember from this chapter are:

- If the medication label does not contain reconstitution directions, these directions may be located on the medication package insert.

- The type and amount of diluent to be used for reconstitution must be exactly as specified in the reconstitution instructions.

- If directions are given for both IM and IV reconstitution, be careful to read the correct set of instructions for the solution you are preparing.

- The person who reconstitutes a drug must initial the vial and print the expiration time and date on the label, unless all of the drug is used immediately.

- If a solution is prepared using multiple-strength medication directions, the strength reconstituted must also be printed on the label.

SUMMARY SELF-TEST

Refer to the ceftriaxone label in **Figure 10-10** to answer the following questions about reconstitution.

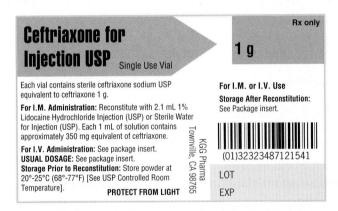

Figure 10-10

1. What is the total dosage of this vial? _____

2. What volume of diluent must be used for reconstitution? _____

3. What will be the dosage strength of 1 mL of reconstituted solution? _____

Refer to the levothyroxine sodium label in **Figure 10-11** to answer the following questions.

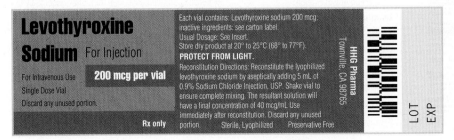

Figure 10-11

4. What is the dosage strength of this vial in mcg? In mg? _____

5. What volume of diluent must you add to prepare the solution for use? _____

6. What kind of diluent must be used? _____

7. How long will this reconstituted solution retain its potency? _____

8. What is the per mL strength of the reconstituted solution? _____

Refer to the voriconazole label in Figure 10-12 to answer the following questions.

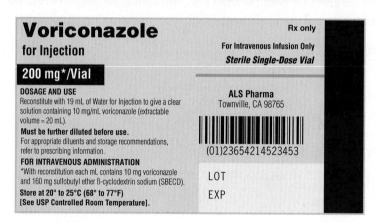

Figure 10-12

9. How much diluent is required to reconstitute this solution? _____

10. What diluent is specified for use? _____

11. What is the strength of each 1 mL of the reconstituted solution? _____

12. What is the total dosage of this vial? _____

Refer to the cefpodoxime proxetil label in Figure 10-13 to answer the following questions.

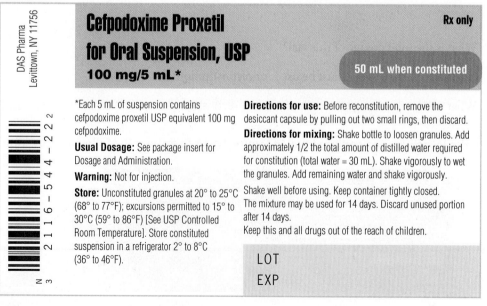

Figure 10-13

13. How much diluent will be required to reconstitute this medication?   _____

14. What type of diluent is listed for reconstitution?   _____

15. How is this diluent to be added?   _____

16. What is the reconstituted dosage strength?   _____

17. How long will the reconstituted cefpodoxime proxetil solution retain
    its potency?   _____

Refer to the acyclovir label in Figure 10-14 to answer the following questions for reconstitution.

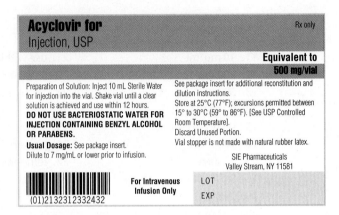

Acyclovir for
Injection, USP   Rx only

Equivalent to
500 mg/vial

Preparation of Solution: Inject 10 mL Sterile Water for injection into the vial. Shake vial until a clear solution is achieved and use within 12 hours. **DO NOT USE BACTERIOSTATIC WATER FOR INJECTION CONTAINING BENZYL ALCOHOL OR PARABENS.**
Usual Dosage: See package insert.
Dilute to 7 mg/mL or lower prior to infusion.

See package insert for additional reconstitution and dilution instructions.
Store at 25°C (77°F); excursions permitted between 15° to 30°C (59° to 86°F). [See USP Controlled Room Temperature].
Discard Unused Portion.
Vial stopper is not made with natural rubber latex.

SIE Pharmaceuticals
Valley Stream, NY 11581

(01)2132312332432   **For Intravenous Infusion Only**   LOT   EXP

Figure 10-14

18. What type of diluent is recommended for reconstitution?   _____

19. How much diluent must be added?   _____

20. What is the total dosage strength of this vial?   _____

21. How soon must this solution be used?   _____

Refer to the penicillin G potassium label in Figure 10-15 to answer the following questions.

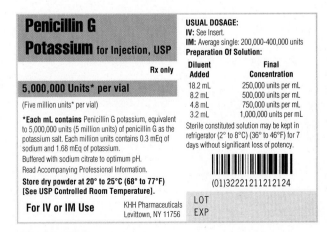

Penicillin G
Potassium for Injection, USP

Rx only

5,000,000 Units* per vial

(Five million units* per vial)

*Each mL contains Penicillin G potassium, equivalent to 5,000,000 units (5 million units) of penicillin G as the potassium salt. Each million units contains 0.3 mEq of sodium and 1.68 mEq of potassium.
Buffered with sodium citrate to optimum pH.
Read Accompanying Professional Information.
Store dry powder at 20° to 25°C (68° to 77°F) [See USP Controlled Room Temperature].

For IV or IM Use   KHH Pharmaceuticals
Levittown, NY 11756

USUAL DOSAGE:
IV: See Insert.
IM: Average single: 200,000-400,000 units
Preparation Of Solution:

Diluent Added	Final Concentration
18.2 mL	250,000 units per mL
8.2 mL	500,000 units per mL
4.8 mL	750,000 units per mL
3.2 mL	1,000,000 units per mL

Sterile constituted solution may be kept in refrigerator (2° to 8°C) (36° to 46°F) for 7 days without significant loss of potency.

(01)32221211212124   LOT   EXP

Figure 10-15

22. What is the total dosage strength of this vial? _____

23. How much diluent must be added to prepare a 250,000 units/mL strength? _____

24. How much diluent must be added to prepare a 500,000 units/mL strength? _____

25. How much diluent must be added to prepare a 750,000 units/mL strength? _____

26. This label has no information on the type of diluent to use. Where will you find this? _____

27. How must this solution be stored? _____

28. If reconstituted at 1:10 am on December 18, what day will it expire? _____

Answers

1. 1 g
2. 2.1 mL
3. 350 mg/mL
4. 200 mcg, 0.2 mg
5. 5 mL
6. 0.9% NaCl
7. use immediately
8. 40 mcg/mL
9. 19 mL
10. Water for Injection
11. 10 mg/mL
12. 200 mg
13. 30 mL
14. distilled water
15. separate halves
16. 100 mg/5 mL
17. 14 days
18. Sterile Water
19. 10 mL
20. 500 mg
21. use within 12 hours
22. 5,000,000 units
23. 18.2 mL
24. 8.2 mL
25. 4.8 mL
26. package insert
27. refrigerate
28. December 25

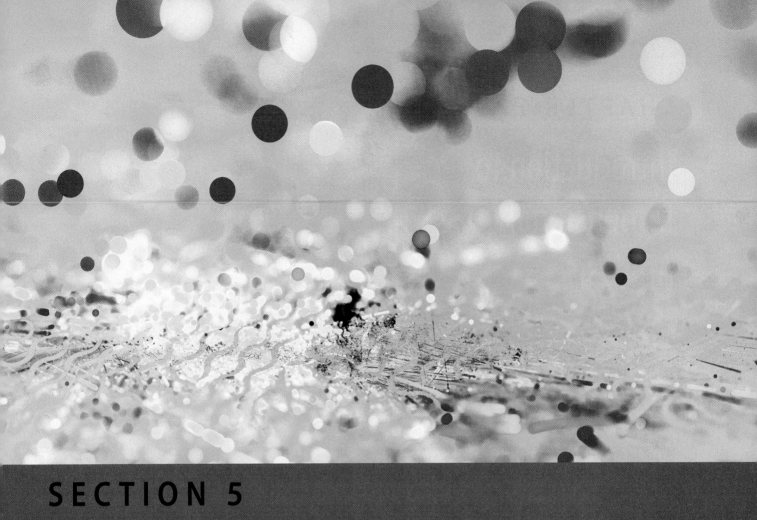

SECTION 5
Dimensional Analysis in Clinical Calculations

CHAPTER 11 Introduction to Dimensional Analysis

CHAPTER 11

Introduction to Dimensional Analysis

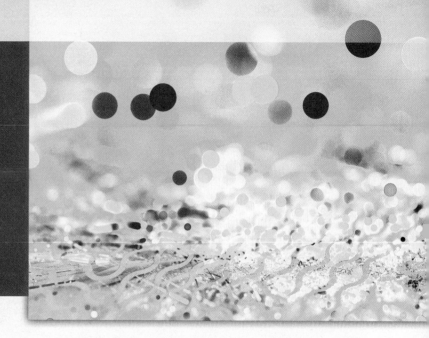

OBJECTIVES

The learner will:

1. Use dimensional analysis to calculate dosages.

PREREQUISITES

Chapters 1–5

INTRODUCTION

Dimensional analysis (**DA**) has been in use in science for almost 2 centuries. You may already be familiar with it under another of its names: the label factor or factor label method, or units conversion.

DA has been used in clinical medical settings for decades. It is actually ratio and proportion made simple. Its great virtue is that **it reduces multiple-step calculations to a single equation**. However, to understand the simplicity of DA, it is necessary to look at clinical ratios from a different perspective.

CLINICAL RATIOS

Clinical ratios provide the components for **all** the calculations you have already learned and will be learning in the remainder of this text. Some examples of ratios you are already familiar with from previous chapters include the following:

> **Oral dosages:** 1 tab = 250 mg; 5 mL = 125 mg
>
> **IM and subcutaneous dosages:** 2 g = 1.5 mL; 1 mL = 10 units; 10 mL = 20 mEq
>
> **Metric conversions:** 1000 mcg = 1 mg; 1 g = 1000 mg

In addition, you will be using the following ratios, although it isn't necessary for you to memorize them at this time:

IV flow rates: 80 gtt per min; 100 mL per hr

IV set calibrations: 10 gtt per mL; 15 gtt per mL; 60 gtt per mL

Time conversions: 60 min = 1 hr; 1 hr = 60 min

In DA, ratios are written as common fractions:

$$\frac{1 \text{ tab}}{250 \text{ mg}} \quad \frac{5 \text{ mL}}{125 \text{ mg}} \quad \frac{2 \text{ g}}{1.5 \text{ mL}}$$

$$\frac{1 \text{ mL}}{10 \text{ units}} \quad \frac{10 \text{ mL}}{20 \text{ mEq}} \quad \frac{1000 \text{ mcg}}{1 \text{ mg}}$$

THE BASIC DA EQUATION

The first step in setting up a DA equation is to **write the unit of measure being calculated**. One commonly calculated measure is mL, so let's begin by using an mL calculation to illustrate the steps involved. Notice that color is used in the first DA examples to help you learn the sequence of ratio entry.

EXAMPLE 1

The available dosage strength is **750 mg in 2.5 mL**. How many mL will be needed to prepare a **600 mg** dosage?

Write the mL unit of measure being calculated, followed by an equal sign:

$$mL =$$

There are two important reasons for identifying the unit of measure being calculated first: It eliminates any confusion over exactly **which** measure is being calculated, and it dictates how the first or "starting" clinical ratio is entered in the equation.

> ⚷ In a DA equation, the unit of measure being calculated is written first, followed by an equal sign.

Next, go back to the problem to **identify the complete clinical ratio that contains mL**. This is provided by the **dosage strength available**, which is **750 mg in 2.5 mL**. Enter this as a common fraction so that **the 2.5 mL *numerator* matches the mL unit of measure being calculated; 750 mg** becomes **the *denominator*.**

$$mL = \frac{2.5 \text{ mL}}{750 \text{ mg}}$$

> ⚷ In a DA equation, the unit of measure being calculated is matched in the numerator of the first clinical ratio entered.

Enter all additional ratios so that **each *denominator* is matched in its successive *numerator*.** In this example, the **denominator in the first ratio is mg**, so the **next numerator must be mg**. Go back to the problem to discover that this is provided by the **600 mg** dosage to be given. Enter this now as the next numerator to complete this single-step equation.

$$mL = \frac{2.5 \text{ mL}}{750 \text{ mg}} \times \frac{600 \text{ mg}}{}$$

🔑 The unit of measure in each denominator of a DA equation is matched in the successive numerator entered.

All the pertinent clinical ratios have now been entered in this one-step DA equation. The next step is to **cancel the alternate denominator/numerator measurement units (but not their quantities) to be sure they match**. This ensures that the clinical ratios were entered correctly. **After cancellation, only the unit of measure being calculated may remain in the equation**. The denominator/numerator mg/mg units cancel, leaving only the mL unit being calculated remaining in the equation.

$$mL = \frac{2.5 \text{ mL}}{750 \text{ mg}} \times \frac{600 \text{ mg}}{}$$

🔑 Only the unit of measure being calculated may remain in the equation after the denominator/numerator units of measure are cancelled.

Only the mL being calculated remains in the equation. You can now do the math. You have two calculation choices: (1) reduce the numbers first as shown in this example or (2) use a calculator.

Reduction Option

$$mL = \frac{2.5 \text{ mL}}{750 \text{ mg}} \times \frac{600 \text{ mg}}{}$$

$$mL = \frac{2.5 \text{ mL}}{\underset{5}{750} \text{ mg}} \times \frac{\overset{4}{600} \text{ mg}}{} \quad \text{Divide by 150}$$

$$mL = \frac{\overset{2}{10}}{\underset{1}{5}} = 2 \text{ mL}$$

Calculator Option

Multiply the numerators 2.5 by 600, then divide by the denominator 750. The answer will be same regardless of the Calculation Option used.

To obtain a dosage of 600 mg from an available dosage strength of 750 mg in 2.5 mL, you would give 2 mL.

DA works exactly the same way for every calculation **regardless of the number of ratios entered**. As you can see, there are no complicated rules to memorize. In these simple steps, you have now learned how to use DA for **all** clinical calculations.

EXAMPLE 2

A dosage of **50,000 units** is ordered to be added to an IV solution. The strength available is **10,000 units in 1.5 mL**. Calculate how many **mL** will contain this dosage.

Reduction Option

Write the mL being calculated to the left of the equation, followed by an equal sign:

$$mL =$$

Locate the complete ratio containing mL, the 10,000 units in 1.5 mL dosage strength available. Enter this value now, with **1.5 mL as the numerator to match the mL being calculated**; 10,000 units becomes the denominator:

$$mL = \frac{1.5 \text{ mL}}{10,000 \text{ units}}$$

The units denominator must be matched in the next numerator. This is provided by the 50,000 units ordered. Enter this now to complete this one-step equation:

$$mL = \frac{1.5 \text{ mL}}{10,000 \text{ units}} \times \frac{50,000 \text{ units}}{}$$

Cancel the alternate denominator/numerator units/units entries to double-check for correct ratio entry. Only the mL being calculated remains in the equation. Do the math:

$$mL = \frac{1.5 \text{ mL}}{10,000 \text{ units}} \times \frac{50,000 \text{ units}}{}$$

$$mL = \frac{1.5 \text{ mL}}{\underset{1}{10,000} \text{ units}} \times \frac{\overset{5}{50,000} \text{ units}}{}$$

Divide 50,000 by 10,000 to obtain 5; multiply 1.5 by 5 to obtain 7.5 mL

$$mL = 1.5 \times 5 = \textbf{7.5 mL}$$

Calculator Option

Multiply the numerators 1.5 by 50,000 and divide by the 10,000 denominator.

It will require a 7.5 mL volume of the 10,000 units in 1.5 mL solution to prepare the 50,000 units ordered for this IV additive.

Let's stop for a moment now and take a look at what happens if you enter the ratios incorrectly in a DA equation. We'll **assume that the units of measure have not been entered with their quantities** and that the **entries have been mixed up**. The correct equation will be shown alongside for comparison.

EXAMPLE 3

A drug label reads **100 mg per 2 mL**. The medication order is for **130 mg**. How many **mL** must you prepare?

Correct	Incorrect
$mL = \dfrac{2 \text{ mL}}{100 \text{ mg}} \times \dfrac{130 \text{ mg}}{} = \textbf{2.6 mL}$	$mL = \dfrac{100}{2} \times \dfrac{130}{} = \textbf{6500 mL}$

In the incorrect equation, the starting ratio is upside down, and since the units of measure were not entered with their quantities, there is no way to catch this error. The safety step of cancellation to check ratio entry cannot be done. But notice something else: The answer, 6500 mL, is impossible. If the entries in a DA equation are mixed up, the numbers are often so outrageous that you will know instantly that you have made a mistake. **But mistakes are not always this obvious, so stick to the step-by-step calculation rules.** There is a reason for every one of them.

Let's look at a few more examples.

EXAMPLE 4

How many **mL** will you draw up to prepare a **1.2 g** dosage if the solution available is labeled **2 g in 3 mL**?

Reduction Option

Write the mL unit being calculated to the left of the equation, followed by an equal sign. Enter the starting ratio, 2 g in 3 mL, with 3 mL as the numerator to match the mL being calculated; 2 g becomes the denominator:

$$mL = \frac{3 \text{ mL}}{2 \text{ g}}$$

Match the g denominator in the next numerator with the 1.2 g ordered to complete the equation:

$$mL = \frac{3\ mL}{2\ g} \times \frac{1.2\ g}{}$$

Cancel the alternate denominator/numerator g units of measure to double-check that the entries are correct. Only the mL being calculated remains:

$$mL = \frac{3\ mL}{2\ \cancel{g}} \times \frac{1.2\ \cancel{g}}{}$$

Do the math, expressing fractional answers to the nearest tenth:

$$mL = \frac{3\ mL}{2\ \cancel{g}} \times \frac{1.2\ \cancel{g}}{} = \textbf{1.8 mL}$$

Calculator Option

The numerators 3 and 1.2 are multiplied and divided by the denominator 2.

The 1.2 g dosage ordered is contained in 1.8 mL of the 2 g in 3 mL solution available.

EXAMPLE 5

Medication with a strength of **0.75 mg per mL** is available to prepare a dosage of **2 mg**. Calculate the number of mL this will require.

Reduction Option

Write the mL being calculated to the left of the equation, followed by an equal sign:

$$mL =$$

The mL being calculated is provided for the first ratio by the 0.75 mg per mL dosage strength available. Enter 1 mL as the numerator and 0.75 mg as the denominator:

$$mL = \frac{1\ mL}{0.75\ mg}$$

The mg denominator must now be matched. This is provided by the 2 mg dosage ordered. Enter this now to complete this one-step equation:

$$mL = \frac{1\ mL}{0.75\ mg} \times \frac{2\ mg}{}$$

Cancel the alternate denominator/numerator mg units of measure to check for correct ratio entry, then do the math:

$$mL = \frac{1\ mL}{0.75\ \cancel{mg}} \times \frac{2\ \cancel{mg}}{} = 2.67 = \textbf{2.7 mL}$$

Calculator Option

Multiply 1 mL and 2 mg numerators, and divide by 0.75 mg denominator. The answers will be identical.

It will require 2.7 mL of the 0.75 mg in 1 mL dosage available to administer the 2 mg ordered.

PROBLEMS 11-1

Calculate these dosages using DA. Express mL answers to the nearest tenth. Use the calculation method you prefer.

1. A dosage of 0.3 g has been ordered. The strength available is 0.4 g in 1.5 mL.   _____

2. A dosage strength of 0.8 mg in 2 mL is to be used to prepare a 0.5 mg dosage.   _____

3. Prepare a 1.8 mg dosage from a solution labeled 2 mg in 3 mL.   _____

4. The order is for 1500 mg. You have available a 1200 mg per mL solution.   _____

5. A dosage strength of 0.2 mg in 1.5 mL is available. Give 0.15 mg.   _____

6. The strength available is 1000 mg in 3.6 mL. Prepare a 600 mg dosage.   _____

7. A 10,000 units dosage has been ordered. The strength available is 8000 units in 1 mL.   _____

8. An IV additive has a dosage strength of 20 mEq per 20 mL. A dosage of 15 mEq has been ordered.   _____

9. A 200,000 units dosage must be prepared from a 150,000 units in 2 mL strength.   _____

10. An IV additive order is for 400 mg. The solution available has a strength of 500 mg in 20 mL.   _____

Answers 1. 1.1 mL   **2.** 1.3 mL   **3.** 2.7 mL   **4.** 1.3 mL   **5.** 1.1 ml   **6.** 2.2 mL   **7.** 1.3 mL   **8.** 15 mL   **9.** 2.7 mL
10. 16 mL

You now know the basics of using DA in calculations. **But how do you know if the answer you obtain is correct?** The answer to this question is provided by the key points already covered:

- **If** the unit being calculated is correctly identified to the left of the equation

- **If** the starting ratio is entered so that its numerator matches the unit of measure being calculated

- **If** the unit of measure in each denominator is matched in each successively entered numerator

- **If** the only unit of measure remaining after cancellation is the same as the unit of measure being calculated

- **If** the quantities have been correctly entered

- **If** the math has been double-checked and is correct

THEN THE ANSWER WILL BE CORRECT.

A tall order? Not really. You are doing a clinical dosage calculation. All you must do is carefully follow each step, and the answer will be correct.

In addition, **don't divorce your previous learning and reasoning from the calculation process**. You already know that **most IM dosages are contained in a 0.5 to 3 mL volume**, that **IV additives may be contained in larger volumes**, and that **dosages rarely include large numbers of tablets and capsules. If you get an unreasonable answer to a calculation, you must question it**. In time, you will know the average dosages of all the drugs you give and another safety component will be added to your repertoire. For now, just concentrate on the simple mechanics of calculation you have just been taught. Don't take shortcuts with these steps, and you'll do just fine.

EQUATIONS REQUIRING METRIC CONVERSIONS

The major advantage of DA is that **it allows you to enter multiple ratios in a single equation**. This offers an option if a drug is ordered in one unit of measure—for example, mg—but is labeled in another—for example, g or mcg.

There are two ways to handle a conversion. Sometimes, it will be easier to do the conversion before setting up the equation. In other instances, you may elect to incorporate the conversion into an equation. For practice purposes, let's look at how **conversion ratios**—for example, **1 g = 1000 mg** or **1 mg = 1000 mcg**—may be entered in a DA equation.

EXAMPLE 1

The IM dosage ordered is **275 mg**. The drug available is labeled **0.5 g per 2 mL**. How many **mL** must you give?

Enter the mL to be calculated to the left of the equation. Locate the ratio containing mL, the 0.5 g per 2 mL dosage strength, and enter it, with 2 mL as the numerator; 0.5 g becomes the denominator:

$$mL = \frac{2 \text{ mL}}{0.5 \text{ g}}$$

When you refer back to the problem, you will not find a g measure to match the starting ratio g denominator. The dosage to be given is in mg. So, a **conversion ratio between g and mg** is needed: 1 g = 1000 mg. Enter this ratio now, with **1 g as the numerator to match the g of the previous denominator**; 1000 mg becomes the new denominator:

$$mL = \frac{2 \text{ mL}}{0.5 \text{ g}} \times \frac{1 \text{ g}}{1000 \text{ mg}}$$

The final entry, the 275 mg dosage to be given, will automatically fall into its correct position as it is entered as the final numerator to match the mg of the previous denominator. The equation is now complete:

$$mL = \frac{2 \text{ mL}}{0.5 \text{ g}} \times \frac{1 \text{ g}}{1000 \text{ mg}} \times \frac{275 \text{ mg}}{}$$

Cancel the alternate denominator/numerator g/g and mg/mg units of measure to double-check the ratio entry. Only the mL being calculated remains. Do the math:

$$mL = \frac{2 \text{ mL}}{0.5 \text{ g}} \times \frac{1 \text{ g}}{1000 \text{ mg}} \times \frac{275 \text{ mg}}{} = 1.1 \text{ mL}$$

To give a dosage of 275 mg, you must prepare 1.1 mL of the 0.5 g in 2 mL strength solution.

EXAMPLE 2

The drug label reads **800 mcg in 1.5 mL**. The IM order is for **0.6 mg**.

Enter the mL to be calculated, followed by an equal sign to the left of the equation. Locate the ratio containing mL, 800 mcg in 1.5 mL. Enter 1.5 mL as the numerator to match the mL being calculated; 800 mcg becomes the denominator:

$$mL = \frac{1.5\ mL}{800\ mcg}$$

There is no mcg measure in the problem, which is your clue to the necessity for a conversion ratio. Enter the 1000 mcg = 1 mg conversion ratio, with 1000 mcg as the numerator to match the mcg of the previous denominator; 1 mg becomes the denominator:

$$mL = \frac{1.5\ mL}{800\ mcg} \times \frac{1000\ mcg}{1\ mg}$$

The mg denominator is now matched by the 0.6 mg dosage to be given, and completes the equation:

$$mL = \frac{1.5\ mL}{800\ mcg} \times \frac{1000\ mcg}{1\ mg} \times \frac{0.6\ mg}{}$$

Cancel the alternate denominator/numerator mcg/mcg and mg/mg units of measure to check for correct ratio entry. Only the mL being calculated should remain in the equation. Do the math:

$$mL = \frac{1.5\ mL}{800\ \cancel{mcg}} \times \frac{1000\ \cancel{mcg}}{1\ \cancel{mg}} \times \frac{0.6\ \cancel{mg}}{} = 1.12 = \textbf{1.1 mL}$$

To give a dosage of 0.6 mg from the available 1.5 mL per 800 mcg strength, you must prepare 1.1 mL.

EXAMPLE 3

Prepare a **0.5 mg** dosage from an available strength of **200 mcg per mL**.

Enter the mL being calculated to the left of the equation, followed by an equal sign. Enter the 1 mL in 200 mcg dosage as the starting ratio, with 1 mL as the numerator to match the mL being calculated; 200 mcg becomes the denominator:

$$mL = \frac{1\ mL}{200\ mcg}$$

A mcg to mg conversion ratio is needed. Enter 1000 mcg as the numerator to match the mcg in the previous denominator; 1 mg becomes the new denominator:

$$mL = \frac{1\ mL}{200\ mcg} \times \frac{1000\ mcg}{1\ mg}$$

The mg denominator is now matched by the 0.5 mg dosage ordered to complete the equation:

$$mL = \frac{1\ mL}{200\ mcg} \times \frac{1000\ mcg}{1\ mg} \times \frac{0.5\ mg}{}$$

Cancel the alternate mcg/mcg and mg/mg units of measure to double-check for correct ratio entry. Only the mL unit being calculated remains in the equation. Do the math:

$$\text{mL} = \frac{1 \text{ mL}}{200 \cancel{\text{ meg}}} \times \frac{1000 \cancel{\text{ meg}}}{1 \cancel{\text{ mg}}} \times \frac{0.5 \cancel{\text{ mg}}}{} = 2.5 \text{ mL}$$

A 0.5 mg dosage requires a 2.5 mL volume of the 200 mcg per mL strength solution available.

EXAMPLE 4

The medication has a strength of **0.5 g in 1.5 mL**. Prepare **750 mg**.
   Enter the mL to be calculated to the left of the equation, followed by an equal sign. Enter the starting ratio, the 1.5 mL in 0.5 g dosage available, with 1.5 mL as the numerator, to match the mL being calculated; 0.5 g becomes the denominator:

$$\text{mL} = \frac{1.5 \text{ mL}}{0.5 \text{ g}}$$

There is no g dosage in the problem, which signals the need for a conversion ratio. Enter the 1 g = 1000 mg conversion ratio, with 1 g as the numerator, to match the g denominator of the starting ratio; 1000 mg becomes the new denominator:

$$\text{mL} = \frac{1.5 \text{ mL}}{0.5 \text{ g}} \times \frac{1 \text{ g}}{1000 \text{ mg}}$$

Enter the dosage ordered, 750 mg, as the final numerator to match the mg in the previous denominator. The equation is complete:

$$\text{mL} = \frac{1.5 \text{ mL}}{0.5 \text{ g}} \times \frac{1 \text{ g}}{1000 \text{ mg}} \times \frac{750 \text{ mg}}{}$$

Cancel the alternate g/g and mg/mg units of measure to check the accuracy of ratio entry, then do the math:

$$\text{mL} = \frac{1.5 \text{ mL}}{0.5 \cancel{\text{ g}}} \times \frac{1 \cancel{\text{ g}}}{1000 \cancel{\text{ mg}}} \times \frac{750 \cancel{\text{ mg}}}{} = 2.25 = 2.3 \text{ mL}$$

A 750 mg dosage requires 2.3 mL of the 0.5 g in 1.5 mL medication.

PROBLEMS 11-2

Calculate these dosages using DA. Express mL answers to the nearest tenth.

1. Prepare 0.1 g of an IM medication from a strength of 200 mg per mL.   _____

2. A drug label reads 0.1 g in 2 mL. Prepare a 130 mg dosage.   _____

3. An oral solution has a strength of 500 mg in 5 mL. Prepare a 0.6 g dosage.   _____

4. Prepare a 0.75 g dosage from a 250 mg per mL strength solution.   _____

5. Prepare 500 mg for IM injection from an available strength of 1 g per 3 mL. _____

6. A dosage of 85 mg is ordered, and the drug available is labeled 0.1 g in 1.5 mL. _____

7. The strength available is 500 mcg in 1.5 mL. Prepare a 0.75 mg dosage. _____

8. A dosage of 1500 mg has been ordered. The solution available is 0.5 g per mL. _____

9. The dosage strength available is 200 mcg per mL. A 0.5 mg dosage has been ordered. _____

10. The dosage ordered is 0.2 g. Tablets available are labeled 80 mg. _____

Answers 1. 0.5 mL **2.** 2.6 mL **3.** 6 mL **4.** 3 mL **5.** 1.5 mL **6.** 1.3 mL **7.** 2.3 mL **8.** 3 mL **9.** 2.5 mL
10. 2½ tab

SUMMARY

This completes your introduction to clinical calculations using dimensional analysis. The important points to remember from this chapter are:

- The unit of measure being calculated is written first to the left of the equation, followed by an equal sign.

- All ratios entered must include the quantity and the unit of measure.

- The numerator in the starting ratio must be in the same measurement unit as the unit of measure being calculated.

- The unit of measure in each denominator must be matched in the numerator of each successive ratio entered.

- Metric system conversions can be made by incorporating a conversion ratio directly into the DA equation.

- The unit of measure in each alternate denominator and numerator must cancel, leaving only the unit of measure being calculated remaining in the equation.

- The numerator of the starting ratio never cancels.

SUMMARY SELF-TEST

Calculate these dosages using DA. Express mL answers to the nearest tenth (or hundredth where indicated) using the medication labels provided. Measure the dosages you calculate on the syringes provided. Have your instructor check your answers to confirm that you have calculated and measured the dosages correctly.

Dosage Ordered

mL Needed

1. terbutaline sulfate 800 mcg

_____

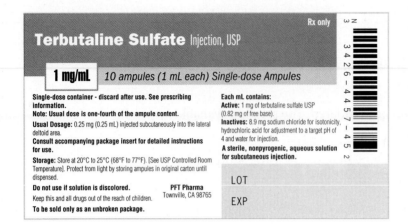

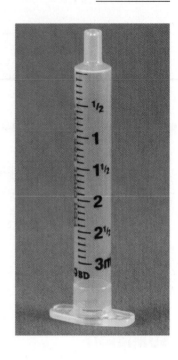

2. furosemide 15 mg

_____

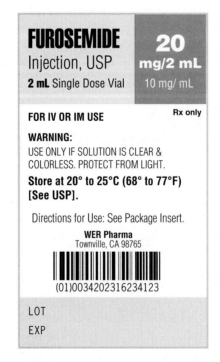

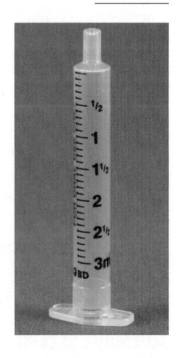

Dosage Ordered   **mL Needed**

3. hydroxyzine HCl 70 mg   _____

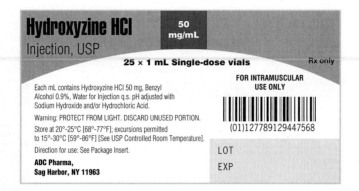

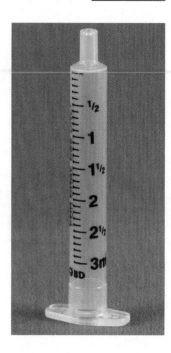

4. fentanyl citrate 0.15 mg   _____

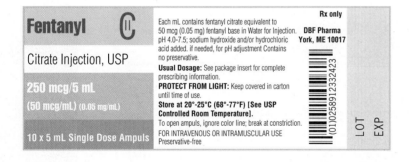

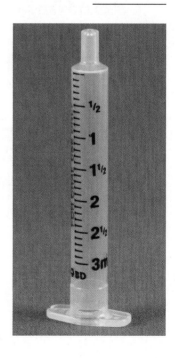

Dosage Ordered

mL Needed

5. naloxone 350 mcg

_____

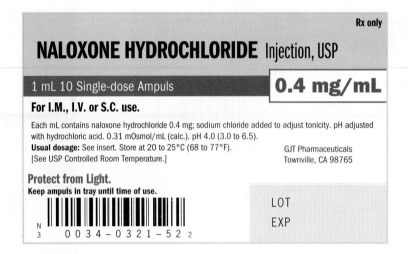

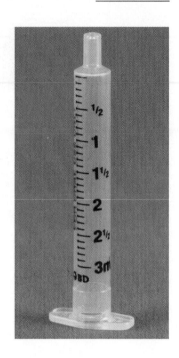

6. clindamycin 225 mg

_____

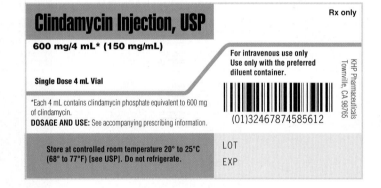

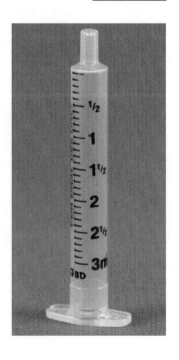

Dosage Ordered   **mL Needed**

7. glycopyrrolate 75 mcg (calculate to the nearest hundredth)   _____

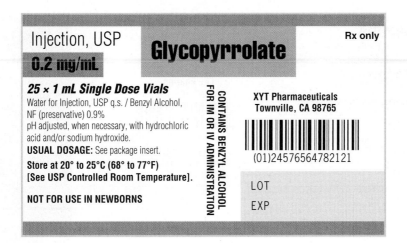

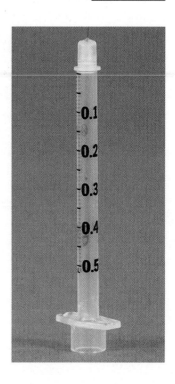

8. midazolam HCl 4 mg   _____

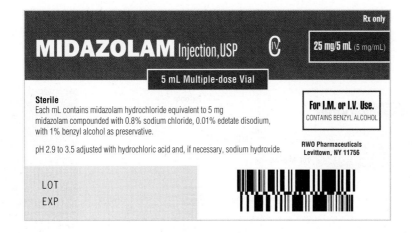

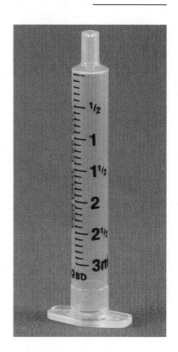

Dosage Ordered

mL Needed

9. droperidol 3 mg

_____

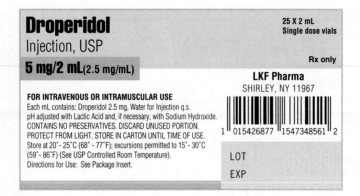

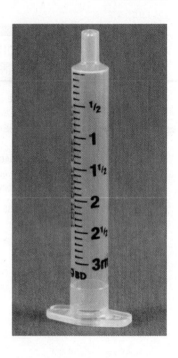

10. cyanocobalamin 0.8 mg

_____

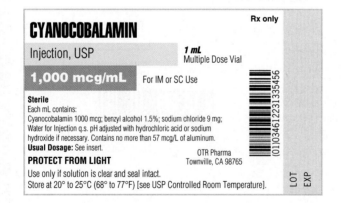

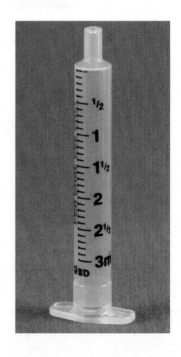

Dosage Ordered   **mL Needed**

11. potassium acetate 30 mEq for IV additive   _____

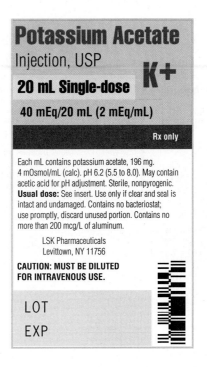

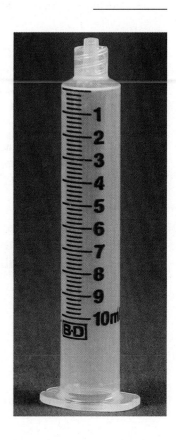

12. calcium gluconate 0.93 mEq   _____

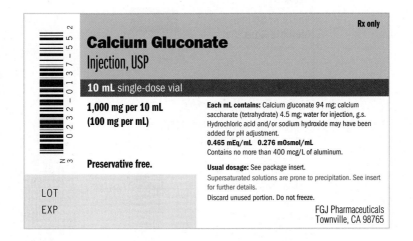

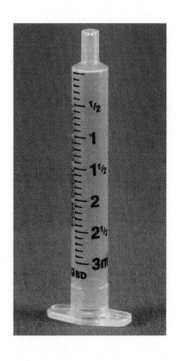

Dosage Ordered   **mL Needed**

13. morphine sulfate 1.5 mg   _____

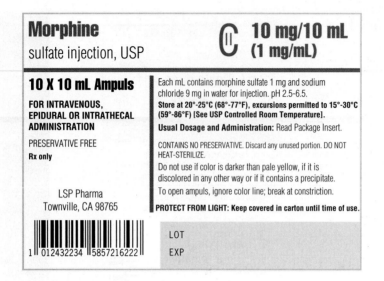

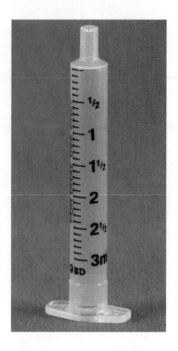

14. heparin sodium 450 units (calculate to the nearest hundredth)   _____

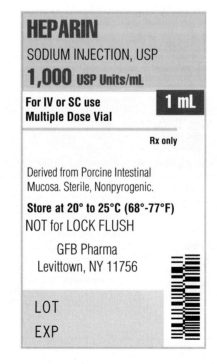

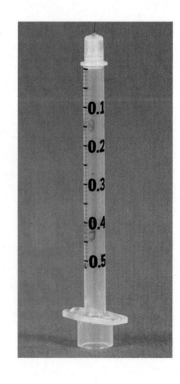

Dosage Ordered

mL Needed

15. droperidol 4 mg

_____

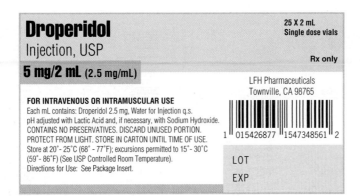

Droperidol
Injection, USP

5 mg/2 mL (2.5 mg/mL)

25 X 2 mL
Single dose vials

Rx only

LFH Pharmaceuticals
Townville, CA 98765

FOR INTRAVENOUS OR INTRAMUSCULAR USE
Each mL contains: Droperidol 2.5 mg, Water for Injection q.s.
pH adjusted with Lactic Acid and, if necessary, with Sodium Hydroxide.
CONTAINS NO PRESERVATIVES. DISCARD UNUSED PORTION.
PROTECT FROM LIGHT. STORE IN CARTON UNTIL TIME OF USE.
Store at 20°- 25°C (68° - 77°F); excursions permitted to 15°- 30°C
(59°- 86°F) (See USP Controlled Room Temperature).
Directions for Use: See Package Insert.

1 015426877 1547348561 2

LOT

EXP

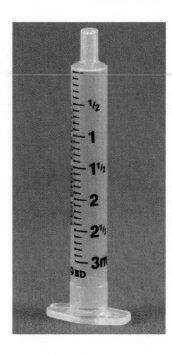

16. phenytoin 0.1 g

_____

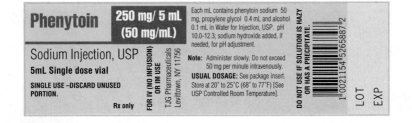

Phenytoin

250 mg/ 5 mL
(50 mg/mL)

Sodium Injection, USP

5mL Single dose vial

SINGLE USE –DISCARD UNUSED
PORTION.

Rx only

FOR IV (NO INFUSION)
OR IM USE

TJG Pharmaceuticals
Levittown, NY 11756

Each mL contains phenytoin sodium 50
mg, propylene glycol 0.4 mL and alcohol
0.1 mL in Water for Injection, USP. pH
10.0-12.3; sodium hydroxide added, if
needed, for pH adjustment.

Note: Administer slowly, Do not exceed
50 mg per minute intravenously.
USUAL DOSAGE: See package insert.
Store at 20° to 25°C (68° to 77°F) [See
USP Controlled Room Temperature].

DO NOT USE IF SOLUTION IS HAZY
OR HAS A PRECIPITATE.

1 0021154 5265887 2

LOT

EXP

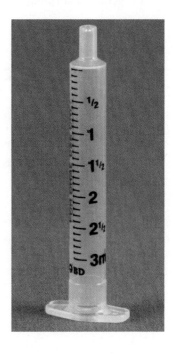

Dosage Ordered

mL Needed

17. medroxyprogesterone 0.9 g

_____

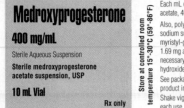

Medroxyprogesterone
400 mg/mL
Sterile Aqueous Suspension
Sterile medroxyprogesterone acetate suspension, USP
10 mL Vial
Rx only

Store at controlled room temperature 15°-30°C (59°-86°F)

Each mL contains: Medroxyprogesterone acetate, 400 mg.
Also, polyethylene glycol 3350, 20.3 mg; sodium sulfate anhydrous, 11 mg; myristyl-gamma-picolinium chloride, 1.69 mg added as preservative, When necessary, pH was adjusted with sodium hydroxide and/or hydrochloric acid.
See package insert for complete product information.
Shake vigorously immediately before each use.

For intramuscular use only
Caution: Federal law prohibits dispensing without prescription.

SDP Pharma
Levittown, NY 11756

LOT
EXP

005826 526598

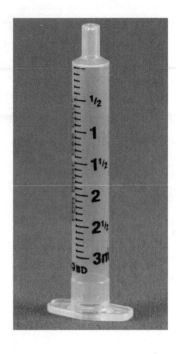

18. gentamicin 70 mg

_____

Rx only

Gentamicin Injection, USP

20 mL Multiple Dose Vial

equivalent to
40 mg/mL

For IM or IV Use.
Must be diluted for IV use.

Sterile
Each mL contains; Gentamicin sulfate equivalent to 40 mg gentamicin; 1.8 mg methylparaben and 0.2 mg propylparaben as preservatives; 3.2 mg sodium metabisulfite, 0.1 mg disodium edetate; water for injection q.s. sodium hydroxide and / or sulfuric acid may have been added for pH adjustment.
Usual Dosage: See insert.
Warning: Patients treated with gentamicin sulfate and other aminoglycosides should be under close observation because of the potential toxicity. See Warnings and Precautions in the insert.

Store at 20°-25°C (68°-77°F) [See USP **NFG Pharmaceuticals**
Controlled Room Temperature]. **Townville, CA 98765**

LOT
EXP

N
3 0172-02515-2 2

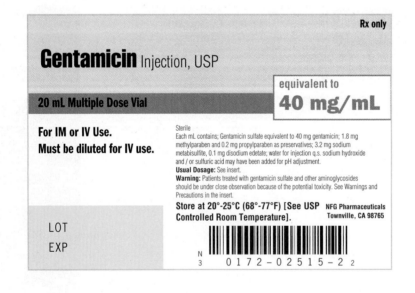

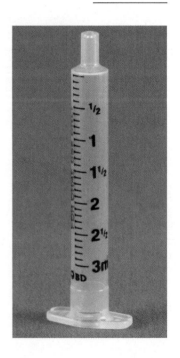

Dosage Ordered

mL Needed

19. hydroxyzine HCl 120 mg

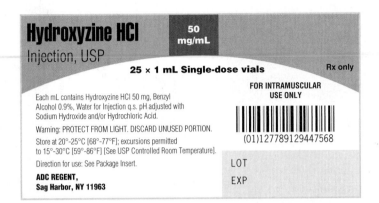

Hydroxyzine HCl
Injection, USP

50 mg/mL

25 × 1 mL Single-dose vials

Rx only

Each mL contains Hydroxyzine HCl 50 mg, Benzyl
Alcohol 0.9%, Water for Injection q.s. pH adjusted with
Sodium Hydroxide and/or Hydrochloric Acid.

Warning: PROTECT FROM LIGHT. DISCARD UNUSED PORTION.

Store at 20°-25°C [68°-77°F]; excursions permitted
to 15°-30°C [59°-86°F] [See USP Controlled Room Temperature].

Direction for use: See Package Insert.

ADC REGENT,
Sag Harbor, NY 11963

FOR INTRAMUSCULAR
USE ONLY

(01)127789129447568

LOT

EXP

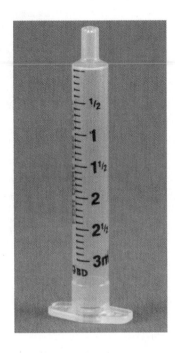

_____

20. sodium chloride 60 mEq for an IV additive

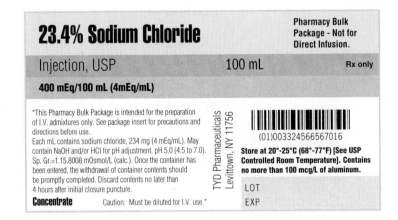

23.4% Sodium Chloride

Injection, USP   100 mL

400 mEq/100 mL (4mEq/mL)

Pharmacy Bulk
Package - Not for
Direct Infusion.

Rx only

*This Pharmacy Bulk Package is intended for the preparation
of I.V. admixtures only. See package insert for precautions and
directions before use.
Each mL contains sodium chloride, 234 mg (4 mEq/mL). May
contain NaOH and/or HCl for pH adjustment. pH 5.0 (4.5 to 7.0).
Sp. Gr.=1.15.8008 mOsmol/L (calc.). Once the container has
been entered, the withdrawal of container contents should
be promptly completed. Discard contents no later than
4 hours after initial closure puncture.

Concentrate   Caution: Must be diluted for I.V. use.*

TYD Pharmaceuticals
Levittown, NY 11756

(01)003324566567016

Store at 20°-25°C (68°-77°F) [See USP
Controlled Room Temperature]. Contains
no more than 100 mcg/L of aluminum.

LOT

EXP

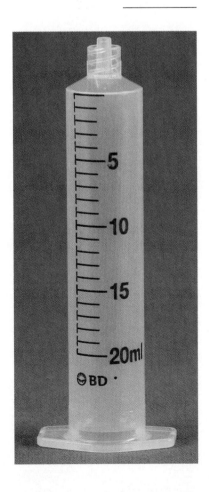

_____

Dosage Ordered   **mL Needed**

21. atropine sulfate 150 mcg   _____

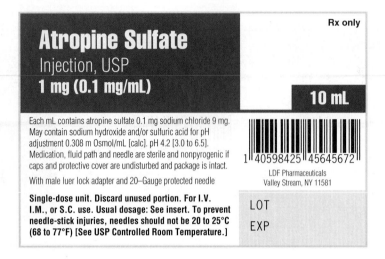

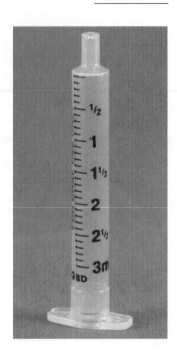

22. meperidine 75 mg   _____

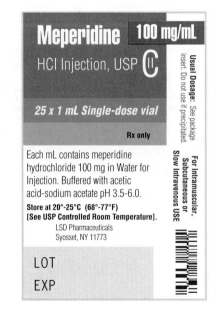

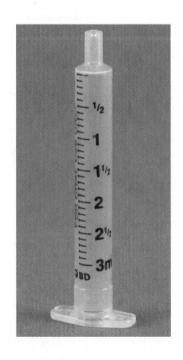

Dosage Ordered   **mL Needed**

23. fentanyl citrate 80 mcg   _____

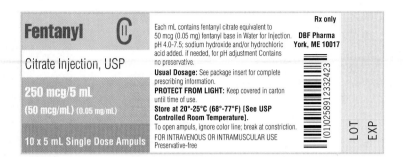

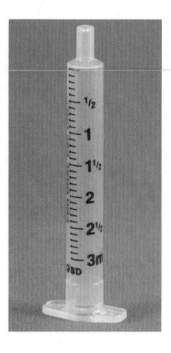

24. betamethasone sodium phosphate and betamethasone acetate 10 mg   _____

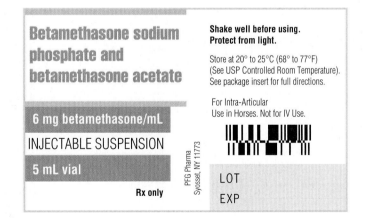

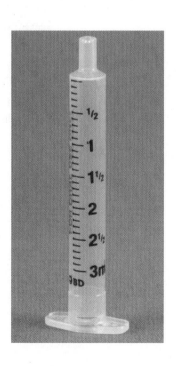

Dosage Ordered

mL Needed

25. morphine sulfate 20 mg

_____

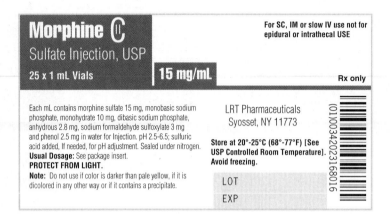

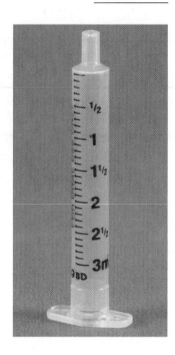

26. gentamicin 0.1 g

_____

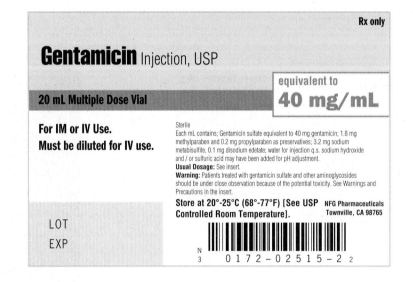

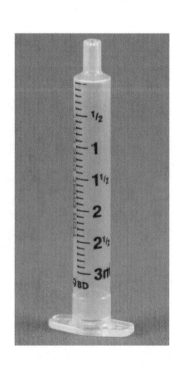

Dosage Ordered | **mL Needed**

27. phenytoin 0.15 g

_____

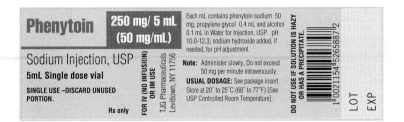

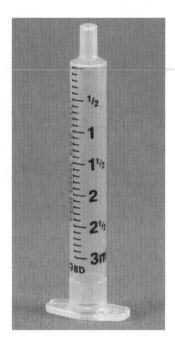

28. doxorubicin HCl 16 mg for an IV additive

_____

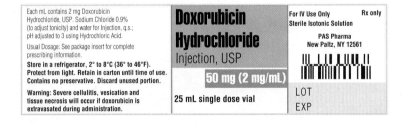

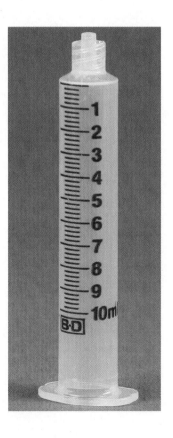

Dosage Ordered

29. meperidine HCl 30 mg

_____

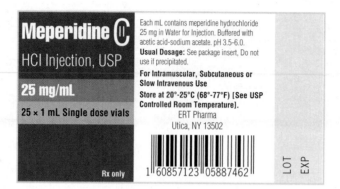

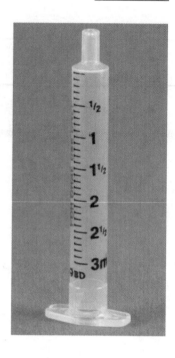

30. methotrexate 40 mg

_____

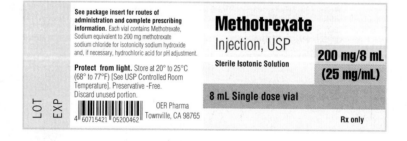

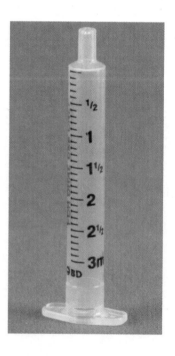

Dosage Ordered

mL Needed

31. midazolam HCl 3 mg

_____

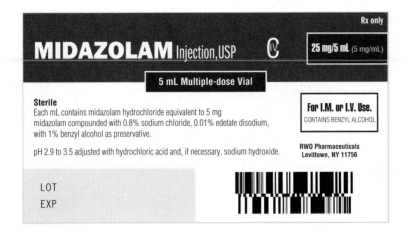

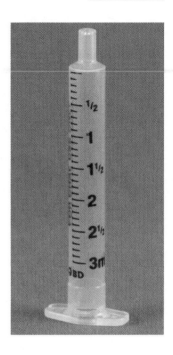

32. ondansetron 3 mg

_____

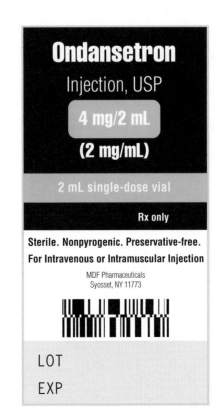

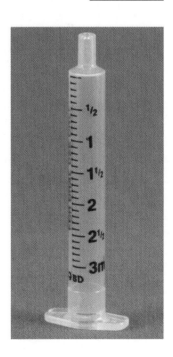

Dosage Ordered   **mL Needed**

33. dexamethasone 5 mg   _____

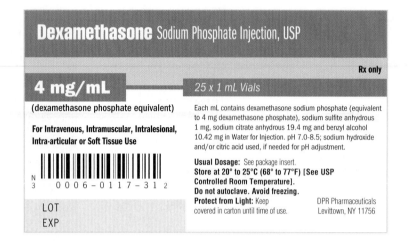

Each mL contains dexamethasone sodium phosphate (equivalent to 4 mg dexamethasone phosphate), sodium sulfite anhydrous 1 mg, sodium citrate anhydrous 19.4 mg and benzyl alcohol 10.42 mg in Water for Injection. pH 7.0-8.5; sodium hydroxide and/or citric acid used, if needed for pH adjustment.

Dexamethasone Sodium Phosphate Injection, USP

Rx only

4 mg/mL

(dexamethasone phosphate equivalent)

25 x 1 mL Vials

For Intravenous, Intramuscular, Intralesional, Intra-articular or Soft Tissue Use

N3 0006-0117-31 2

LOT
EXP

Usual Dosage: See package insert.
Store at 20° to 25°C (68° to 77°F) [See USP Controlled Room Temperature].
Do not autoclave. Avoid freezing.
Protect from Light: Keep covered in carton until time of use.

DPR Pharmaceuticals
Levittown, NY 11756

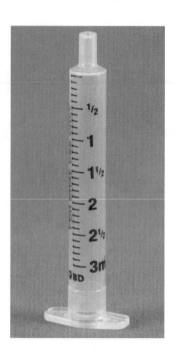

34. hydroxyzine HCl 40 mg   _____

Hydroxyzine hydrochloride

Rx only

Intramuscular Solution

25 mg/mL

ABC Pharmaceuticals
Levittown, NY 11756

(01)38723723478234

LOT
EXP

Each mL contains **25 mg** of hydroxyzine, hydrochloride 0.9% benzyl alcohol and sodium hydroxide to adjust to optimum pH. To avoid discoloration, protect from prolonged exposure to light

FOR INTRAMUSCULAR USE ONLY

USUAL ADULT DOSE: Intramuscularly: 25-100 mg stat repeat every 4 to 6 hours, as needed. See accompanying prescribing information.

CAUTION: Federal law prohibits dispensing without prescription

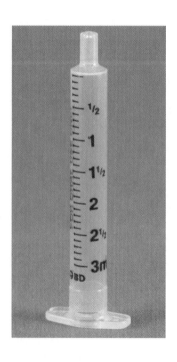

Dosage Ordered

mL Needed

35. ketorolac tromethamine 20 mg

_____

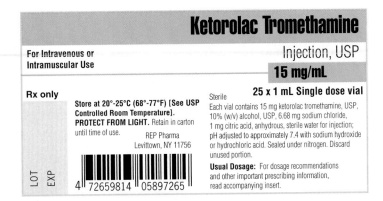

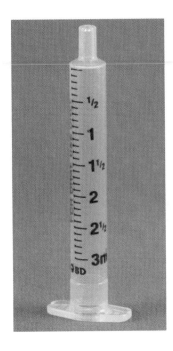

36. nalbuphine HCl 30 mg

_____

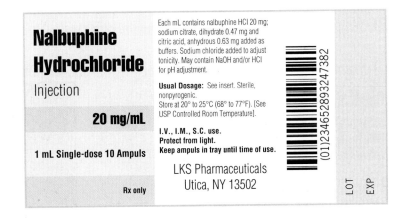

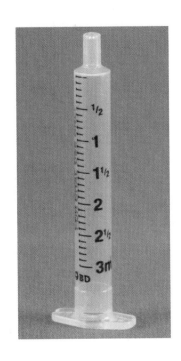

Dosage Ordered

mL Needed

37. morphine 15 mg

_____

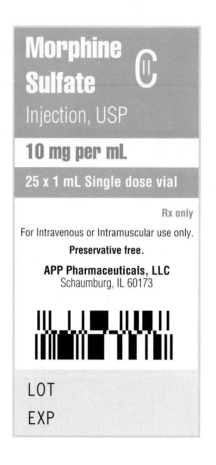

Morphine Sulfate Injection, USP
C II
10 mg per mL
25 x 1 mL Single dose vial

Rx only

For Intravenous or Intramuscular use only.

Preservative free.

APP Pharmaceuticals, LLC
Schaumburg, IL 60173

LOT

EXP

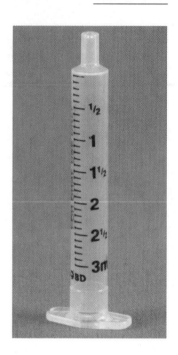

38. cyanocobalamin 750 mcg

_____

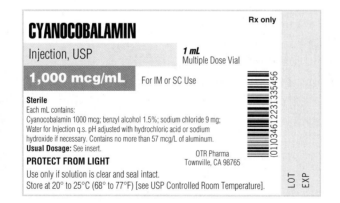

CYANOCOBALAMIN

Rx only

Injection, USP

1 mL
Multiple Dose Vial

1,000 mcg/mL   For IM or SC Use

Sterile
Each mL contains:
Cyanocobalamin 1000 mcg; benzyl alcohol 1.5%; sodium chloride 9 mg;
Water for Injection q.s. pH adjusted with hydrochloric acid or sodium
hydroxide if necessary. Contains no more than 57 mcg/L of aluminum.
Usual Dosage: See insert.

OTR Pharma
Townville, CA 98765

PROTECT FROM LIGHT

Use only if solution is clear and seal intact.
Store at 20° to 25°C (68° to 77°F) [see USP Controlled Room Temperature].

(01)03461223133 5456

LOT
EXP

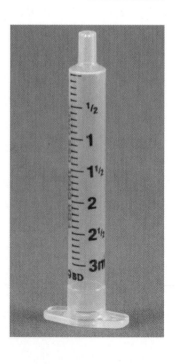

Dosage Ordered

mL Needed

39. aminophylline 0.4 g for an IV additive

_____

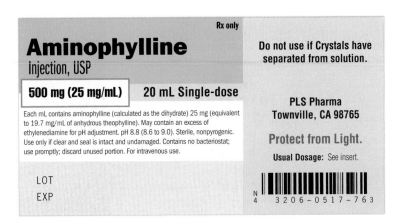

Rx only

Aminophylline
Injection, USP

500 mg (25 mg/mL) | **20 mL Single-dose**

Each mL contains aminophylline (calculated as the dihydrate) 25 mg (equivalent to 19.7 mg/mL of anhydrous theophylline). May contain an excess of ethylenediamine for pH adjustment. pH 8.8 (8.6 to 9.0). Sterile, nonpyrogenic. Use only if clear and seal is intact and undamaged. Contains no bacteriostat; use promptly; discard unused portion. For intravenous use.

LOT
EXP

Do not use if Crystals have separated from solution.

PLS Pharma
Townville, CA 98765

Protect from Light.

Usual Dosage: See insert.

N
4   3 2 0 6 – 0 5 1 7 – 7 6 3

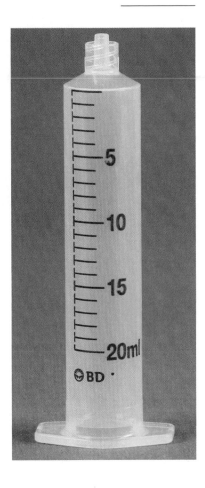

40. phenytoin 125 mg

_____

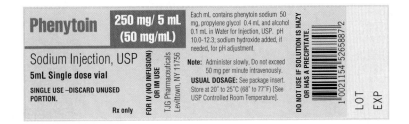

Phenytoin | **250 mg/ 5 mL** **(50 mg/mL)**

Sodium Injection, USP

5mL Single dose vial

SINGLE USE –DISCARD UNUSED PORTION.

Rx only

FOR IV (NO INFUSION) OR IM USE
TJG Pharmaceuticals
Levittown, NY 11756

Each mL contains phenytoin sodium 50 mg, propylene glycol 0.4 mL and alcohol 0.1 mL in Water for Injection, USP. pH 10.0-12.3; sodium hydroxide added, if needed, for pH adjustment.

Note: Administer slowly, Do not exceed 50 mg per minute intravenously.

USUAL DOSAGE: See package insert. Store at 20° to 25°C (68° to 77°F) [See USP Controlled Room Temperature].

DO NOT USE IF SOLUTION IS HAZY OR HAS A PRECIPITATE.

0021154 5265887 2

LOT
EXP

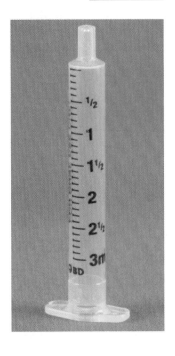

Dosage Ordered

mL Needed

41. ketorolac 25 mg

_____

Ketorolac Tromethamine

For Intravenous or Intramuscular Use	Injection, USP
	15 mg/mL
Rx only	**25 x 1 mL Single dose vial**

Store at 20°-25°C (68°-77°F) [See USP Controlled Room Temperature]. **PROTECT FROM LIGHT.** Retain in carton until time of use.
REP Pharma
Levittown, NY 11756

LOT
EXP

4 72659814 05897265

Sterile
Each vial contains 15 mg ketorolac tromethamine, USP, 10% (w/v) alcohol, USP, 6.68 mg sodium chloride, 1 mg citric acid, anhydrous, sterile water for injection; pH adjusted to approximately 7.4 with sodium hydroxide or hydrochloric acid. Sealed under nitrogen. Discard unused portion.

Usual Dosage: For dosage recommendations and other important prescribing information, read accompanying insert.

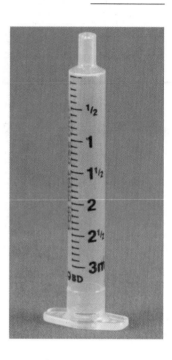

42. hydroxyzine hydrochloride 50 mg

_____

Hydroxyzine hydrochloride   Rx only

Intramuscular Solution	**25 mg/mL**

ABC Pharmaceuticals
Levittown, NY 11756

(01)38723723478234

LOT

EXP

Each mL contains **25 mg** of hydroxyzine, hydrochloride 0.9% benzyl alcohol and sodium hydroxide to adjust to optimum pH. To avoid discoloration, protect from prolonged exposure to light

FOR INTRAMUSCULAR USE ONLY
USUAL ADULT DOSE: Intramuscularly: 25-100 mg stat repeat every 4 to 6 hours, as needed. See accompanying prescribing information.

CAUTION: Federal law prohibits dispensing without prescription

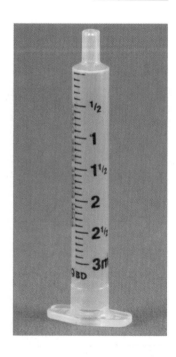

Dosage Ordered | **mL Needed**

43. gentamicin 0.1 g _____

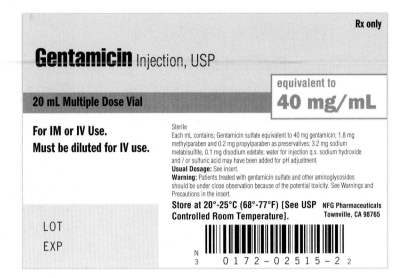

Rx only

Gentamicin Injection, USP

equivalent to
40 mg/mL

20 mL Multiple Dose Vial

For IM or IV Use.
Must be diluted for IV use.

Sterile
Each mL contains; Gentamicin sulfate equivalent to 40 mg gentamicin; 1.8 mg
methylparaben and 0.2 mg propylparaben as preservatives; 3.2 mg sodium
metabisulfite, 0.1 mg disodium edetate; water for injection q.s. sodium hydroxide
and / or sulfuric acid may have been added for pH adjustment.
Usual Dosage: See insert.
Warning: Patients treated with gentamicin sulfate and other aminoglycosides
should be under close observation because of the potential toxicity. See Warnings and
Precautions in the insert.
Store at 20°-25°C (68°-77°F) [See USP NFG Pharmaceuticals
Controlled Room Temperature]. Townville, CA 98765

LOT
EXP

N
3   0172-02515-2 2

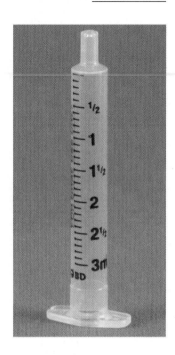

44. glycopyrrolate 180 mcg _____

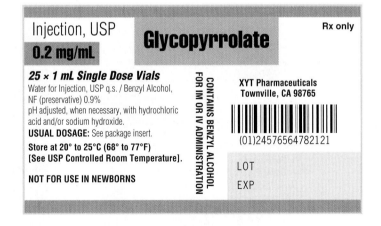

Injection, USP

Glycopyrrolate

Rx only

0.2 mg/mL

25 × 1 mL Single Dose Vials
Water for Injection, USP q.s. / Benzyl Alcohol,
NF (preservative) 0.9%
pH adjusted, when necessary, with hydrochloric
acid and/or sodium hydroxide.
USUAL DOSAGE: See package insert.
Store at 20° to 25°C (68° to 77°F)
[See USP Controlled Room Temperature].

NOT FOR USE IN NEWBORNS

CONTAINS BENZYL ALCOHOL
FOR IM OR IV ADMINISTRATION

XYT Pharmaceuticals
Townville, CA 98765

(01)24576564782121

LOT
EXP

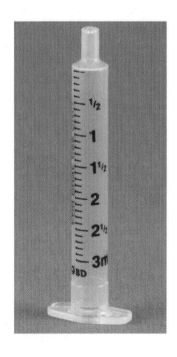

Dosage Ordered   **mL Needed**

45. penicillin G benzathine and procaine 600,000 units   _____

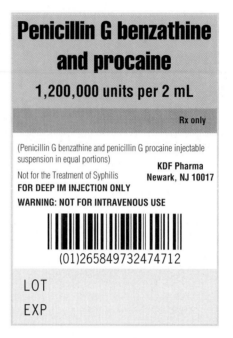

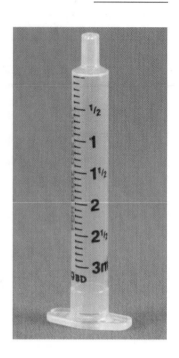

46. heparin sodium 1500 units   _____

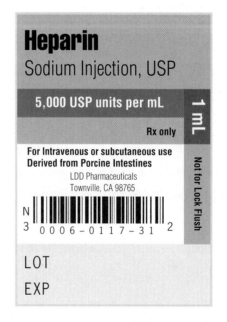

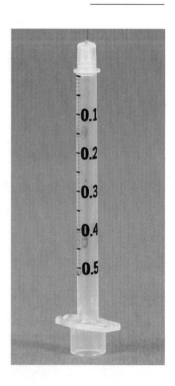

Dosage Ordered

mL Needed

47. potassium chloride 2 mEq for an IV additive

_____

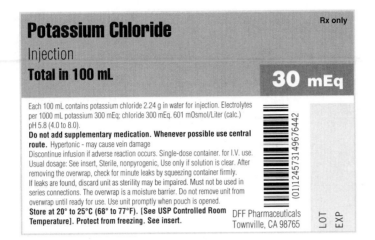

Potassium Chloride
Injection
Total in 100 mL

Rx only

30 mEq

Each 100 mL contains potassium chloride 2.24 g in water for injection. Electrolytes per 1000 mL potassium 300 mEq; chloride 300 mEq. 601 mOsmol/Liter (calc.) pH 5.8 (4.0 to 8.0).
Do not add supplementary medication. Whenever possible use central route. Hypertonic - may cause vein damage
Discontinue infusion if adverse reaction occurs. Single-dose container. for I.V. use. Usual dosage: See insert, Sterile, nonpyrogenic, Use only if solution is clear. After removing the overwrap, check for minute leaks by squeezing container firmly. If leaks are found, discard unit as sterility may be impaired. Must not be used in series connections. The overwrap is a moisture barrier. Do not remove unit from overwrap until ready for use. Use unit promptly when pouch is opened.
Store at 20° to 25°C (68° to 77°F). [See USP Controlled Room Temperature]. Protect from freezing. See insert.

DFF Pharmaceuticals
Townville, CA 98765

LOT
EXP

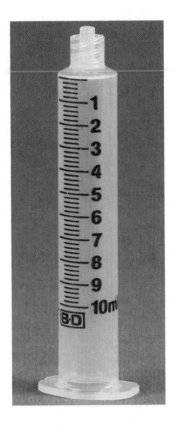

48. ketorolac 10 mg

_____

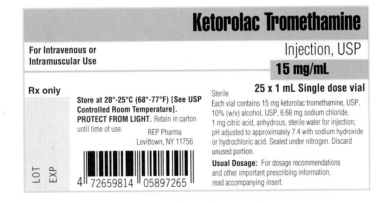

Ketorolac Tromethamine

For Intravenous or
Intramuscular Use

Injection, USP
15 mg/mL

25 x 1 mL Single dose vial

Rx only

Store at 20°-25°C (68°-77°F) [See USP Controlled Room Temperature].
PROTECT FROM LIGHT. Retain in carton until time of use.

REP Pharma
Levittown, NY 11756

LOT
EXP

4 72659814 05897265

Sterile
Each vial contains 15 mg ketorolac tromethamine, USP, 10% (w/v) alcohol, USP, 6.68 mg sodium chloride, 1 mg citric acid, anhydrous, sterile water for injection; pH adjusted to approximately 7.4 with sodium hydroxide or hydrochloric acid. Sealed under nitrogen. Discard unused portion.

Usual Dosage: For dosage recommendations and other important prescribing information, read accompanying insert.

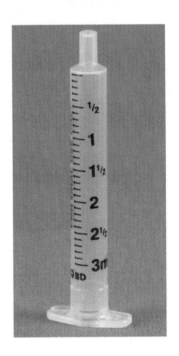

Dosage Ordered

mL Needed

49. hydroxyzine hydrochloride 14 mg

_____

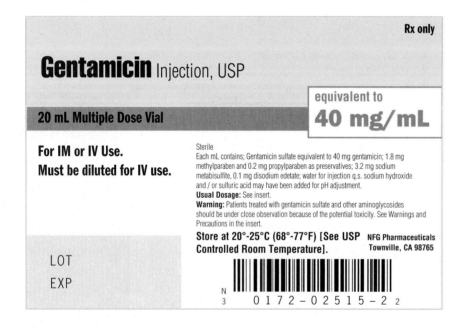

Hydroxyzine hydrochloride	Rx only
Intramuscular Solution	**25 mg/mL**

ABC Pharmaceuticals
Levittown, NY 11756

(01)38723723478234

LOT

EXP

Each mL contains **25 mg** of hydroxyzine hydrochloride 0.9% benzyl alcohol and sodium hydroxide to adjust to optimum pH. To avoid discoloration, protect from prolonged exposure to light

FOR INTRAMUSCULAR USE ONLY

USUAL ADULT DOSE: Intramuscularly: 25-100 mg stat repeat every 4 to 6 hours, as needed. See accompanying prescribing information.

CAUTION: Federal law prohibits dispensing without prescription

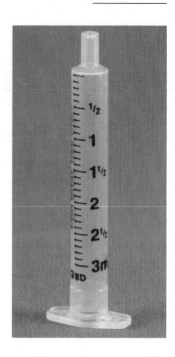

50. gentamicin 70 mg

_____

Gentamicin Injection, USP

Rx only

20 mL Multiple Dose Vial

equivalent to
40 mg/mL

For IM or IV Use.
Must be diluted for IV use.

Sterile
Each mL contains; Gentamicin sulfate equivalent to 40 mg gentamicin; 1.8 mg methylparaben and 0.2 mg propylparaben as preservatives; 3.2 mg sodium metabisulfite, 0.1 mg disodium edetate; water for injection q.s. sodium hydroxide and / or sulfuric acid may have been added for pH adjustment.
Usual Dosage: See insert.
Warning: Patients treated with gentamicin sulfate and other aminoglycosides should be under close observation because of the potential toxicity. See Warnings and Precautions in the insert.

Store at 20°-25°C (68°-77°F) [See USP Controlled Room Temperature]. **NFG Pharmaceuticals**
Townville, CA 98765

LOT

EXP

N
3   0172-02515-2 2

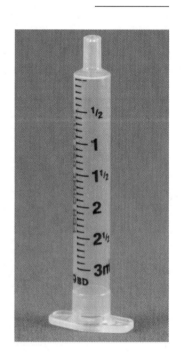

Dosage Ordered   **mL Needed**

51. glycopyrrolate 450 mcg   _____

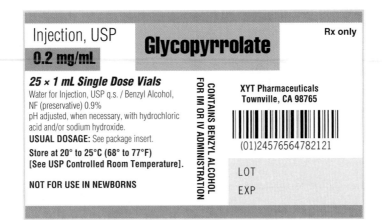

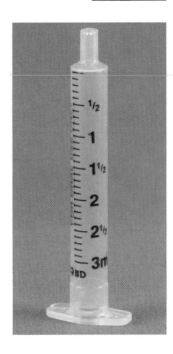

52. heparin 3500 units   _____

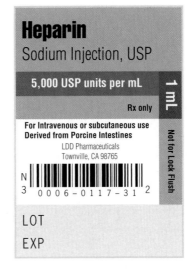

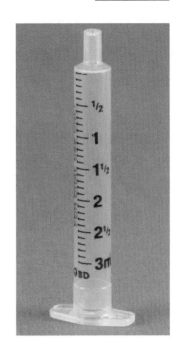

Answers

1. 0.8 mL	**14.** 0.45 mL	**27.** 3 mL	**40.** 2.5 mL
2. 1.5 mL	**15.** 1.6 mL	**28.** 8 mL	**41.** 1.7 mL
3. 1.4 mL	**16.** 2 mL	**29.** 1.2 mL	**42.** 2 mL
4. 3 mL	**17.** 2.3 mL	**30.** 1.6 mL	**43.** 2.5 mL
5. 0.9 mL	**18.** 1.8 mL	**31.** 0.6 mL	**44.** 0.9 mL
6. 1.5 mL	**19.** 2.4 mL	**32.** 1.5 mL	**45.** 1 mL
7. 0.38 mL	**20.** 15 mL	**33.** 1.3 mL	**46.** 0.3 mL
8. 0.8 mL	**21.** 1.5 mL	**34.** 1.6 mL	**47.** 6.7 mL
9. 1.2 mL	**22.** 0.8 mL	**35.** 1.3 mL	**48.** 0.7 mL
10. 0.8 mL	**23.** 1.6 mL	**36.** 1.5 mL	**49.** 0.6 mL
11. 15 mL	**24.** 1.7 mL	**37.** 1.5 mL	**50.** 1.8 mL
12. 2 mL	**25.** 1.3 mL	**38.** 0.8 mL	**51.** 2.3 mL
13. 1.5 mL	**26.** 2.5 mL	**39.** 16 mL	**52.** 0.7 mL

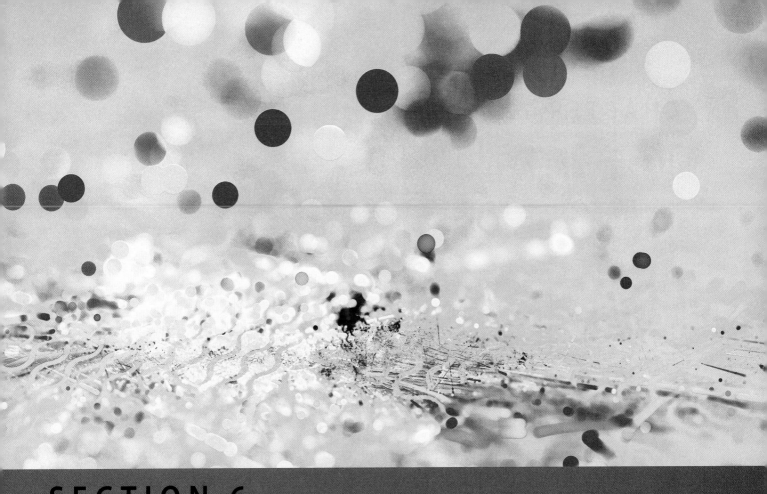

SECTION 6
Intravenous Calculations

CHAPTER 12

IV Flow Rate Calculations

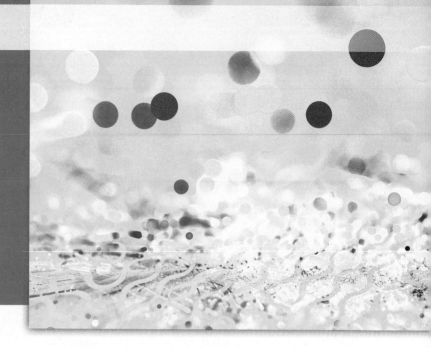

The learner will:

1. Identify the calibrations in gtt/mL on IV administration sets.

2. Calculate flow rates using dimensional analysis.

3. Recalculate flow rates to correct off-schedule infusions.

INTRODUCTION

This chapter presents two ways to calculate IV flow rates: (1) using dimensional analysis and (2) using a specific IV formula/division factor calculation.

Intravenous fluids are ordered on the basis of **mL/hr** to be administered—for example, 125 mL/hr. With the widespread use of electronic infusion devices that can be **set to deliver a mL/hr rate**, simply setting the rate ordered on the device and making sure it is working properly is all that is required for many infusions.

The most common flow rate calculation is necessary **when an infusion device is not being used**. It involves **converting a mL/hr order to the gtt/min rate necessary to infuse it**—for example, **1000 mL to infuse at 125 mL/hr or 3000 mL/24 hr**.

Monitoring IV therapy in the clinical setting is the primary responsibility of staff nurses. Your responsibility, as you care for your patients, is to be careful not to dislodge the IV setup and to check that the IV is running, because a patient's positional changes can occasionally kink the line and stop the flow.

You will need to use DA when you assume calculation and monitoring responsibilities, and this chapter includes the necessary instruction in all IV-related calculations.

IV TUBING CALIBRATION

The size of IV drops is regulated by the type of IV set being used, which is **calibrated in number of gtt/mL**. Unfortunately, not all sets, nor their drop size, are the same. Each clinical facility uses at least two sizes of infusion sets: a standard **macrodrip set calibrated at 10, 15, or 20 gtt/mL**, which is used for routine adult IV administrations, and a **microdrip set calibrated at 60 gtt/mL**, which is used when more exact measurements are needed. For example, a microdrip set may be used to infuse medications or in critical care and pediatric infusions. **Figure 12-1** depicts the various drop/gtt sizes.

🔑 IV administration sets are calibrated in gtt/mL.

The **gtt/mL calibration of each IV infusion set is clearly printed on each package**. The first step in calculating flow rates, then, is to identify the gtt/mL calibration of the set to be used for an infusion.

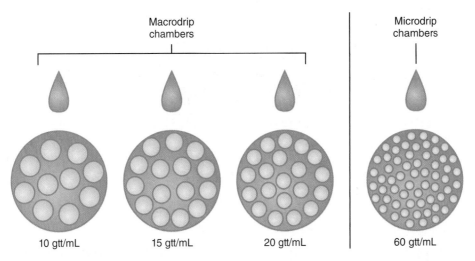

Figure 12-1 Comparative IV drop sizes.

PROBLEMS 12-1

Identify the calibration in gtt/mL for each IV infusion set.

1. **Figure 12-2** _____

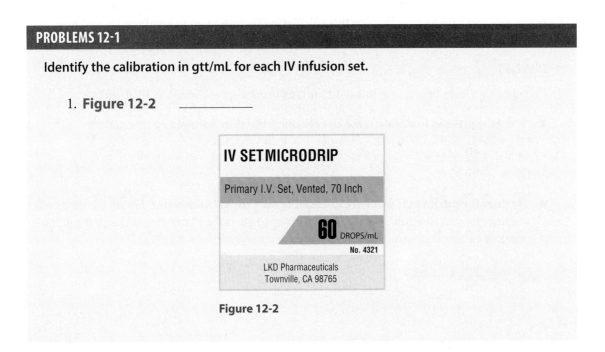

Figure 12-2

2. **Figure 12-3** _____

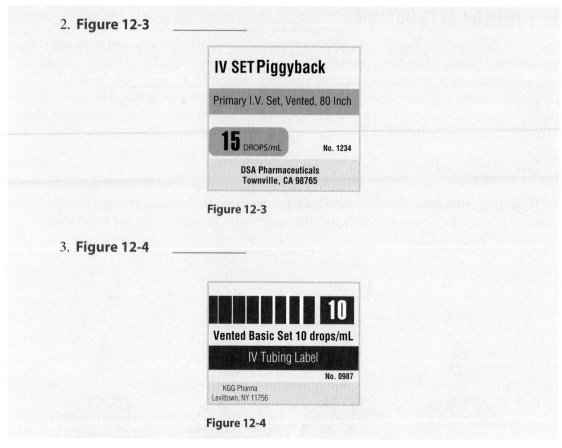

Figure 12-3

3. **Figure 12-4** _____

Figure 12-4

Answers 1. 60 gtt/mL   **2.** 15 gtt/mL   **3.** 10 gtt/mL

CALCULATING gtt/min FLOW RATES FOR MACRODRIP SETS

The flow rate in **gtt/min** is calculated from the **calibration of the IV set being used** (either 10, 15, or 20 gtt/mL) and the **mL/hr ordered**. You will immediately notice a difference from the previous DA calculations you have learned because **this calculation includes two new values: gtt and min**. However, the DA calculation steps are identical.

EXAMPLE 1

Calculate a **gtt/min** flow rate to infuse **125 mL/hr** using a set calibrated at **10 gtt/mL**.

■ Enter the **gtt/min** to be calculated as a **common fraction**, followed by an equal sign:

$$\frac{\text{gtt}}{\text{min}} =$$

■ **Begin ratio entries as if you were calculating only the gtt numerator**. Locate the ratio containing gtt—the 10 gtt/mL set calibration. Enter 10 gtt as the numerator to match the gtt numerator being calculated; 1 mL becomes the denominator:

$$\frac{\text{gtt}}{\text{min}} = \frac{10 \text{ gtt}}{1 \text{ mL}}$$

- Match the mL denominator with the 125 mL of the 125 mL/hr ordered; 1 hr becomes the denominator:

$$\frac{\text{gtt}}{\text{min}} = \frac{10\ \text{gtt}}{1\text{mL}} \times \frac{125\ \text{mL}}{1\ \text{hr}}$$

- **Enter a "1 hr equals 60 min" conversion ratio**, with 1 hr as the numerator and 60 min as the denominator. Notice that **the min being calculated falls automatically into place** as the final denominator to complete the equation:

$$\frac{\text{gtt}}{\text{min}} = \frac{10\ \text{gtt}}{1\ \text{mL}} \times \frac{125\ \text{mL}}{1\ \text{hr}} \times \frac{1\ \text{hr}}{60\ \text{min}}$$

- Cancel the mL, mL and hr, and hr denominator/numerators to check for correct ratio entry. Do the math using your preferred Calculator or Reduction Option choice:

$$\frac{\text{gtt}}{\text{min}} = \frac{10\ \text{gtt}}{1\ \cancel{\text{mL}}} \times \frac{125\ \cancel{\text{mL}}}{1\ \cancel{\text{hr}}} \times \frac{1\ \cancel{\text{hr}}}{60\ \text{min}} = 20.8 = \textbf{21 gtt/min}$$

To infuse 125 mL/hr using a 10 gtt/mL infusion set, the flow rate is 21 gtt/min.

🔑 Flow rates are rounded to the nearest whole gtt.

EXAMPLE 2

A **20 gtt/mL** set is used to infuse **90 mL/hr**. Calculate the **gtt/min** flow rate.

- Enter the gtt/min to be calculated, followed by an equal sign:

$$\frac{\text{gtt}}{\text{min}} =$$

- Enter the 20 gtt/mL infusion set ratio with 20 gtt to match the gtt numerator being calculated; 1 mL becomes the denominator:

$$\frac{\text{gtt}}{\text{min}} = \frac{20\ \text{gtt}}{1\ \text{mL}}$$

- Match the mL denominator with the 90 mL of the mL/hr ordered; 1 hr is the new denominator:

$$\frac{\text{gtt}}{\text{min}} = \frac{20\ \text{gtt}}{1\ \text{mL}} \times \frac{90\ \text{mL}}{1\ \text{hr}}$$

- Enter a "1 hr equals 60 min" conversion ratio, with 1 hr as the numerator and 60 min as the denominator, to complete the equation:

$$\frac{\text{gtt}}{\text{min}} = \frac{20\ \text{gtt}}{1\ \text{mL}} \times \frac{90\ \text{mL}}{1\ \text{hr}} \times \frac{1\ \text{hr}}{60\ \text{min}}$$

- Cancel the mL, mL and hr, and hr denominator/numerators to check for correct ratio entry. Do the math using your preferred Calculator or Reduction Option choice:

$$\frac{gtt}{min} = \frac{20\ gtt}{1\ \cancel{mL}} \times \frac{90\ \cancel{mL}}{1\ \cancel{hr}} \times \frac{1\ \cancel{hr}}{60\ min} = \textbf{30 gtt/min}$$

To infuse 90 mL/hr using a set calibrated at 20 gtt/mL, the rate is 30 gtt/min.

EXAMPLE 3

Calculate the **gtt/min** rate to infuse **2500 mL** in **24 hr** using a **15 gtt/mL** infusion set.

- Enter the gtt/min to be calculated, followed by an equal sign:

$$\frac{gtt}{min} =$$

- Enter the 15 gtt/mL infusion set ratio with 15 gtt to match the gtt numerator being calculated; 1 mL becomes the denominator:

$$\frac{gtt}{min} = \frac{15\ gtt}{1\ mL}$$

- Enter the 2500 mL/24 hr ordered with 2500 mL as the numerator to match the previous mL denominator. Enter 24 hr as the new denominator:

$$\frac{gtt}{min} = \frac{15\ gtt}{1\ mL} \times \frac{2500\ mL}{24\ hr}$$

- Enter a "1 hr equals 60 min" conversion ratio, with 1 hr as the numerator and 60 min as the denominator, to complete the equation:

$$\frac{gtt}{min} = \frac{15\ gtt}{1\ mL} \times \frac{2500\ mL}{24\ hr} \times \frac{1\ hr}{60\ min}$$

- Cancel the mL, mL and hr, and hr denominator/numerators to check for correct ratio entry. Do the math using your preferred Calculator or Reduction Option choice:

$$\frac{gtt}{min} = \frac{15\ gtt}{1\ \cancel{mL}} \times \frac{2500\ \cancel{mL}}{24\ \cancel{hr}} \times \frac{1\ \cancel{hr}}{60\ min} = 26.04 = \textbf{26 gtt/min}$$

To infuse 2500 mL in 24 hr using a 15 gtt/mL calibrated infusion set, the rate is 26 gtt/min.

EXAMPLE 4

Calculate the **gtt/min** rate to infuse **2000 mL** in **10 hr** using a **10 gtt/mL** IV infusion set.

- Enter the gtt/min to be calculated, followed by an equal sign:

$$\frac{gtt}{min} =$$

- Enter the 10 gtt/mL infusion set ratio with 10 gtt as the numerator to match the gtt numerator being calculated; 1 mL becomes the denominator:

$$\frac{gtt}{min} = \frac{10\ gtt}{1\ mL}$$

■ Enter the 2000 mL in 10 hr ordered with 2000 mL as the numerator to match the previous mL denominator; 10 hr is the next denominator to be matched:

$$\frac{gtt}{min} = \frac{10 \, gtt}{1 \, mL} \times \frac{2000 \, mL}{10 \, hr}$$

■ Enter a "1 hr equals 60 min" conversion ratio, with 1 hr as the numerator and 60 min as the denominator, to complete the equation:

$$\frac{gtt}{min} = \frac{10 \, gtt}{1 \, mL} \times \frac{2000 \, mL}{10 \, hr} \times \frac{1 \, hr}{60 \, min}$$

■ Cancel the mL, mL and hr, and hr denominator/numerators to check for correct ratio entry. Do the math using your preferred Calculator or Reduction Option choice:

$$\frac{gtt}{min} = \frac{10 \, gtt}{1 \, \cancel{mL}} \times \frac{2000 \, \cancel{mL}}{10 \, \cancel{hr}} \times \frac{1 \, \cancel{hr}}{60 \, min} = 33.3 = \mathbf{33 \, gtt/min}$$

To infuse 2000 mL in 10 hr using a 10 gtt/mL calibrated infusion set, the rate is 33 gtt/min.

PROBLEMS 12-2

Calculate gtt/min flow rates. Round to the nearest whole gtt.

1. An IV of 2000 mL is to infuse in 12 hr using a 10 gtt/mL set.   _____

2. The order is for 3500 mL to infuse in 24 hr using a set calibrated at 20 gtt/mL.   _____

3. Infuse 500 mL in 3 hr using a 15 gtt/mL set.   _____

4. A volume of 1500 mL is to infuse in 5 hr using a 15 gtt/mL set.   _____

5. The order is for 1750 mL to infuse in 9 hr using a 20 gtt/mL set.   _____

6. An IV of 2500 mL is to infuse in 18 hr on a set calibrated at 10 gtt/mL.   _____

7. A 3000 mL volume is to infuse in 24 hr on a set calibrated at 20 gtt/mL.   _____

8. A volume of 2750 mL is to infuse in 22 hr on a 15 gtt/mL set.   _____

9. An IV of 750 mL is ordered to infuse in 8 hr on a 10 gtt/mL set.   _____

10. A volume of 1250 mL is to infuse in 12 hr using a 15 gtt/mL set.   _____

Answers 1. 28 gtt/min   **2.** 49 gtt/min   **3.** 42 gtt/min   **4.** 75 gtt/min   **5.** 65 gtt/min   **6.** 23 gtt/min
7. 42 gtt/min   **8.** 31 gtt/min   **9.** 16 gtt/min   **10.** 26 gtt/min

FORMULA/DIVISION FACTOR METHODS OF FLOW RATE CALCULATION

The information on these two calculation methods is included primarily for your information. The truth is that as an undergraduate you will not be assuming responsibility for calculating flow rates. These are ordered by physicians, and your nursing responsibility will be to monitor the infusion rate ordered. As a graduate these are methods that, with clinical IV experience, you will use on a regular basis. It will be helpful for you to return to this content for an update as you move ahead in your clinical career.

The **formula** and **division factor** methods are intrinsically related because **the division factor is derived from the formula method**. Let's start by looking at the formula method.

The formula method has a limitation in that it can **only be used if the flow rate is expressed as mL per hr, or 60 min**. For example, 150 mL/hr or 110 mL/60 min. It is especially suitable for small-volume infusions to be completed in less than 60 min—for example, 30 mL in 20 min.

$$\text{Flow rate} = \frac{\text{mL/hr volume} \times \text{set calibration}}{\text{time (60 min or less)}}$$

EXAMPLE 1

An IV of 500 mL is ordered to infuse at **125 mL/hr**. Calculate the **gtt/min** rate for a set calibrated at **10 gtt/mL**.

■ **Convert the hr rate to 60 min:**

$$\frac{125 \, (\text{mL}) \times 10 \, (\text{gtt/mL})}{60 \, (\text{min})}$$

■ **Calculate the gtt/min rate:**

$$\frac{125 \times 10}{60} = 20.8 = \textbf{21 gtt/min}$$

EXAMPLE 2

Administer an IV medication of **100 mL** in **40 min** using a set calibrated at **15 gtt/mL**.

$$\frac{100 \, \text{mL} \times 15 \, \text{gtt/mL}}{40 \, \text{min}} = 37.5 = \textbf{38 gtt/min}$$

EXAMPLE 3

A **75 mL** volume of IV medication is ordered to infuse in **45 min**. The set is calibrated at **20 gtt/mL**.

$$\frac{75 \, \text{mL} \times 20 \, \text{gtt/mL}}{45 \, \text{min}} = 33.3 = \textbf{33 gtt/min}$$

PROBLEMS 12-3

Calculate the flow rate in gtt/min to the nearest whole drop using the formula method.

1. Administer an IV of 110 mL/hr using a set calibrated at 20 gtt/mL. _____

2. A 500 mL IV solution is ordered to infuse at 200 mL/hr using a set calibrated at 15 gtt/mL. _____

3. A volume of 80 mL is to be infused in 20 min using a 10 gtt/mL set. _____

4. An IV of 1000 mL is ordered to infuse at 150 mL/hr using a 10 gtt/mL calibrated set. _____

5. An IV rate of 90 mL/hr is ordered using a 15 gtt/mL calibrated set. _____

6. An IV of 500 mL is to infuse at 120 mL/hr using a 20 gtt/mL calibrated set. _____

7. A total of 90 mL is to infuse at 100 mL/hr using a 20 gtt/mL set. _____

8. A 15 gtt/mL set is used to infuse 120 mL at 80 mL/hr. _____

9. A rate of 60 mL/hr is ordered for a volume of 250 mL using a 10 gtt/mL set. _____

10. A medication volume of 50 mL is to infuse at 20 mL/hr using a 20 gtt/mL set. _____

Answers 1. 37 gtt/min **2.** 50 gtt/min **3.** 40 gtt/min **4.** 25 gtt/min **5.** 23 gtt/min **6.** 40 gtt/min
7. 33 gtt/min **8.** 20 gtt/min **9.** 10 gtt/min **10.** 7 gtt/min

When an IV is ordered to infuse in **more than 1 hour**, the formula method can still be used. However, it is necessary to add a preliminary step and determine the **mL/hr** that the ordered volume will represent.

EXAMPLE 1

Calculate the gtt/min flow rate for an IV of **1000 mL** to infuse in **8 hr** on a set calibrated at **20 gtt/mL**.

- **Convert 1000 mL/8 hr to mL/hr:**

  100 mL/8 hr = 1000 ÷ 8 = **125 mL/hr (60 min)**

- **Calculate the gtt/min flow rate:**

$$\frac{125 \ (mL) \times 20 \ (gtt/mL)}{60 \ (min)} = 41.6 = \textbf{42 gtt/min}$$

EXAMPLE 2

Calculate the gtt/min flow rate for a volume of **2500 mL** to infuse in **24 hr** on a set calibrated at **10 gtt/mL.**

- ■ **Convert 2500 mL/24 hr to mL/hr:**

$$2500 \text{ mL/24 hr} = 2500 \div 24 = \textbf{104 mL/hr (60 min)}$$

- ■ **Calculate the gtt/min flow rate:**

$$\frac{104 \text{ mL} \times 10 \text{ gtt/mL}}{60 \text{ min}} = 17.3 = \textbf{17 gtt/min}$$

EXAMPLE 3

An IV of **1200 mL** is to infuse in **16 hr** on a set calibrated at **15 gtt/mL.**

$$1200 \text{ mL/16hr} = 1200 \div 16 = \textbf{75mL/hr (60 min)}$$

$$\frac{75 \text{ mL} \times 15 \text{ gtt/mL}}{60 \text{ min}} = 18.7 = \textbf{19 gtt/min}$$

PROBLEMS 12-4

Calculate the gtt/min flow rate using the formula method.

1. A volume of 2000 mL to infuse in 24 hr on a set calibrated at 15 gtt/mL   _____

2. A volume of 300 mL to infuse in 6 hr on a 60 gtt/mL microdrip set   _____

3. A volume of 500 mL to infuse in 4 hr on a 15 gtt/mL calibrated set   _____

4. A 10 hr infusion of 1200 mL using a 20 gtt/mL set   _____

5. An infusion of 500 mL in 5 hr on a set calibrated at 10 gtt/mL   _____

6. A 2000 mL volume to infuse in 18 hr using a 20 gtt/mL set   _____

7. A 10 gtt/mL set to infuse 400 mL in 4 hr   _____

8. An 8 hr infusion of 1500 mL to use a set calibrated at 15 gtt/mL   _____

9. A volume of 250 mL to infuse in 2 hr using a 20 gtt/mL set   _____

10. A 5 hr infusion of 750 mL using a 10 gtt/mL set.   _____

Answers **1.** 21 gtt/min   **2.** 50 gtt/min   **3.** 31 gtt/min   **4.** 40 gtt/min   **5.** 17 gtt/min   **6.** 37 gtt/min
7. 17 gtt/min   **8.** 47 gtt/min   **9.** 42 gtt/min   **10.** 25 gtt/min

DIVISION FACTOR METHOD FOR MACRODRIP SETS

The **division factor** is derived from the formula method, and it is invaluable for use in clinical facilities where **all the macrodrip infusion sets have the same calibration**—either 10, 15, or 20 gtt/mL. Once again, **this method can only be used if the rate is expressed in mL/hr (60 min)**. Let's start by looking at how the division factor is obtained.

EXAMPLE

Administer an IV at **125 mL/hr**. The set calibration is **10 gtt/mL**. Calculate the gtt/min rate. Enter 60 min instead of 1 hr.

$$\frac{125 \text{ (mL)} \times \overset{1}{\cancel{10}} \text{ (gtt/mL)}}{\underset{6}{\cancel{60}} \text{ (min)}} = 20.8 = \textbf{21 gtt/min}$$

Look at the completed equation, and notice that because the time is restricted to 60 min, **the set calibration (10) will be divided into 60 (min) to obtain a constant number (6). This constant (6) is the division factor for a 10 gtt/mL calibrated set.**

🔑 The division factor can be obtained for any macrodrip set by dividing 60 by the calibration of the set.

PROBLEMS 12-5

Determine the division factor for these IV sets.

1. 20 gtt/mL   _____

2. 15 gtt/mL   _____

3. 60 gtt/mL   _____

4. 10 gtt/mL   _____

Answers 1. 3   2. 4   3. 1   4. 6

Once you know the division factor, you can **calculate the gtt/min rate in one step by dividing the mL/hr rate by the division factor**. Look again at the example:

$$\frac{125 \text{ (mL)} \times \overset{1}{\cancel{10}} \text{ (gtt/mL)}}{\underset{6}{\cancel{60}} \text{ (min)}} = 20.8 = \textbf{21 gtt/min}$$

or 125 (mL/hr) ÷ 6 = 20.8 = **21 gtt/min**

The 125 mL/hr flow rate divided by the division factor 6 gives the same 21 gtt/min rate.

🔑 The gtt/min flow rate can be calculated for mL/hr IV orders in one step by dividing the mL/hr to be infused by the division factor of the administration set.

EXAMPLE 1

Infuse an IV at **100 mL/hr** using a set calibrated at **10 gtt/mL**.

> **Determine the division factor** : $60 \div 10 = 6$
> **Calculate the flow rate** : $100 \text{ mL} \div 6 = 16.6 = \mathbf{17 \text{ gtt/min}}$

EXAMPLE 2

Infuse an IV at **125 mL/hr** using a set calibrated at **15 gtt/mL**.

> $60 \div 15 = 4$ $125 \text{ mL} \div 4 = 31.2 = \mathbf{31 \text{ gtt/min}}$

EXAMPLE 3

A set calibrated at **20 gtt/mL** is used to infuse **90 mL per hr**.

> $60 \div 20 = 3$ $90 \text{ mL} \div 3 = \mathbf{30 \text{ gtt/min}}$

PROBLEMS 12-6

Calculate the flow rates in gtt/min using the division factor method.

1. A rate of 110 mL/hr via a set calibrated at 20 gtt/mL   _____

2. A set is calibrated at 15 gtt/mL; infuse at 130 mL/hr   _____

3. To infuse 150 mL/hr using a 10 gtt/mL set   _____

4. A set calibrated at 20 gtt/mL to infuse 45 mL/hr   _____

5. A 75 mL/hr volume with a set calibrated at 15 gtt/mL   _____

6. A rate of 130 mL/hr using a 10 gtt/mL set   _____

7. A 200 mL rate using a 15 gtt/mL set   _____

8. A rate of 120 mL/hr using a 10 gtt/mL set   _____

9. A 100 mL/hr rate using a 20 gtt/mL set   _____

10. A rate of 125 mL/hr using a 15 gtt/mL set   _____

Answers 1. 37 gtt/min   **2.** 33 gtt/min   **3.** 25 gtt/min   **4.** 15 gtt/min   **5.** 19 gtt/min   **6.** 22 gtt/min
7. 50 gtt/min   **8.** 20 gtt/min   **9.** 33 gtt/min   **10.** 31 gtt/min

All the preceding examples and problems using the division factor were for **macrodrip** sets. Let's now look at what happens when we use a **microdrip** set calibrated at **60 gtt/mL**.

EXAMPLE

Infuse at **50 mL/hr** using a **60 gtt/mL** microdrip.

> $60 \div 60 = 1$ $50 \text{ mL} \div 1 = \mathbf{50 \text{ gtt/min}}$

Because the set calibration is 60 and the division factor is based on 60 min (1 hr), the division factor is 1. So, **for microdrip sets, the gtt/min flow rate will be identical to the mL/hr ordered**.

🗝 When a 60 gtt/mL microdrip set is used, the flow rate in gtt/min is identical to the volume in mL/hr to be infused.

PROBLEMS 12-7

Calculate gtt/min rates for a microdrip.

1. 120 mL/hr _____

2. 90 mL/hr _____

3. 100 mL/hr _____

4. 75 mL/hr _____

5. 80 mL/hr _____

6. 110 mL/hr _____

7. 60 mL/hr _____

8. 45 mL/hr _____

9. 70 mL/hr _____

10. 130 mL/hr _____

Answers 1. 120 gtt/min   **2.** 90 gtt/min   **3.** 100 gtt/min   **4.** 75 gtt/min   **5.** 80 gtt/min   **6.** 110 gtt/min   **7.** 60 gtt/min   **8.** 45 gtt/min   **9.** 70 gtt/min   **10.** 130 gtt/min

The division factor can also be used to calculate the flow rate of **any volume that can be expressed in mL/hr**. Larger volumes can be divided, and smaller volumes can be multiplied and expressed in mL/hr. This requires the conversion step you learned earlier.

EXAMPLE 1

$$2400 \text{ mL}/24 \text{ hr} = 2400 \div 24 = \textbf{100 mL/hr}$$

EXAMPLE 2

$$1800 \text{ mL}/8 \text{ hr} = 1800 \div 8 = \textbf{225 mL/hr}$$

EXAMPLE 3

$$10 \text{ mL}/30 \text{ min} = 10 \times 2 \, (2 \times 30 \text{ min}) = \textbf{20 mL/hr}$$

EXAMPLE 4

$$15 \text{ mL}/20 \text{ min} = 15 \times 3 \, (3 \times 20 \text{ min}) = \textbf{45 mL/hr}$$

REGULATING FLOW RATE

To regulate a manual flow rate, **count the number of drops falling in the drip chamber**. The standard procedure for counting is to hold a watch next to the drip chamber and actually **count the number of drops falling**. You would adjust the roller clamp during the count until the required rate has been set. A 15 sec count is most commonly used because there is less chance of attention wandering during the count. To do this, divide the ordered gtt/min (60 sec) rate by 4 to obtain the 15 sec drip count (60 sec ÷ 4 = 15 sec).

EXAMPLE 1

An IV is to run at a rate of **60 gtt/min**. What will the 15 sec count be?

$$60 \text{ gtt/min} \div 4 = \textbf{15 gtt}$$

Adjust the rate to 15 gtt/15 sec.

EXAMPLE 2

A 70 **gtt/min** IV rate is ordered. What will the 15 sec count be?

$$70 \text{ gtt/min} \div 4 = 17.5 = \textbf{18 gtt}$$

Adjust the rate to 18 gtt/15 sec.

EXAMPLE 3

Adjust an IV to a rate of **50 gtt/min** using a 15 sec count.

$$50 \text{ gtt/min} \div 4 = \textbf{13 gtt}$$

Adjust the rate to 13 gtt/15 sec.

PROBLEMS 12-8

Answer the questions about 15 sec drip rates.

1. The 15 sec count of an IV flow rate is 7 gtt. A 29 gtt/min rate is required. Is this rate correct? _____

2. You are to regulate a newly started IV to deliver 67 gtt/min. Using a 15 sec count, how would you set the flow rate? _____

3. An IV is to run at 48 gtt/min. What must the 15 sec drip rate be? _____

4. How many gtt will you count in 15 sec if the rate is 55 gtt/min? _____

5. An IV is to run at 84 gtt/min. What will the 15 sec rate be? _____

6. What must the 15 sec count be to infuse 80 gtt/min? _____

7. A 110 gtt/min rate is ordered. What must the 15 sec count be? _____

8. A 100 gtt/min rate is ordered. What must the 15 sec count be? _____

9. A rate of 90 gtt/min is ordered. Is a count of 15 gtt in 15 sec correct? _____

10. An IV is infusing at a rate of 30 gtt in 15 sec. A rate of 120 gtt/min was ordered. Is this rate correct? _____

Answers **1.** Yes **2.** 17 gtt/15 sec **3.** 12 gtt/15 sec **4.** 14 gtt/15 sec **5.** 21 gtt/15 sec **6.** 20 gtt/15 sec **7.** 28 gtt/15 sec **8.** 25 gtt/15 sec **9.** No, too slow **10.** Yes

Individual clinical facilities and states/provinces may require a 30 or 60 sec (1 min) count. When a 60 sec count is required, take particular care not to let your attention wander during the count, which can easily happen in this longer time frame. A 60 sec count will require a 1 min count, whereas a 30 sec count will require the gtt/min rate to be divided by 2 (60 sec ÷ 2 = 30 sec).

EXAMPLE 1

An IV is to be infused at 56 gtt/min. What is the 30 sec rate?

$$56 \text{ gtt/min} \div 2 = 28 \text{ gtt}$$

Adjust the rate to 28 gtt/30 sec.

EXAMPLE 2

A rate of 72 gtt/min has been ordered. What will the 30 sec count be?

$$72 \text{ gtt/min} \div 2 = 36 \text{ gtt}$$

Adjust the rate to 36 gtt/30 sec.

PROBLEMS 12-9

Calculate the 30 sec flow rate count.

1. An IV to be run at a rate of 48 gtt/min   _____

2. An IV ordered to infuse at 52 gtt/min   _____

3. An IV to infuse at 120 gtt/min   _____

4. An infusion rate of 90 gtt/min   _____

5. An IV to infuse at 100 gtt/min   _____

Answers 1. 24 gtt/30 sec   2. 26 gtt/30 sec   3. 60 gtt/30 sec   4. 45 gtt/30 sec   5. 50 gtt/30 sec

CORRECTING OFF-SCHEDULE RATES

Because a patient's positional changes can alter the infusion rate slightly, IVs occasionally infuse ahead of or behind schedule. When this occurs, the usual procedure is to **recalculate the flow rate using the volume and time remaining** and to **adjust the flow rate accordingly**. Once again, this is a staff nurse responsibility. Each situation must be individually evaluated, especially if the discrepancy is large. **If too much fluid has infused, immediately assess the patient's response** to the increased intake and take appropriate action. **If too little fluid has infused, assess his or her ability to tolerate an increased rate** because many medications and fluids have restrictions on the rate of administration. Both of these factors must be considered before rates can be increased to "catch up." In addition, **most clinical facilities will have specific policies to cover over- or under-infusion due to altered flow rates, and you will be responsible for knowing these policies**.

The following are some examples of how the rate can be recalculated. Because IVs are usually checked hourly, the focus will first be on recalculation using exact hours. Some recalculations have also been included using fractions of hours rounded to the nearest quarter hour: 15 min = 0.25 hr, 30 min = 0.5 hr, and 45 min = 0.75 hr. These equivalents are close enough for uncomplicated infusions because the exact time of completion is not totally predictable. IVs needing exact infusion would be monitored by electronic infusion devices.

EXAMPLE 1

An IV of **1000 mL** was ordered to infuse over **10 hr** at a rate of **25 gtt/min**. The set calibration is **15 gtt/mL**. After **5 hr**, a total of 650 mL has infused instead of the **500 mL** ordered. Recalculate the new gtt/min flow rate to complete the infusion on schedule.

> **Time remaining:** 10 hr − 5 hr = **5 hr**
> **Volume remaining:** 1000 mL − 650 mL = **350 mL**
> 350 mL ÷ 5 hr = **70 mL/hr**
>
> Set calibration is **15 gtt/mL**.
> 70 ÷ 4 (division factor) = 17.5 = **18 gtt/min**
> **Slow the rate from 25 gtt/min to 18 gtt/min.**

EXAMPLE 2

An IV of **800 mL** was to infuse over **8 hr** at **20 gtt/min**. After **4 hr 15 min**, only **300 mL** has infused. Recalculate the **gtt/min** rate to complete on schedule. The set calibration is **15 gtt/mL**.

> **Time remaining:** 8 hr − 4.25 hr = **3.75 hr**
> **Volume remaining:** 800 mL − 300 mL = **500 mL**
> 500 mL ÷ 3.75 hr = 133.3 = **133 mL/hr**
>
> Set calibration is **15 gtt/mL**.
> 133 ÷ 4 (division factor) = 33.2 = **33 gtt/min**
> **Increase the rate to 33 gtt/min.**

EXAMPLE 3

An IV of **500 mL** is infusing at **28 gtt/min**. It was to complete in **3 hr**, but after **1½ hr**, only **175 mL** has infused. Recalculate the **gtt/min** rate to complete the infusion on schedule. Set calibration is **10 gtt/mL**.

> **Time remaining:** 3 hr − 1.5 hr = **1.5 hr**
> **Volume remaining:** 500 mL − 175 mL = **325 mL**
> 325 mL ÷ 1.5 hr = 216.6 = **217 mL/hr**
>
> Set calibration is **10 gtt/mL**.
> 217 ÷ 6 (division factor) = 36.1 = **36 gtt/min**
> **Increase the rate to 36 gtt/min.**

EXAMPLE 4

A volume of **250 mL** was to infuse **56 gtt/min** in **1½ hr** using a set calibrated at **20 gtt/mL**. After **30 min**, **175 mL** has infused. Recalculate the flow rate.

> **Time remaining:** 1.5 hr − 30 min = **1 hr**
> **Volume remaining:** 250 mL − 175 mL = **75 mL**
>
> Set calibration is **20 gtt/mL**.
> 75 ÷ 3 (division factor) = **25 gtt/min**
> **Decrease the rate to 25 gtt/min.**

PROBLEMS 12-10

Recalculate flow rates for infusions to complete on schedule.

1. An IV of 500 mL was ordered to infuse in 3 hr using a 15 gtt/mL set. With 1½ hr remaining, you discover that only 150 mL is left in the bag. At what rate will you need to reset the flow?   _____

2. An IV of 1000 mL was scheduled to run in 12 hr. After 4 hr, only 220 mL has infused. The set calibration is 20 gtt/mL. Recalculate the rate for the remaining solution.   _____

3. An IV of 1000 mL was ordered to infuse in 8 hr. With 3 hr of infusion time left, you discover that 600 mL has infused. The set delivers 20 gtt/mL. Recalculate the drip rate, and indicate how many drops you will count in 15 sec to set the new rate.   _____

4. An IV of 750 mL was ordered to run in 6 hr with a set calibrated at 10 gtt/mL. After 2 hr, you notice that 300 mL has infused. Recalculate the flow rate, and indicate how many drops you will count in 15 sec to reset the rate.   _____

5. An IV of 800 mL was started at 9 am to infuse in 4 hr. At 10 am, 150 mL has infused. The set is calibrated at 15 gtt/mL. Recalculate the flow rate in gtt/min.   _____

6. An IV of 600 mL was to infuse in 5 hr. After 2 hr, 400 mL has infused. Recalculate the gtt/min rate to complete on time. A 20 gtt/mL set is being used.   _____

7. A volume of 250 mL was to infuse in 2 hr. With 1 hr left, 70 mL has infused. Calculate a new gtt/min rate to complete on time using a 15 gtt/mL set.   _____

8. An infiltrated IV is restarted with a volume of 420 mL to complete in 3 hr. Calculate the gtt/min rate for a 20 gtt/mL set. What will the new 30 sec count be?   _____

9. After 1 hr 30 min, 350 mL of a 1000 mL IV has infused. It was ordered to complete in 4 hr using a set calibrated at 15 gtt/mL. Calculate the gtt/min rate to complete on time.   _____

10. A total of 300 mL of an ordered 1000 mL in 10 hr infusion has completed in 4.5 hr. The set calibration is 15 gtt/mL. What gtt/min rate is necessary to complete on time? Calculate the 15 sec count to deliver this rate.   _____

Answers 1. 25 gtt/min   **2.** 33 gtt/min   **3.** 44 gtt/min; 11 gtt/15 sec   **4.** 19 gtt/min; 4–5 gtt/15 sec
5. 54 gtt/min   **6.** 22 gtt/min   **7.** 45 gtt/min   **8.** 47 gtt/min; 23–24 gtt/30 sec   **9.** 65 gtt/min
10. 32 gtt/min; 8 gtt/15 sec

SUMMARY

This concludes the chapter on IV flow rate calculation and monitoring. The important points to remember from this chapter are:

- IVs are ordered as mL/hr to be administered.

- Manual flow rates are counted in gtt/min.

- IV tubing is calibrated in gtt/mL.

- Macrodrip IV sets have a calibration of 10, 15, or 20 gtt/mL.

- Microdrip sets have a calibration of 60 gtt/mL.

- The formula for calculating flow rates is

$$\frac{\text{mL/hr volume} \times \text{set calibration}}{\text{time (60 min or less)}}$$

- The division factor method can be used to calculate flow rates only if the volume to be administered is specified in mL/hr (60 min).

- The division factor is obtained by dividing 60 by the set calibration.

- To determine flow rate by the division factor method, divide the mL/hr to be administered by the division factor.

- Because microdrip sets have a calibration of 60 gtt/mL, their division factor is 1, and the flow rate in gtt/min is the same as the mL/hr ordered.

- If an IV runs ahead of or behind schedule, a possible procedure is to use the time and mL remaining to calculate a new flow rate.

- If an IV is determined to have infused ahead of schedule, immediately assess the patient's tolerance to the excess fluid and take appropriate action.

- If a rate must be increased to compensate for the infusion running behind schedule, the type of fluid being infused and his or her ability to tolerate an increased rate must be assessed.

SUMMARY SELF-TEST

Answer as briefly as possible.

1. Determine the division factor for the following IV sets.
   a) 60 gtt/mL   _____
   b) 15 gtt/mL   _____
   c) 20 gtt/mL   _____
   d) 10 gtt/mL   _____

2. How is the flow rate determined in the division factor method?   _____

3. The division factor method can only be used if the volume to be administered is expressed in . . .   _____

4. An IV is to infuse at 50 gtt/min. How will you set it using a 15 sec count?   _____

5. You are to adjust an IV at a rate of 60 gtt/min. What will the 15 sec count be?   _____

Calculate the flow rate in gtt/min.

6. An infusion of 2000 mL has been ordered to run 16 hr. The set calibration is 10 gtt/mL.

7. The order is for 500 mL in 8 hr. The set is calibrated at 15 gtt/mL.

8. Administer 150 mL in 3 hr. A microdrip is used.

9. A total of 1500 mL has been ordered to infuse in 12 hr. Set calibration is 20 gtt/mL.

10. An IV medication of 30 mL is to be administered in 30 min using a 15 gtt/mL set.

11. Administer 100 mL in 1 hr using a 15 gtt/mL set.

12. Infuse 500 mL in 6 hr. Set calibration is 10 gtt/mL.

13. The order is to infuse 1 liter in 10 hr. At the end of 8 hr, you notice that there is 500 mL left. What would the new flow rate need to be to finish on schedule if the set calibration is 10 gtt/mL?

14. An IV was started at 9 am with orders to infuse 500 mL in 6 hr. At noon, the IV infiltrated with 350 mL left in the bag. At 1 pm, the IV was restarted. The set calibration is 20 gtt/mL. Calculate the new flow rate to deliver the infusion on time.

15. A 50 mL IV is to infuse in 15 min. The set calibration is 15 gtt/mL. After 5 min, the IV contains 40 mL. Calculate the flow rate to deliver the volume on time.

16. An IV of 1000 mL is ordered to run at 25 mL/hr using a microdrip set.

17. An infusion of 800 mL has been ordered to run in 5 hr. Set calibration is 10 gtt/mL.

18. Administer 1500 mL in 8 hr using a set calibrated at 20 gtt/mL.

19. The order is for 750 mL to run in 6 hr. Set calibration is 15 gtt/mL.

20. An IV of 1000 mL was ordered to run in 8 hr. After 4 hr, only 250 mL has infused. The set calibration is 20 gtt/mL. Recalculate the rate for the remaining solution to complete on time.

21. The order is to infuse 50 mL in 1 hr. The set calibration is a microdrip.

22. An IV of 500 mL is to infuse in 6 hr using a set calibrated at 10 gtt/mL.

23. Infuse 120 mL in 1 hr. Set calibration is 10 gtt/mL.

24. Administer 12 mL in 22 min using a microdrip set.

25. A patient is to receive 3000 mL in 20 hr. Set is calibrated at 20 gtt/mL.

26. Infuse 1 liter in 5 hr using a set calibration of 15 gtt/mL.

27. A total of 1180 mL is to infuse in 12 hr using a set calibrated at 20 gtt/mL.

28. A volume of 150 mL is to infuse in 30 min. At the end of 20 min, you discover that 100 mL has infused. The set calibration is 10 gtt/mL. Should you adjust the flow rate? If so, what is the new rate? _____

29. The order is for 1000 mL in 5 hr. The set calibration is 20 gtt/mL. _____

30. Infuse 15 mL in 14 min using a 20 gtt/mL set. _____

31. The order is for 1000 mL in 10 hr using a 20 gtt/mL calibration. _____

32. A microdrip is used to administer 12 mL in 17 min. _____

33. Infuse 2750 mL in 20 hr using a 10 gtt/mL set. _____

34. An IV of 1800 mL is to infuse in 15 hr using a 15 gtt/mL set. _____

35. Infuse 600 mL in 6 hr with a 10 gtt/mL set. _____

36. Administer 22 mL in 18 min using a microdrip set. _____

37. An order of 1800 mL is to infuse in 10 hr. Set calibration is 20 gtt/mL. _____

38. Infuse 8 mL in 9 min using a microdrip. _____

39. Infuse 4000 mL in 20 hr. A 20 gtt/mL set is used. _____

40. An IV of 500 mL that was to infuse in 2 hr is discovered to have only 150 mL left after 30 min. Recalculate the flow rate. Set calibration is 15 gtt/mL. _____

Answers

1. (a) 1 (b) 4	9. 42 gtt/min	20. 63 gtt/min	30. 21 gtt/min
(c) 3 (d) 6	10. 15 gtt/min	21. 50 gtt/min	31. 33 gtt/min
2. mL/hr ÷ division	11. 25 gtt/min	22. 14 gtt/min	32. 42 gtt/min
factor	12. 14 gtt/min	23. 20 gtt/min	33. 23 gtt/min
3. mL/hr	13. 42 gtt/min	24. 33 gtt/min	34. 30 gtt/min
(mL/60 min)	14. 58 gtt/min	25. 50 gtt/min	35. 17 gtt/min
4. 13 gtt/15 sec	15. 60 gtt/min	26. 50 gtt/min	36. 73 gtt/min
5. 15 gtt/15 sec	16. 25 gtt/min	27. 33 gtt/min	37. 60 gtt/min
6. 21 gtt/min	17. 27 gtt/min	28. No, the rate is cor-	38. 53 gtt/min
7. 16 gtt/min	18. 63 gtt/min	rect at 50 gtt/min	39. 67 gtt/min
8. 50 gtt/min	19. 31 gtt/min	29. 67 gtt/min	40. 25 gtt/min

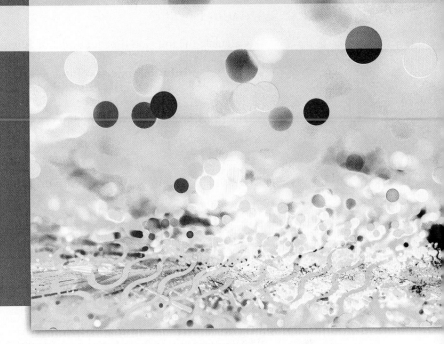

CHAPTER 13

IV Infusion and Completion Time Calculations

OBJECTIVES

The learner will calculate:

1. Infusion times.

2. Completion times using international/military and standard time.

3. Infusion time, so as to label the IV bag/bottle with the start, progress, and completion times.

INTRODUCTION

There are a number of reasons for calculating IV infusion and completion times: to know when an IV solution will complete so that additional solutions ordered can be prepared in advance and ready to hang; to discontinue an IV when it has completed; and to label an IV bag with start, progress, and completion times so that the infusion can be monitored and adjusted to keep it on schedule. Knowing the infusion time is also important because laboratory studies are sometimes made before, during, or after specified amounts of IV solutions have infused. The infusion time may be calculated in hours and/ or minutes, depending on the type and amount of solution ordered.

CALCULATING INFUSION TIME FROM mL/hr ORDERED

The infusion time is calculated for each bag/bottle to be hung and infused. The largest-capacity IV solution bag or bottle is 1000 mL, but 500 mL, 250 mL, and 50 mL bags are also commonly used. Calculations for odd-numbered volumes remaining when an IV infiltrates are also routinely done.

Infusion time is calculated by dividing the volume being infused by the mL/hr rate ordered.

Because most IVs take several hours to infuse, the unit of time being calculated most often includes hours (hr) and minutes (min).

EXAMPLE 1

Calculate the infusion time for an IV of **500 mL** to infuse at **50 mL/hr**.

$$\textbf{Infusion time = volume} \div \textbf{mL/hr rate}$$
$$= 500 \text{ mL} \div 50 \text{ mL/hr} = \textbf{10 hr}$$

The infusion time for an IV of 500 mL infusing at 50 mL/hr is 10 hr.

EXAMPLE 2

The order is to infuse **1000 mL** at **75 mL/hr**. Calculate the infusion time.

$$1000 \text{ mL} \div 75 \text{ mL/hr} = \textbf{13.33 hr}$$

In this example, the 13 represents the number of hours, whereas the .33 **represents the fraction of an additional hour.**

🗝 Fractional hours are converted to minutes by multiplying 60 min by the fraction obtained.

Calculate the number of minutes by multiplying 60 min by the fractional .33 hr:

$$60 \text{ min/hr} \times .33 \text{ hr} = 19.8 = \textbf{20 min}$$

The infusion time is 13 hr 20 min.

EXAMPLE 3

An IV of **1000 mL** is to infuse at **90 mL/hr**. Calculate the infusion time.

$$1000 \text{ mL} \div 90 \text{ mL/hr} = \textbf{11.11 hr}$$

Remember that .11 represents the fraction of an additional hour. Convert this to minutes by multiplying 60 min by .11:

$$60 \text{ min/hr} \times .11 \text{ hr} = 6.6 = \textbf{7 min}$$

The infusion time is 11 hr 7 min.

EXAMPLE 4

Calculate the infusion time for **750 mL** at a rate of **80 mL/hr**.

$$750 \text{ mL} \div 80 \text{ mL/hr} = \textbf{9.38 hr}$$

$$60 \text{ min/hr} \times .38 \text{ hr} = 22.8 = \textbf{23 min}$$

The infusion time is 9 hr 23 min.

EXAMPLE 5

A rate of **75 mL/hr** is ordered for a volume of **500 mL**. Calculate the infusion time.

$$500 \text{ mL} \div 75 \text{ mL/hr} = \textbf{6.67 hr}$$

$$60 \text{ min/hr} \times .67 \text{ hr} = 40.2 = \textbf{40 min}$$

The infusion time is 6 hr 40 min.

PROBLEMS 13-1

Calculate the infusion times.

1. An IV of 900 mL to infuse at 80 mL/hr   _____

2. A volume of 250 mL to infuse at 30 mL/hr   _____

3. An infusion of 180 mL to run at 25 mL/hr   _____

4. A volume of 1000 mL ordered at 60 mL/hr   _____

5. An IV of 150 mL to infuse at 80 mL/hr   _____

6. An infusion of 1000 mL at 125 mL/hr   _____

7. A rate of 120 mL/hr for 500 mL   _____

8. A volume of 800 mL at 60 mL/hr   _____

9. An IV of 250 mL at 80 mL/hr   _____

10. A rate of 135 mL/hr for 750 mL   _____

Answers   1. 11 hr 15 min   **2.** 8 hr 20 min   **3.** 7 hr 12 min   **4.** 16 hr 40 min   **5.** 1 hr 53 min   **6.** 8 hr
7. 4 hr 10 min   **8.** 13 hr 20 min   **9.** 3 hr 8 min   **10.** 5 hr 34 min

Note: Answers may vary due to rounding or calculator setting, so variations of 1–2 min may be considered correct.

CALCULATING INFUSION COMPLETION TIMES

The completion time is the actual hour and/or minute an infusion bag or bottle will complete or empty. Completion times are calculated in either **international/military time** using the 24-hour clock, or **standard time**, depending on individual clinical facility policy.

> 🔑 The completion time is calculated by adding the infusion time to the time the IV was started.

An example is the addition of an infusion time of 90 min to a 0515 international/military time or 5:15 am standard time when an IV was started.

INTERNATIONAL/MILITARY TIME CALCULATIONS

EXAMPLE 1

An IV started at **0400** is to complete in **2 hr 30 min**. Calculate the completion time.

- **Add the 2 hr 30 min infusion time to the 0400 start time:**

$$
\begin{array}{r}
0400 \\
+\ \underline{230} \\
0630
\end{array}
$$

- **The completion time is 0630.**

EXAMPLE 2

An IV started at **0750** is to complete in **5 hr 10 min**. Calculate the completion time.

- **Add the 5 hr 10 min infusion time to the 0750 start time:**

$$
\begin{array}{r}
0750 \\
+ \ 510 \\
\hline
1260
\end{array}
$$

- **Change the 60 min to 1 hr and add to 1200 = 1300.**

- **The completion time is 1300.**

EXAMPLE 3

An IV started at **2250** is to complete in **4 hr 20 min**. Calculate the completion time.

- **Add the infusion time to the start time:**

$$
\begin{array}{r}
2250 \\
+ \ 420 \\
\hline
2670
\end{array}
$$

- **Change the 70 min to 1 hr 10 min = 2710.**

- **Deduct 24 hr from 2710 = 0310.**

- **The completion time is 0310.**

PROBLEMS 13-2

Calculate the international/military completion times.

1. An IV started at 0415 to infuse in 1 hr 30 min _____

2. An infusion started at 1735 to complete in 2 hr 40 min _____

3. An IV to complete in 1 hr 14 min that was started at 0025 _____

4. An IV started at 2300 to complete in 3 hr 40 min _____

5. An infusion time of 6 hr 20 min for an infusion started at 0325 _____

6. An IV started at 0445 to complete in 3 hr 20 min _____

7. A medication infusion started at 0740 to complete in 90 min _____

8. An IV medication started at 1247 to complete in 45 min _____

9. An IV started at 1430 to complete in 4 hr _____

10. An IV started at 1605 to complete in 3 hr 30 min _____

Answers **1.** 0545 **2.** 2015 **3.** 0139 **4.** 0240 **5.** 0945 **6.** 0805 **7.** 0910 **8.** 1332 **9.** 1830 **10.** 1935

STANDARD TIME CALCULATIONS

EXAMPLE 1

An IV medication will infuse in **20 minutes**. It is now **6:14 pm**. When will it complete?

- **Add the 20 minutes infusion time to the 6:14 pm start time:**

    6:14 pm + **20 min = 6:34 pm**

- **The completion time will be at 6:34 pm.**

EXAMPLE 2

An IV is to infuse in **2 hr 33 min**. It is now **4:43 pm**. When will it complete?

- **Add the 2 hr 33 min infusion time to the 4:43 start time:**

    4:43 pm
    + 2:33
    ‾‾‾‾‾
    6:76

- **Change the 76 min to 1 hr 16 min to make the completion time 7:16 pm.**

- **The infusion will complete at 7:16 pm.**

EXAMPLE 3

An IV infusion time is **13 hr 20 min**. What is its completion time if it was started at **10:45 am**?

- **Add the 13 hr 20 min infusion time to the 10:45 am start time:**

    10:45 am
    + 13:20
    ‾‾‾‾‾
    23:65

- **Change the 65 min to 1 hr 5 min = 24:05. Subtract 12 hr.**

- **The completion time will be 12:05 am.**

EXAMPLE 4

An IV with an infusion time of **10 hr 7 min** is started at **9:42 am**. When will it complete?

- **Add the 10 hr 7 min infusion time to the 9:42 am start time:**

    9:42 am
    + 10:07
    ‾‾‾‾‾
    19:49

- **Subtract 12 hr to make the completion time 7:49 pm.**

- **The completion time will be 7:49 pm.**

EXAMPLE 5

An IV with an infusion time of **12 hr 30 min** is started at **2:10 am**. When will it complete?

■ **Add the 12 hr 30 min infusion time to the 2:10 am start time:**

$$
\begin{array}{r}
2{:}10\ \text{am} \\
+\ \underline{12{:}30} \\
14{:}40
\end{array}
$$

■ **Subtract 12 hr to make the time 2:40 pm.**

■ **The completion time will be 2:40 pm.**

PROBLEMS 13-3

Calculate IV completion using standard time.

1. An IV started at 4:40 am that has an infusion time of 9 hr 42 min _____

2. An IV medication started at 7:30 am that has an infusion time of 45 min _____

3. An IV with an infusion time of 7 hr 7 min that was restarted at 10:42 am _____

4. An IV with a restart time of 9:07 pm that has an infusion time of 6 hr 27 min _____

5. An IV with an infusion time of 3 hr 30 min that was started at 11:49 pm _____

6. An IV started at 2:43 pm to infuse in 40 min _____

7. An IV medication started at 10:15 am to complete in 90 min _____

8. An infusion started at 7:05 pm to complete in 8 hr _____

9. An IV started at 5:47 am to complete in 5 hr _____

10. An IV started at 4:20 am to complete in 12 hr _____

Answers 1. 2:22 pm **2.** 8:15 am **3.** 5:49 pm **4.** 3:34 am **5.** 3:19 am **6.** 3:23 pm **7.** 11:45 am **8.** 3:05 am **9.** 10:47 am **10.** 4:20 pm

LABELING SOLUTION BAGS WITH INFUSION AND COMPLETION TIMES

In many clinical facilities, it is routine to label bags when they are hung with start, progress, and finish times to provide a visual reference of the status of the infusion. This allows the infusion to be regulated visually at any time. Where the rate of infusion of IV fluids is critical, monitors are routinely used to guarantee accuracy.

Refer to **Figure 13-1**, where you can see close-up the calibrations on a 1000 mL bag. Notice that each 50 mL is calibrated but that only the 100 mL calibrations are numbered: 1, 2, 3 (for 100, 200, 300), etc. Also notice that the calibrations on the IV bag are not all the same width. They are somewhat wider at the bottom because gravity and the pressure of the solution force more fluid to the bottom of the bag.

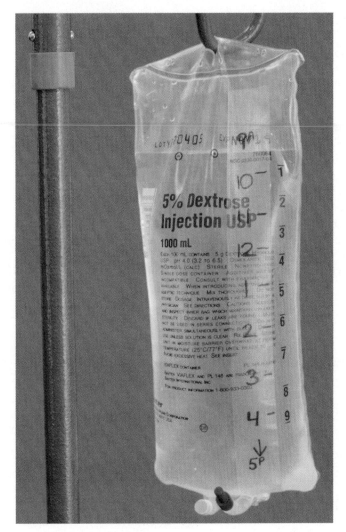

Figure 13-1

SUMMARY

This concludes the chapter on calculation of infusion and completion times and labeling of IV bags/bottles with start, progress, and completion times. The important points to remember from this chapter are:

- The infusion time is the time required for an IV to infuse completely.

- The infusion time is calculated by dividing the total volume to infuse by the mL/hr rate ordered.

- The completion time is calculated by adding the infusion time to the start time.

- When the minutes calculated is 60 or more, an additional hour is added to the completion time and 60 min are subtracted from the total minutes.

- Calculating completion times provides an opportunity to plan ahead and have the next solution ordered ready to hang or to discontinue an IV when it has completed.

- Most clinical facilities label IV solution bags/bottles with start, progress, and finish times to provide a visual record of the infusion status.

SUMMARY SELF-TEST

Calculate the infusion and completion times.

1. The order is for 50 mL to infuse at 50 mL/hr. The infusion was started at 10:10 am.

    Infusion time _____   Completion time _____

2. An infusion of 950 mL is ordered at 80 mL/hr. It was started at 8:02 am.

    Infusion time _____   Completion time _____

3. A total of 280 mL remains in an IV bag. The flow rate is 70 mL/hr. It is now 11:03 am.

    Infusion time _____   Completion time _____

4. The order is to infuse 500 mL at 90 mL/hr. The IV was started at 2:40 pm.

    Infusion time _____   Completion time _____

5. An infiltrated IV with 850 mL remaining is restarted at 10 am at a rate of 150 mL/hr.

    Infusion time _____   Completion time _____

6. At 4:04 am, an IV of 500 mL is started at a rate of 50 mL/hr.

    Infusion time _____   Completion time _____

7. An IV medication with a volume of 150 mL is started at 1:45 pm to infuse at 60 mL/hr.

    Infusion time _____   Completion time _____

8. An IV of 520 mL is restarted at 0420 at a rate of 125 mL/hr.

    Infusion time _____   Completion time _____

9. It is 12:00 pm, and an IV of 900 mL is to infuse at a rate of 100 mL/hr.

    Infusion time _____   Completion time _____

10. An IV of 1000 mL is started at 0550 to infuse at 130 mL/hr.

    Infusion time _____   Completion time _____

11. An infusion of 250 mL is started at 11:20 am to infuse at a rate of 20 mL/hr.

    Infusion time _____   Completion time _____

12. The flow rate ordered for 1 L is 80 mL/hr. It was started at 8:07 pm.

    Infusion time _____   Completion time _____

13. A 250 mL volume is started at 3:40 pm to be infused at 90 mL/hr.

    Infusion time _____   Completion time _____

14. A medication volume of 100 mL is started at 4:00 pm to infuse at 42 mL/hr.

    Infusion time _____   Completion time _____

15. At 11:00 pm, 200 mL remain in an IV. The rate is 120 mL/hr.

    Infusion time _____   Completion time _____

16. An infusion of 350 mL is to run at 150 mL/hr. It is now 9:47 am.

    Infusion time _____   Completion time _____

17. An IV medication of 25 mL is started at 8:17 am to run at 25 mL/hr.

    Infusion time _____   Completion time _____

18. An IV of 425 mL is restarted at 0814 to infuse at 90 mL/hr.

    Infusion time _____   Completion time _____

19. At 10:30 pm, there is 180 mL left in an IV that is infusing at 25 mL/hr.

        Infusion time _____   Completion time _____

20. At 1400, 500 mL is started to run at a rate of 60 mL/hr.

        Infusion time _____   Completion time _____

21. An infusion of 250 mL is started at 3:04 am to run at 100 mL/hr.

        Infusion time _____   Completion time _____

22. With 525 mL remaining, a rate change to 108 mL/hr is ordered. It is 2:10 am.

        Infusion time _____   Completion time _____

23. A liter is started at 8:42 am at a rate of 120 mL/hr.

        Infusion time _____   Completion time _____

24. An infusion of 1000 mL is to run at 200 mL/hr. It is started at 6:40 pm.

        Infusion time _____   Completion time _____

25. An IV medication of 100 mL is started at 7:50 am to run at 150 mL/hr.

        Infusion time _____   Completion time _____

26. A volume of 500 mL is started at 4:04 pm at a rate of 75 mL/hr.

        Infusion time _____   Completion time _____

27. An IV of 950 mL is restarted at 2:10 am at 100 mL/hr.

        Infusion time _____   Completion time _____

28. An IV medication of 30 mL is started at 0915 at a rate of 60 mL/hr.

        Infusion time _____   Completion time _____

29. A medication volume of 90 mL is started at 6:15 am to be infused at 90 mL/hr.

        Infusion time _____   Completion time _____

30. A rate of 80 mL/hr is set at 4:20 pm to infuse a medication with a volume of 100 mL.

        Infusion time _____   Completion time _____

31. A volume of 750 mL is started at 0303 at a rate of 96 mL/hr.

        Infusion time _____   Completion time _____

Answers

1. 1 hr; 11:10 am
2. 11 hr 53 min; 7:55 pm
3. 4 hr; 3:03 pm
4. 5 hr 34 min; 8:14 pm
5. 5 hr 40 min; 3:40 pm
6. 10 hr; 2:04 pm
7. 2 hr 30 min; 4:15 pm
8. 4 hr 10 min; 0830

9. 9 hr; 9 pm
10. 7 hr 41 min; 1331
11. 12 hr 30 min; 11:50 pm
12. 12 hr 30 min; 8:37 am
13. 2 hr 47 min; 6:27 pm
14. 2 hr 23 min; 6:23 pm
15. 1 hr 40 min; 12:40 am

16. 2 hr 20 min; 12:07 pm
17. 1 hr; 9:17 am
18. 4 hr 43 min; 1257
19. 7 hr 12 min; 5:42 am
20. 8 hr 20 min; 2220
21. 2 hr 30 min; 5:34 am
22. 4 hr 52 min; 7:02 am
23. 8 hr 20 min; 5:02 pm

24. 5 hr; 11:40 pm
25. 40 min; 8:30 am
26. 6 hr 40 min; 10:44 pm
27. 9 hr 30 min; 11:40 am
28. 30 min; 0945
29. 1 hr; 7:15 am
30. 1 hr 15 min; 5:35 pm
31. 7 hr 49 min; 1052

Note: Answers may vary slightly due to rounding.

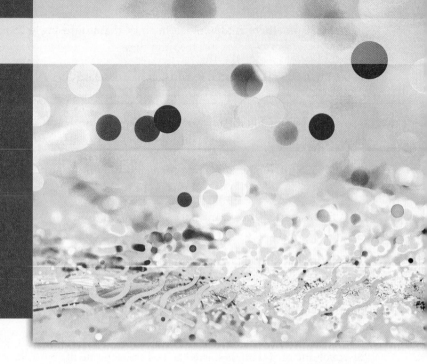

CHAPTER 14

IV Medication and Titration Calculations

OBJECTIVES

The learner will calculate:

1. Flow rates to infuse ordered dosages.

2. Dosages and flow rates based on kg body weight.

3. Dosage and flow rate ranges for titrated medications.

INTRODUCTION

Many IV drugs are used in critical and life-threatening situations to alter or maintain vital physiologic functions—for example, heart rate, cardiac output, blood pressure (BP), and respiration. In general, these drugs have a very rapid action and short duration. They are frequently administered diluted in 250–500 mL of IV solution, most commonly D5W.

Intravenous medications may be ordered by dosage (mcg/mg/units per min/hr) or based on body weight (mcg/mg/units per kg per min/hr). They may also be ordered to infuse within a specific dosage range—for example, 1–3 mcg/min—to elicit a measurable physiologic response; an example would be to maintain a systolic BP above 100 mm Hg.

    IV drugs require close and continuous monitoring, and an electronic infusion device (EID) is most often used for their administration.

Dosage increments or reductions are made within the ordered range until the desired response has been established.

If an EID is not used, a microdrip set calibrated at 60 gtt/mL or a dosage-controlled Soluset®/Buretrol®/Volutrol® burette is used.

🔑 All calculations in this chapter are for an EID or microdrip, so the mL/hr and gtt/min rates are interchangeable.

Calculations include converting ordered dosages to the flow rates necessary to administer them, and using flow rates to calculate the dosage infusing at any given moment. **Body weight is often a critical factor in IV dosages, and its use in calculations is also covered**. A number of EIDs display, and can be set to deliver, dosage and flow rate equivalents, but you must know how to do these calculations in case you encounter a situation in which you will have to do one. IV drugs that alter a basic physiologic function generally have narrow margins of safety, and accuracy is imperative in calculations involving these medications. Double-checking of math is both mandatory and routine. As a general rule, you will calculate dosages to the nearest tenth and round flow rates to the nearest mL or gtt. When an EID is used, flow rates can be programmed to deliver tenths of a mL.

🔑 All calculations assume the use of an EID or microdrip infusion set, so the mL/hr and gtt/min rates are identical and interchangeable.

CALCULATING mL/hr RATE FOR DOSAGE ORDERED

One common IV critical care calculation is to determine the mL/hr flow rate for a specific drug dosage ordered. Let's start by looking at some examples of these calculations.

EXAMPLE 1

A cardiac medication with a strength of **125 mg/100 mL** is to infuse at a rate of **20 mg/hr**. Calculate the **mL/hr** flow rate.

$$\frac{mL}{hr} = \frac{100\ mL}{125\ mg} \times \frac{20\ mg}{1\ hr}$$

$$= \frac{100\ mL}{125\ mg} \times \frac{20\ mg}{1\ hr}$$

$$= 16\ \mathbf{mL/hr}$$

To infuse 20 mg/hr, set the flow rate at 16 mL/hr.

EXAMPLE 2

A dosage of **2 mcg/min** has been ordered using an **8 mg in 250 mL** solution. Calculate the **mL/hr** flow rate.

- This equation will need a 60 min = 1 hr and a 1 mg = 1000 mcg conversion.

$$\frac{mL}{hr} = \frac{250\ mL}{8\ mg} \times \frac{1\ mg}{1000\ mcg} \times \frac{2\ mcg}{1\ min} \times \frac{60\ min}{1\ hr}$$

$$= \frac{250\ mL}{8\ mg} \times \frac{1\ mg}{1000\ mcg} \times \frac{2\ mcg}{1\ min} \times \frac{60\ min}{1\ hr}$$

$$= 3.75 = 4\ \mathbf{mL/hr}$$

- **To infuse 2 mcg/min, set the flow rate at 4 mL/hr.**

EXAMPLE 3

A medication with a strength of **50 mg in 250 mL** is used to infuse a dosage of **200 mcg/min**. Calculate the flow rate in **mL/hr**.

- This equation will need a 60 min = 1 hr and 1 mg = 1000 mcg conversion.

$$\frac{mL}{hr} = \frac{250\ mL}{50\ mg} \times \frac{1\ mg}{1000\ mcg} \times \frac{200\ mcg}{1\ min} \times \frac{60\ min}{1\ hr}$$

$$= \frac{250\ mL}{50\ \cancel{mg}} \times \frac{1\ \cancel{mg}}{1000\ \cancel{mcg}} \times \frac{200\ \cancel{mcg}}{1\ \cancel{min}} \times \frac{60\ \cancel{min}}{1\ hr}$$

$$= \textbf{60 mL/hr}$$

- To infuse 200 mcg/min, set the flow rate at 60 mL/hr.

PROBLEMS 14-1

Calculate the mL/hr flow rates. Express answers to the nearest whole mL/hr.

1. A 20 mg/hr dosage is ordered using a 100 mg/100 mL solution.   _____

2. A medication is ordered at the rate of 3 mcg/min. The solution strength is 8 mg in 250 mL.   _____

3. A solution of 2 g medication in 500 mL is used to administer a dosage of 2 mg/min.   _____

4. A 2 mcg/min infusion is ordered. The solution strength is 1 mg/250 mL.   _____

5. An initial dose of a drug is ordered at 25 mg/hr. The solution strength is 125 mg/100 mL.   _____

6. A 100 mg/250 mL solution strength is ordered at a rate of 15 mg/hr.   _____

7. A solution strength of 10 mg/250 mL is to infuse at 5 mcg/min.   _____

8. A 500 mL/1.5 g solution is to infuse at 3 mg/min.   _____

9. A 10 mg/250 mL solution is to infuse at 20 mcg/min.   _____

10. A 250 mg/100 mL solution is to infuse at 30 mg/hr.   _____

Answers 1. 20 mL/hr   **2.** 6 mL/hr   **3.** 30 mL/hr   **4.** 30 mL/hr   **5.** 20 mL/hr   **6.** 38 mL/hr   **7.** 8 mL/hr   **8.** 60 mL/hr   **9.** 30 mL/hr   **10.** 12 mL/hr

CALCULATING mL/hr RATE FOR DOSAGE FOR mL/kg ORDERED

Many IV medication infusions are calculated based on body weight—for example, 95.9 mcg/kg/hr. **Body weight to the nearest tenth kg** is used for the calculations. There are two ways the flow rate can be calculated. The first method requires two steps.

TWO-STEP FLOW RATE CALCULATION FOR DOSAGE PER kg ORDERED

The dosage for the body weight is calculated to the nearest tenth, then used to determine the flow rate.

EXAMPLE 1

Medication is ordered at the rate of **3 mcg/kg/min** for an adult weighing **95.9 kg**. The solution strength is **400 mg** in **250 mL**. Calculate the flow rate.

- **Calculate the 3 mcg/min dosage for 95.9 kg.**

  $$3 \text{ mcg/kg/min} \times 95.9 \text{ kg} = \textbf{287.7 mcg/min}$$

- **Calculate the mL/hr flow rate for 287.7 mcg/min.**

  $$\frac{\text{mL}}{\text{hr}} = \frac{250 \text{ mL}}{400 \text{ mg}} \times \frac{1 \text{ mg}}{1000 \text{ mcg}} \times \frac{287.7 \text{ mcg}}{1 \text{ min}} \times \frac{60 \text{ min}}{1 \text{ hr}}$$

  $$= \frac{250 \text{ mL}}{400 \text{ mg}} \times \frac{1 \text{ mg}}{1000 \text{ mcg}} \times \frac{287.7 \text{ mcg}}{1 \text{ min}} \times \frac{60 \text{ min}}{1 \text{ hr}}$$

  $$= 10.79 = \textbf{11 mL/hr}$$

To infuse 3 mcg/kg/min, set the flow rate at 11 mL/hr.

EXAMPLE 2

A solution strength of **2.5 g in 250 mL** has been ordered at a rate of **100 mcg/kg/min** for an adult weighing **104.6 kg**. Calculate the flow rate.

- **Calculate the dosage for 104.6 kg.**

  $$100 \text{ mcg/kg/min} \times 104.6 \text{ kg} = 10{,}460 \text{ mcg/min} = \textbf{10.5 mg/min}$$

- **Calculate the flow rate for 10.5 mg/min.**

  $$\frac{\text{mL}}{\text{hr}} = \frac{250 \text{ mL}}{2.5 \text{ g}} \times \frac{1 \text{ g}}{1000 \text{ mg}} \times \frac{10.5 \text{ mg}}{1 \text{ min}} \times \frac{60 \text{ min}}{1 \text{ hr}}$$

  $$= \frac{250 \text{ mL}}{2.5 \text{ g}} \times \frac{1 \text{ g}}{1000 \text{ mg}} \times \frac{10.5 \text{ mg}}{1 \text{ min}} \times \frac{60 \text{ min}}{1 \text{ hr}}$$

  $$= 63 = \textbf{63 mL/hr}$$

To infuse 100 mcg/kg/min, set the flow rate at 63 mL/hr.

EXAMPLE 3

A medication has been ordered at **4 mcg/kg/min** from a solution of **50 mg in 250 mL**. The patient's weight is **107.3 kg**.

- **Calculate the dosage for 107.3 kg.**

  $$4 \text{ mcg/kg/min} \times 107.3 \text{ kg} = \textbf{429.2 mcg/min}$$

■ **Calculate the flow rate for 429.2 mcg/min.**

$$\frac{mL}{hr} = \frac{250 \text{ mL}}{50 \text{ mg}} \times \frac{1 \text{ mg}}{1000 \text{ mcg}} \times \frac{429.5 \text{ mcg}}{1 \text{ min}} \times \frac{60 \text{ min}}{1 \text{ hr}}$$

$$= \frac{250 \text{ mL}}{50 \text{ mg}} \times \frac{1 \text{ mg}}{1000 \text{ mcg}} \times \frac{429.5 \text{ mcg}}{1 \text{ min}} \times \frac{60 \text{ min}}{1 \text{ hr}}$$

$$= 128.7 = \textbf{129 mL/hr}$$

To infuse 4 mcg/kg/min, set the flow rate at 129 mL/hr.

PROBLEMS 14-2

Calculate the mcg/min and mL/hr flow rates.

	mcg/min	mL/hr
1. A 3 mcg/kg/min dosage has been ordered for an adult weighing 87.4 kg. The solution being used has a strength of 50 mg in 250 mL.	_____	_____
2. IV medication has been ordered to infuse at 4 mcg/kg/min using a 400 mg/250 mL solution. The body weight is 92.4 kg.	_____	_____
3. A 2.5 mcg/kg/min dosage has been ordered. The solution strength is 0.5 g/250 mL. The body weight is 80.7 kg.	_____	_____
4. A rate of 150 mcg/kg/min has been ordered for a body weight of 92.1 kg. The solution strength is 2.5 g in 250 mL.	_____	_____
5. A 5 mcg/kg/min infusion has been ordered for a body weight of 80.3 kg. The solution to be used contains 1 g in 500 mL.	_____	_____
6. A 2 mcg/kg/min dosage has been ordered for an adult weighing 79.9 kg. The solution strength available is 50 mg/250 mL.	_____	_____
7. A dosage of 3 mcg/kg/min has been ordered using a 350 mg/250 mL solution strength. The body weight is 86.9 kg.	_____	_____
8. An adult weighing 84.3 kg has a dosage of 3 mcg/kg/min ordered. The solution to be used is 0.75 g/300 mL.	_____	_____

	mcg/min	mL/hr

9. A 4.5 mcg/kg/min dosage is ordered for an 84.9 kg adult. The solution strength is 1.2 g/500 mL. _____ _____

10. A 6 mcg/kg/min dosage is ordered for an adult weighing 85.8 kg. The solution strength is 800 mg/500 mL. _____ _____

Answers 1. 262.2 mcg/min; 79 mL/hr   **2.** 369.6 mcg/min; 14 mL/hr   **3.** 201.8 mcg/min; 6 mL/hr
4. 13,815 mcg/min; 83 mL/hr   **5.** 401.5 mcg/min; 12 mL/hr   **6.** 159.8 mcg/min; 48 mL/hr   **7.** 260.7 mcg/min;
11 mL/hr   **8.** 252.9 mcg/min; 6 mL/hr   **9.** 382.1 mcg/min; 10 mL/hr   **10.** 514.8 mcg/min; 19 mL/hr

ONE-STEP mL/hr FLOW RATE CALCULATION FOR DOSAGE PER kg ORDERED

The one-step method of flow rate calculation requires very careful entry of ratios and equally careful cancellation of measurement units to verify accuracy in ratio entry. Let's look at the entire equation step by step. Express flow rates to the nearest mL.

EXAMPLE 1

Medication is ordered at the rate of **3 mcg/kg/min** for an adult weighing **95.9 kg**. The solution strength is **400 mg** in **250 mL**. Calculate the flow rate.

- The first two ratios entered are the same as in the two-step method:

$$\frac{mL}{hr} = \frac{250\ mL}{400\ mg} \times \frac{1\ mg}{1000\ mcg}$$

- The denominator to be matched next is mcg. This is provided by the 3 mcg/kg/min dosage. Enter this with 3 mcg as the numerator; two measures, kg and min, become the new denominators:

$$\frac{mL}{hr} = \frac{250\ mL}{400\ mg} \times \frac{1\ mg}{1000\ mcg} \times \frac{3\ mcg}{kg/min}$$

- Both kg and min must be matched in the next numerators. Either can be entered first, but min is the best choice because a conversion ratio is needed to change min to the hr being calculated. Enter the 60 min = 1 hr conversion, with 60 min as the numerator, to match the previous min denominator:

$$\frac{mL}{hr} = \frac{250\ mL}{400\ mg} \times \frac{1\ mg}{1000\ mcg} \times \frac{3\ mcg}{kg/min} \times \frac{60\ min}{1\ hr}$$

- Only one measure remains to be entered: the 95.9 kg body weight. Enter this value as the final numerator to match the remaining kg denominator, which completes the equation:

$$\frac{mL}{hr} = \frac{250\ mL}{400\ mg} \times \frac{1\ mg}{1000\ mcg} \times \frac{3\ mcg}{kg/min} \times \frac{60\ min}{1\ hr} \times \frac{95.9\ kg}{}$$

- Cancel the alternate denominator/numerator measures. Only mL and hr remain in the equation. Do the math:

$$\frac{mL}{hr} = \frac{250 \text{ mL}}{400 \text{ mg}} \times \frac{1 \text{ mg}}{1000 \text{ mcg}} \times \frac{3 \text{ mcg}}{\text{kg/min}} \times \frac{60 \text{ min}}{1 \text{ hr}} \times \frac{95.9 \text{ kg}}{}$$

$$= 10.79 = \textbf{11 mL/hr}$$

The 11 mL/hr answer is identical to the 11 mL/hr answer obtained in the two- step calculation previously demonstrated.

EXAMPLE 2

A dosage of **2.5 g in 250 mL** has been ordered at a rate of **100 mcg/kg/min** for an adult weighing **104.6 kg**. Calculate the flow rate.

- Enter the mL/hr being calculated. The first mL numerator is provided by the 250 mL containing 2.5 g medication. Enter it now:

$$\frac{mL}{hr} = \frac{250 \text{ mL}}{2.5 \text{ g}}$$

- The dosage ordered is in mcg, so g-to-mg and mg-to-mcg conversion ratios are needed. Enter these now:

$$\frac{mL}{hr} = \frac{250 \text{ mL}}{2.5 \text{ g}} \times \frac{1 \text{ g}}{1000 \text{ mg}} \times \frac{1 \text{ mg}}{1000 \text{ mcg}}$$

- Enter the 100 mcg/kg/min dosage next, with mcg as the numerator to match the previous mcg denominator:

$$\frac{mL}{hr} = \frac{250 \text{ mL}}{2.5 \text{ g}} \times \frac{1 \text{ g}}{1000 \text{ mg}} \times \frac{1 \text{ mg}}{1000 \text{ mcg}} \times \frac{100 \text{ mcg}}{\text{kg/min}}$$

- Enter the min/hr conversion ratio:

$$\frac{mL}{hr} = \frac{250 \text{ mL}}{2.5 \text{ g}} \times \frac{1 \text{ g}}{1000 \text{ mg}} \times \frac{1 \text{ mg}}{1000 \text{ mcg}} \times \frac{100 \text{ mcg}}{\text{kg/min}} \times \frac{60 \text{ min}}{1 \text{ hr}}$$

- Enter the 104.6 kg body weight to complete the equation:

$$\frac{mL}{hr} = \frac{250 \text{ mL}}{2.5 \text{ g}} \times \frac{1 \text{ g}}{1000 \text{ mg}} \times \frac{1 \text{ mg}}{1000 \text{ mcg}} \times \frac{100 \text{ mcg}}{\text{kg/min}} \times \frac{60 \text{ min}}{1 \text{ hr}} \times \frac{104.6 \text{ kg}}{}$$

- Cancel the alternate denominator/numerator entries to double-check the accuracy of ratio entry. Do the math:

$$\frac{mL}{hr} = \frac{250 \text{ mL}}{2.5 \text{ g}} \times \frac{1 \text{ g}}{1000 \text{ mg}} \times \frac{1 \text{ mg}}{1000 \text{ mcg}} \times \frac{100 \text{ mcg}}{\text{kg/min}} \times \frac{60 \text{ min}}{1 \text{ hr}} \times \frac{104.6 \text{ kg}}{}$$

$$= 62.76 = \textbf{63 mL/hr}$$

The 63 mL/hr answer is identical to the 63 mL/hr answer obtained in the two-step calculation.

EXAMPLE 3

A medication has been ordered at **4 mcg/kg/min** from a solution of **50 mg** in **250 mL**. The body weight is **107.3 kg**.

$$\frac{mL}{hr} = \frac{250\ mL}{50\ mg}$$

$$\frac{mL}{hr} = \frac{250\ mL}{50\ mg} \times \frac{1\ mg}{1000\ mcg}$$

$$\frac{mL}{hr} = \frac{250\ mL}{50\ mg} \times \frac{1\ mg}{1000\ mcg} \times \frac{4\ mcg}{kg/min}$$

$$\frac{mL}{hr} = \frac{250\ mL}{50\ mg} \times \frac{1\ mg}{1000\ mcg} \times \frac{4\ mcg}{kg/min} \times \frac{60\ min}{1\ hr}$$

$$\frac{mL}{hr} = \frac{250\ mL}{50\ mg} \times \frac{1\ mg}{1000\ mcg} \times \frac{4\ mcg}{kg/min} \times \frac{60\ min}{1\ hr} \times \frac{107.3\ kg}{}$$

$$= 128.76 = \textbf{129 mL/hr}$$

The 129 mL/hr answer is identical to the 129 mL/hr rate calculated in the two-step method.

PROBLEMS 14-3

Calculate the mL/hr flow rates. Express answers to the nearest whole mL/hr.

1. A 3.5 mcg/kg/min dosage has been ordered for an adult weighing 90.3 kg. The solution being used has a strength of 40 mg in 150 mL.   _____

2. IV medication has been ordered to infuse at 3 mcg/kg/min using a 250 mg/250 mL solution. The body weight is 87.3 kg.   _____

3. A 4 mcg/kg/min dosage has been ordered. The solution strength is 600 mg/250 mL. The body weight is 90.3 kg.   _____

4. A rate of 200 mcg/kg/min has been ordered for a 83.3 kg body weight. The solution strength is 3.5 g in 250 mL.   _____

5. A 4.5 mcg/kg/min infusion has been ordered for a 79.9 kg body weight. The solution to be used contains 1.5 g in 200 mL.   _____

6. A 4 mcg/kg/min dosage has been ordered for an adult weighing 83.8 kg. The solution strength available is 50 mg/150 mL.   _____

7. A dosage of 5 mcg/kg/min has been ordered using a 300 mg/250 mL solution strength. The body weight is 86.6 kg.   _____

8. An adult weighing 91.4 kg has a dosage of 4 mcg/kg/min ordered. The solution to be used is 700 mg/500 mL.   _____

9. A 175 mcg/kg/min dosage is ordered for an 84.9 kg adult. The solution strength is 4 g/250 mL.

_____

10. A 5 mcg/kg/min dosage is ordered for an adult weighing 78.9 kg. The solution strength is 2 g/250 mL.

_____

Answers 1. 71 mL/hr   **2.** 16 mL/hr   **3.** 9 mL/hr   **4.** 71 mL/hr   **5.** 3 mL/hr   **6.** 60 mL/hr   **7.** 22 mL/hr   **8.** 16 mL/hr   **9.** 56 mL/hr   **10.** 3 mL/hr

IV TITRATION CALCULATIONS

Titration refers to the **adjustment of dosage within a specific range to obtain a measurable physiologic response**—for example, a drug at 2–4 mcg/min to maintain systolic BP above 100 mm Hg. The dosage is increased or decreased within the ordered range until the desired response is obtained. The **lowest dosage is set first and adjusted upward and downward as necessary**. The **upper dosage is never exceeded** unless a new order is obtained.

Volumetric or syringe pumps are used for administration. Flow rates are calculated in mL/hr for the lowest and highest dosages ordered, and adjusted within this range to elicit the desired physiologic response. Let's look at some examples.

EXAMPLE 1

A 2–4 mcg/min dosage has been ordered. The solution being titrated contains **8 mg** in **250 mL**. Calculate the flow rate of medication for the **2–4 mcg range**.

- Calculate the lower 2 mcg/min flow rate first:

$$\frac{mL}{hr} = \frac{250\ mL}{8\ mg} \times \frac{1\ mg}{1000\ mcg} \times \frac{2\ mcg}{1\ min} \times \frac{60\ min}{1\ hr}$$

$$= \frac{250\ mL}{8\ mg} \times \frac{1\ mg}{1000\ mcg} \times \frac{2\ mcg}{1\ min} \times \frac{60\ min}{1\ hr}$$

$$= 3.75 = \textbf{4 mL/hr}$$

- **The upper 4 mcg/min flow rate is exactly double the 2 mcg/min rate:**

$$4\ mL/hr \times 2 = \textbf{8 mL/hr}$$

- **A dosage of 2–4 mcg/min is delivered by a flow rate of 4–8 mL/hr.**

EXAMPLE 2

A medication is to be titrated between **415 and 830 mcg/min**. The solution concentration is **100 mg** in **40 mL**. Calculate the **mL/hr** flow rate range.

- Calculate the flow rate for the lower 415 mcg/min dosage:

$$\frac{mL}{hr} = \frac{40\ mL}{100\ mg} \times \frac{1\ mg}{1000\ mcg} \times \frac{415\ mcg}{1\ min} \times \frac{60\ min}{1\ hr}$$

$$= \frac{40\ mL}{100\ mg} \times \frac{1\ mg}{1000\ mcg} \times \frac{415\ mcg}{1\ min} \times \frac{60\ min}{1\ hr}$$

$$= 9.96 = \textbf{10 mL/hr}$$

■ The 830 mcg dosage is exactly double 415 mcg:

10 mL/hr × 2 = **20 mL/hr**

■ **A dosage of 415–830 mcg/min requires a flow rate of 10–20 mL/hr.**

EXAMPLE 3

An adult weighing **103.1 kg** has dosage orders for **0.3–3 mcg/kg/min**. The solution concentration is **50 mg in 250 mL**.

■ Calculate the dosage range for 103.1 kg.

Lower dosage: 0.3 mcg/kg/min × 103.1 kg = 30.93 = **30.9 mcg/min**

Upper dosage: 3 mcg/kg/min × 103.1 kg = **309.3 mcg/min**

■ **The dosage range for this 103.1 kg adult is 30.9–309.3 mcg/min.**

■ Calculate the flow rate for the lower 30.9 mcg/min dosage:

$$\frac{mL}{hr} = \frac{250\ mL}{50\ mg} \times \frac{1\ mg}{1000\ mcg} \times \frac{30.9\ mcg}{1\ min} \times \frac{60\ min}{1\ hr}$$

$$= \frac{250\ mL}{50\ \cancel{mg}} \times \frac{1\ \cancel{mg}}{1000\ \cancel{mcg}} \times \frac{30.9\ \cancel{mcg}}{1\ \cancel{min}} \times \frac{60\ \cancel{min}}{1\ hr}$$

$$= 9.2 = \textbf{9 mL/hr}$$

■ Calculate the flow rate for the upper 309.3 mcg/min dosage:

$$\frac{mL}{hr} = \frac{250\ mL}{50\ mg} \times \frac{1\ mg}{1000\ mcg} \times \frac{309.3\ mcg}{1\ min} \times \frac{60\ min}{1\ hr}$$

$$= \frac{250\ mL}{50\ \cancel{mg}} \times \frac{1\ \cancel{mg}}{1000\ \cancel{mcg}} \times \frac{309.3\ \cancel{mcg}}{1\ \cancel{min}} \times \frac{60\ \cancel{min}}{1\ hr}$$

$$= 92.7 = \textbf{93 mL/hr}$$

■ **To deliver 0.3–3 mcg/kg/min, the flow rate must be titrated from 9 to 93 mL/hr.**

PROBLEMS 14-4

Calculate the mL/hr flow rate ranges. Express answers to the nearest whole mL/hr.

1. A 2 g in 500 mL solution is ordered to titrate at 1–2 mg/min. _____

2. A drug is ordered to titrate between 1 mcg/min and 3 mcg/min. The solution strength is 1 mg per 250 mL. _____

3. The dosage range is 5–8 mcg/kg/min. The body weight is 103.7 kg, and the solution strength is 100 mg in 40 mL. _____

4. A drug is to titrate between 50 mcg/kg/min and 100 mcg/kg/min. The body weight is 78.7 kg, and the solution strength is 2500 mg in 250 mL. _____

5. An adult weighing 73.2 kg has a solution of 500 mg medication in 250 mL ordered to titrate between 3 mcg/kg/min and 10 mcg/kg/min.   _____

6. A 2–3 mg/min dosage has been ordered. The solution strength available is 1.5 g/400 mL.   _____

7. A dosage of 6–7 mcg/min has been ordered using a 5 mg/500 mL solution strength.   _____

8. An adult weighing 101.6 kg has a dosage of 4–7 mcg/kg/min ordered. The solution to be used is 75 mg/50 mL.   _____

9. A 30–70 mcg/kg/min dosage is ordered for an 80.4 kg adult. The solution strength is 3 g/250 mL.   _____

10. A 4–8 mcg/kg/min dosage is ordered for an adult weighing 72.1 kg. The solution strength is 400 mg/250 mL.   _____

Answers 1. 15–30 mL/hr   **2.** 15–45 mL/hr   **3.** 12–20 mL/hr   **4.** 24–47 mL/hr   **5.** 7–22 mL/hr
6. 32–48 mL/hr   **7.** 36–42 mL/hr   **8.** 16–28 mL/hr   **9.** 12–28 mL/hr   **10.** 11–22 mL/hr

SUMMARY

This concludes the chapter on titration of IV medications. The important points to remember about these medications are:

- They have a rapid action and short duration.

- They have a narrow margin of safety, and continuous monitoring is required in their use.

- They are frequency-titrated within a specific dosage/flow rate to elicit a measurable physiologic response.

- When titrated, they are initiated at the lowest dosage ordered and increased or decreased slowly to obtain the desired response.

- They are infused using an EID or 60 gtt/mL microdrip set.

- The mL/hr flow rate for EIDs and the gtt/min microdrip rate are identical and interchangeable.

SUMMARY SELF-TEST

Calculate dosages to the nearest tenth, and flow rates to the nearest whole number.

1. A 6 mcg/kg/min dosage is ordered for an adult weighing 75.4 kg. The solution available is 500 mg in 250 mL.

    mcg/min dosage _____ mL/hr flow rate _____

2. The order is to infuse a solution of 50 mg in 250 mL at 0.8 mcg/kg/min. Calculate the dosage and flow rate for a 65.9 kg adult.

    mcg/min dosage _____ mL/hr flow rate _____

3. A solution of 250 mg in 500 mL is to infuse between 0.5 and 0.7 mg/kg/hr.
   The adult weighs 82.4 kg.

   mg/hr dosage range _____ mL/hr flow rate range _____

4. A solution of 400 mg in 250 mL is infusing at 20 mL/hr.

   mcg/min dosage _____

5. A 1–6 mg/min dosage is ordered. The solution strength is 2 g/500 mL.

   mL/hr flow rate range _____

6. An infusion of 2 g in 500 mL is ordered at 60 mL/hr.

   mg/min dosage _____ mg/hr dosage _____

7. The solution available is 25 mg in 50 mL. The order is to infuse at 8 mg/hr.

   mL/hr flow rate _____

8. A solution of 100 mg in 40 mL is ordered to infuse at 5 mcg/kg/min for an adult
   weighing 77.1 kg.

   mL/hr flow rate _____

9. A drug is ordered at 4 mcg/min. The solution available is 1 mg in 250 mL.

   mL/hr flow rate _____

10. An adult weighing 80 kg has an infusion ordered at 8 mcg/kg/min. The solution strength is
    800 mg in 500 mL.

    mcg/min dosage _____ mL/hr flow rate _____

11. A dosage of 400 mg is added to 250 mL and infused at 45 mL/hr. Calculate the mcg/min
    and mg/hr infusing.

    mcg/min dosage _____ mg/hr dosage _____

12. An adult has orders for a dosage of 1 mg/min. The solution strength is 250 mg in 250 mL.

    mL/hr flow rate _____

13. An adult weighing 77.9 kg is to receive 80 mcg/kg/min. The solution strength is 2.5 g
    in 250 mL.

    mcg/min dosage _____ mL/hr flow rate _____

14. A dosage of 4 mcg/min has been ordered using an 8 mg in 250 mL solution.

    mL/hr flow rate _____

15. An adult who weighs 81.7 kg has orders for 8–10 mcg/kg/min. The solution strength
    is 400 mg in 250 mL.

    mcg/min dosage range _____

16. A 6 mcg/kg/min dosage has been ordered for a 90.7 kg adult. The solution strength
    is 50 mg in 250 mL.

    mcg/min dosage _____ mL/hr flow rate _____

17. A dosage of 5 mcg/kg/min is ordered. The solution available is 400 mg in 250 mL.
    The adult weighs 70.7 kg.

    mcg/min dosage _____ mL/hr flow rate _____

18. A 3 mg/min dosage is ordered. The solution strength is 2 g in 500 mL.

    mL/hr flow rate _____

19. A solution of 50 mg/250 mL is infusing at 15 mL/hr.

    mcg/min infusing _____

20. A 2 g in 500 mL solution is to infuse at a rate of 2 mg/min.

    mL/hr flow rate _____

21. An adult whose weight is 102.4 kg is to receive a dosage of 2 mg/kg/hr. The solution strength is 1 g in 500 mL.

    mg/hr dosage _____ mL/hr flow rate _____

22. A solution strength of 1 g in 100 mL is to infuse at a rate of 15 mcg/kg/min. The body weight is 94.4 kg.

    mcg/min dosage _____ mL/hr flow rate _____

23. An adult is receiving 4 mL/hr of a solution that contains 8 mg in 250 mL.

    mcg/min infusing _____

24. A drug is ordered to titrate between 5 and 10 mcg/kg/min. The body weight is 97.1 kg, and the solution strength is 100 mg/40 mL.

    mcg/min range _____ mL/hr flow rate range _____

25. A 500 mg in 250 mL solution is ordered for a 101.2 kg adult to titrate between 3 and 10 mcg/kg/min.

    mcg/min dosage range _____ mL/hr flow rate range _____

26. An infusion of 500 mg in 250 mL is infusing at a rate of 14 mL/hr.

    mcg/min infusing _____

27. A 5–10 mcg/kg/min dosage is to be titrated for an adult patient weighing 79.6 kg. The solution strength is 100 mg in 40 mL.

    mcg/min dosage range _____ mL/hr flow rate range _____

28. A 400 mg in 250 mL solution is to be titrated at 2–20 mcg/kg/min. The body weight is 62.3 kg.

    mcg/min dosage range _____ mL/hr flow rate range _____

29. A drug has been ordered for an adult weighing 84.9 kg to titrate at 2.5–10 mcg/kg/min. The solution strength is 500 mg in 250 mL.

    mcg/min dosage range _____ mL/hr flow rate range _____

30. A drug is ordered at a rate of 1–4 mg/min. The solution strength is 2 g in 500 mL.

    mL/hr flow rate range _____

31. A 10 mcg/min dosage is ordered using an 8 mg/250 mL solution.

    mL/hr flow rate _____

32. A 2 g in 500 mL dosage is to infuse at 3 mg/min.

    mL/hr flow rate _____

33. A 250 mL solution containing 1 mg of medication is to be infused at 5 mcg/min.

    mL/hr flow rate _____

34. A 4 mcg/min dosage is ordered. The solution is 250 mL with 8 mg of medication.

    mL/hr flow rate _____

35. A 2 g in 500 mL solution is ordered to infuse at a rate of 6 mg/min.

    mL/hr flow rate _____

36. A 2 g in 500 mL solution is ordered to infuse at 4 mg/min.

mL/hr flow rate _____

37. A 12 mcg/min dosage using an 8 mg in 250 mL of solution is ordered.

mL/hr flow rate _____

38. A 40 mg/hr dosage is ordered, and a 100 mg in 100 mL solution is ordered.

mL/hr flow rate _____

39. The order is to infuse 4 mcg/min from a 250 mL solution containing 1 mg of medication.

mL/hr flow rate _____

40. Infuse 10 mg/hr from a 125 mg/100 mL solution.

mL/hr flow rate _____

Answers

1. 452.4 mcg/min;
   14 mL/hr
2. 52.7 mcg/min;
   16 mL/hr
3. 41.2–57.7 mg/hr;
   82–115 mL/hr
4. 533.3 mcg/min
5. 15–90 mL/hr
6. 4 mg/min;
   240 mg/hr
7. 16 mL/hr
8. 9 mL/hr
9. 60 mL/hr
10. 640 mcg/min;
    24 mL/hr

11. 1200 mcg/min;
    72 mg/hr
12. 60 mL/hr
13. 6232 mcg/min;
    37 mL/hr
14. 8 mL/hr
15. 653.6–817 mcg/min
16. 544.2 mcg/min;
    163 mL/hr
17. 353.5 mcg/min;
    13 mL/hr
18. 45 mL/hr
19. 50 mcg/min
20. 30 mL/hr

21. 204.8 mg/hr;
    102 mL/hr
22. 1416 mcg/min;
    8 mL/hr
23. 2.1 mcg/min
24. 485.5–971 mcg/min;
    12–23 mL/hr
25. 303.6–1012 mcg/
    min; 9–30 mL/hr
26. 466.7 mcg/min
27. 398–796 mcg/min;
    10–19 mL/hr
28. 124.6–1246 mcg/
    min; 5–47 mL/hr

29. 212.3–849 mcg/min;
    6–25 mL/hr
30. 15–60 mL/hr
31. 19 mL/hr
32. 45 mL/hr
33. 75 mL/hr
34. 8 mL/hr
35. 90 mL/hr
36. 60 mL/hr
37. 23 mL/hr
38. 40 mL/hr
39. 60 mL/hr
40. 8 mL/hr

CHAPTER 15

Heparin Infusion Calculations

INTRODUCTION

Heparin is a powerful anticoagulant drug that inhibits new blood clot formation, or the extension of existing clots. Heparin is commonly mixed in IV solutions for administration, especially postoperatively to prevent clot formation from venous stasis. Heparin IV use is so frequent that it is prepared in ready-to-hang IV bags, such as the **1000 units strength illustrated** in **Figure 15-1**.

Heparin can also be administered subcutaneously in small dosages. Subcutaneous injections require **deep injection at a 45° angle** to discourage bleeding from medication leaking through the injection tract. Also, **subcutaneous sites are not massaged after injection**, again to prevent bleeding at the site.

Heparin dosages may be based on body weight in kg, or on a patient's clotting time. Because of heparin's potent anticoagulant action, clotting times are checked frequently during its administration.

There is no essential difference in the calculations you have already practiced for critical care dosages and those for heparin dosages, except that heparin dosages for subcutaneous injection are measured using a tuberculin (TB) syringe. However, heparin's action is so critical that it deserves to be addressed separately. In this chapter, you will be introduced to labels of a variety of heparin dosages, practice measuring heparin dosages for addition to IV solutions, calculate units per hour infusing from mL/hr flow rates, and be reminded of the precautions used to maintain patency of intravenous injection ports.

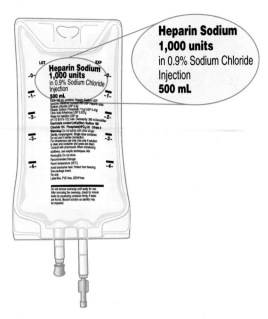

Figure 15-1

HEPARIN IV LABELS

If a commercially prepared IV heparin dosage strength that you require is not available, you may need to prepare the solution yourself from **a number of available vial dosage strengths**. Let's stop and look at some vial labels, so that you can refresh your memory with some typical calculations.

PROBLEMS 15-1

Read the heparin labels provided to determine how many mL of heparin will be necessary to prepare the solutions indicated. Many calculations are simple and do not require the use of dimensional analysis.

1. Refer to the label in **Figure 15-2** to determine how many mL will be required to add 4000 units to an IV solution. _____

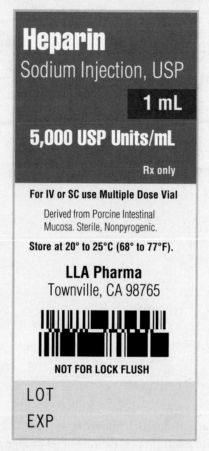

Figure 15-2

2. Refer to the label in **Figure 15-3** to determine how many mL will be required to add 4000 units to an IV solution. _____

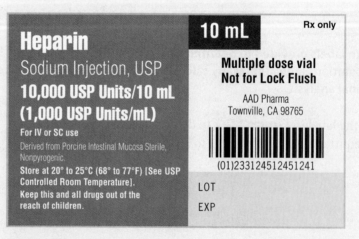

Figure 15-3

3. Refer to the label in **Figure 15-4** to determine how many mL of heparin will be required to add 1800 units to an IV solution. _____

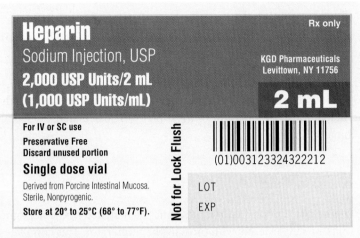

Figure 15-4

4. Refer to the label in **Figure 15-5** to determine how many mL will be required to add 900 units to an IV solution. _____

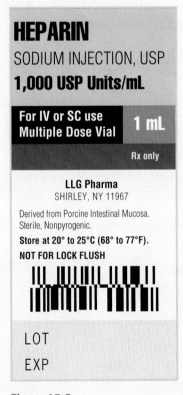

Figure 15-5

Answers 1. 0.8 mL   **2.** 4 mL   **3.** 1.8 mL   **4.** 0.9 mL

CALCULATING mL/hr IV FLOW RATE FROM units/hr ORDERED

Because heparin is most frequently ordered in units/hr to be administered—for example, 1000 units/hr—and infused using an electronic infusion device (EID), a common calculation will be for the mL/hr flow rate needed for this dosage. Let's look at these calculations first, keeping in mind that **the mL/hr flow rate for an EID is identical to the gtt/min rate for a microdrip**.

EXAMPLE 1

The order is to infuse heparin **1000 units/hr** from a solution of **20,000 units in 500 mL** D5W. Calculate the **mL/hr** flow rate.

- Enter the mL/hr being calculated first. Locate the ratio containing mL—in this case, the 20,000 units/500 mL strength—and enter this as the starting ratio with mL as the numerator, to match the mL numerator of the units being calculated; 20,000 units becomes the denominator:

$$\frac{mL}{hr} = \frac{500 \text{ mL}}{20,000 \text{ units}}$$

- The starting ratio denominator, units, must be matched in the next numerator. Enter the 1000 units/hr rate ordered, with units as the numerator. This completes the equation:

$$\frac{mL}{hr} = \frac{500 \text{ mL}}{20,000 \text{ units}} \times \frac{1000 \text{ units}}{1 \text{ hr}}$$

- Cancel alternate denominator/numerator units in the equation to double-check that the ratios have been entered correctly. Only mL and hr should remain. Do the math:

$$\frac{mL}{hr} = \frac{500 \text{ mL}}{20,000 \text{ units}} \times \frac{1000 \text{ units}}{1 \text{ hr}} = 25 \text{ mL/hr}$$

A rate of 25 mL/hr is required to infuse 1000 units/hr from a solution strength of 20,000 units in 500 mL.

EXAMPLE 2

The order is for heparin **800 units/hr**. The solution available is **40,000 units in 1000 mL** D5W. Calculate the **mL/hr** flow rate.

- Enter the mL/hr being calculated. Enter the 1000 mL/40,000 units ratio, with mL as the numerator:

$$\frac{mL}{hr} = \frac{1000 \text{ mL}}{40,000 \text{ units}}$$

- Enter the next ratio, 800 units/hr, with 800 units as the numerator to match the starting ratio denominator:

$$\frac{mL}{hr} = \frac{1000 \text{ mL}}{40,000 \text{ units}} \times \frac{800 \text{ units}}{1 \text{ hr}}$$

- Cancel to double-check for correct ratio entry, and do the math:

$$\frac{mL}{hr} = \frac{1000 \text{ mL}}{40,000 \text{ units}} \times \frac{800 \text{ units}}{1 \text{ hr}} = 20 \text{ mL/hr}$$

A rate of 20 mL/hr is required to infuse 800 units/hr from a solution strength of 40,000 units in 1000 mL.

EXAMPLE 3

The order is to infuse heparin **1100 units/hr** from a solution strength of **60,000 units in 1 L** D5W. Calculate the **mL/hr** flow rate.

$$\frac{mL}{hr} = \frac{1000\ mL}{60,000\ units} \times \frac{1100\ units}{1\ hr}$$

$$\frac{mL}{hr} = \frac{1000\ mL}{60,000\ \cancel{units}} \times \frac{1100\ \cancel{units}}{1\ hr} = 18.33 = \textbf{18 mL/hr}$$

A rate of 18 mL/hr is required to infuse 1100 units per hour from a 60,000 units in 1 L solution.

PROBLEMS 15-2

Calculate the mL/hr flow rates.

1. The order is to infuse 1000 units heparin per hour from an available solution strength of 25,000 units in 500 mL D5W.   _____

2. Heparin has been ordered at 2500 units per hour. The solution strength is 50,000 units in 1000 mL D5W.   _____

3. The order is to infuse 1100 units per hour from a 15,000 units in 1 L D5W solution.   _____

4. An adult patient has orders for 50,000 units of heparin in 1000 mL D5W to infuse at a rate of 2000 units per hour.   _____

5. Administer 1500 units per hour of heparin from an available strength of 40,000 units in 1 L.   _____

Answers 1. 20 mL/hr   **2.** 50 mL/hr   **3.** 73 mL/hr   **4.** 40 mL/hr   **5.** 38 mL/hr

CALCULATING units/hr INFUSING FROM mL/hr FLOW RATE

On occasion, it may be necessary to calculate the units/hr of heparin infusing from the mL/hr flow rate. This is done using the units/mL solution strength and mL/hr rate of infusion.

EXAMPLE 1

An IV of **1000 mL** containing **40,000 units** of heparin is running at **30 mL/hr**. Calculate the **units/hr** infusing.

$$\frac{units}{hr} = \frac{40,000\ units}{1000\ mL} \times \frac{30\ mL}{1\ hr}$$

$$\frac{units}{hr} = \frac{40,000\ units}{1000\ \cancel{mL}} \times \frac{30\ \cancel{mL}}{1\ hr} = \textbf{1200 units/hr}$$

A 1000 mL solution containing 40,000 units heparin running at 30 mL/hr is infusing 1200 units/hr.

EXAMPLE 2

A solution of **1 L** of D5W with **20,000 units** heparin is running at **80 mL/hr**. Calculate the **units/hr** infusing.

$$\frac{\text{units}}{\text{hr}} = \frac{20{,}000 \text{ units}}{1000 \text{ mL}} \times \frac{80 \text{ mL}}{1 \text{ hr}}$$

$$\frac{\text{units}}{\text{hr}} = \frac{20{,}000 \text{ units}}{1000 \text{ mL}} \times \frac{80 \text{ mL}}{1 \text{ hr}} = \textbf{1600 units/hr}$$

A 1 L (1000 mL) solution containing 20,000 units heparin running at 80 mL/hr is infusing 1600 units/hr.

EXAMPLE 3

An IV of D5W **500 mL** containing **10,000 units** heparin is running at **40 mL/hr**. Calculate the **units/hr** infusing.

$$\frac{\text{units}}{\text{hr}} = \frac{10{,}000 \text{ units}}{500 \text{ mL}} \times \frac{40 \text{ mL}}{1 \text{ hr}}$$

$$\frac{\text{units}}{\text{hr}} = \frac{10{,}000 \text{ units}}{500 \text{ mL}} \times \frac{40 \text{ mL}}{1 \text{ hr}} = \textbf{800 units/hr}$$

A 500 mL solution containing 10,000 units heparin running at 40 mL/hr is infusing 800 units/hr.

PROBLEMS 15-3

Calculate the units/hr of heparin infusing in the IV administrations.

1. An IV of 750 mL containing 30,000 units heparin running at 25 mL/hr _____

2. A solution of 20,000 units in 500 mL running at 30 mL/hr _____

3. A 1 L volume of D5W containing heparin 30,000 units running at 40 mL/hr _____

4. An IV of 1 L DNS containing 20,000 units heparin running at 30 mL/hr. _____

5. A 25,000 units heparin in a 500 mL solution running at 30 mL/hr _____

6. An IV of 1000 mL containing 40,000 units heparin running at 25 mL/hr _____

7. A 1000 mL solution with 45,000 units heparin running at 25 mL/hr _____

8. A solution of 1000 mL containing 25,000 units heparin running at 30 mL/hr _____

9. A 1 L solution with 35,000 units heparin running at 45 mL/hr _____

10. A 20,000 units in 500 mL solution running at 20 mL/hr _____

Answers 1. 1000 units/hr   **2.** 1200 units/hr   **3.** 1200 units/hr   **4.** 600 units/hr   **5.** 1500 units/hr   **6.** 1000 units/hr   **7.** 1125 units/hr   **8.** 750 units/hr   **9.** 1575 units/hr   **10.** 800 units/hr

HEPARIN FLUSH DOSAGE

Heparin flush solutions used to maintain patent (open) indwelling IV infusion ports come in **two dosage strengths: 10 units/mL and 100 units/mL. Misreading heparin labels can be life-threatening**. Too large a dosage used for a flush will cause systemic hemorrhage; too small a dosage added to an IV can lead to death from venous stasis and clot emboli.

> ⚷ The average IV port heparin flush dosage is 10 units, and never exceeds 100 units.

SUMMARY

This concludes the chapter on heparin administration. The important points to remember are:

- Heparin is a potent anticoagulant that is frequently added to IV solutions. It is measured in USP units.

- Heparin therapy requires a frequent check of coagulation times.

- Subcutaneous heparin injections are given deep subcutaneously at a 45° angle in an attempt to reduce medication leakage through the injection tract.

- Heparin injection sites are never massaged.

- IV heparin may be ordered by mL/hr flow rate or by units/hr to infuse.

- An EID or microdrip is used for heparin infusion.

- Commercially prepared IV heparin solutions are available in several strengths.

- Additional IV solution strengths may require the preparation of heparin from available 1000 to 50,000 units/mL vial strengths.

- Frequent blood tests for clotting time are required to monitor heparin dosage.

- Heparin IV port flushes never exceed 100 units.

SUMMARY SELF-TEST

Calculate the mL/hr heparin flow rates.

1. An adult is to receive heparin 1000 units/hr. The IV solution available has 25,000 units in 1 L D5W, and a pump will be used.   _____

2. A solution of 35,000 units heparin in 1 L D5W is to infuse via volumetric pump at 1200 units/hr.   _____

3. The order is for 1000 units heparin per hour. The solution strength is 20,000 units in 500 mL D5NS.   _____

4. The order is for 1250 units/hr heparin from a solution strength of 15,000 units in 500 mL D5W. A pump is used to monitor the infusion.   _____

5. A solution of 10,000 units heparin in 500 mL D5W is ordered to infuse at 1000 units/hr.   _____

6. An IV of 1000 mL D5W with 40,000 units heparin is to infuse at 1200 units/hr via a pump.   _____

7. The order is to infuse 500 mL D5W with 25,000 units heparin at 1500 units/hr.   _____

8. 500 mL D5W with 30,000 units of heparin is to infuse via a pump at 1500 units/hr.   _____

9. The order is to infuse 1 L D5W with 45,000 units of heparin at 1875 units/hr.   _____

10. A rate of 500 units/hr is ordered using a 250 mL with 10,000 units IV solution.   _____

11. A solution of 40,000 units in 1000 mL is to be used to infuse 1500 units/hr.   _____

12. A rate of 1500 units/hr is ordered using a 30,000 units in 500 mL solution.   _____

13. Heparin 750 units/hr is ordered using an IV solution of 500 mL containing 5000 units heparin.   _____

14. An IV solution of 10,000 units in 1000 mL heparin is to infuse 500 units/hr.   _____

15. Heparin 1500 units per hour is to be infused using a solution strength of 15,000 units in 500 mL.   _____

Answers

1. 40 mL/hr	5. 50 mL/hr	9. 41.6 or 42 mL/hr	13. 75 mL/hr
2. 34 mL/hr	6. 30 mL/hr	10. 12.5 or 13 mL/hr	14. 50 mL/hr
3. 25 mL/hr	7. 30 mL/hr	11. 37.5 or 38 mL/hr	15. 50 mL/hr
4. 41.6 or 42 mL/hr	8. 25 mL/hr	12. 25 mL/hr	

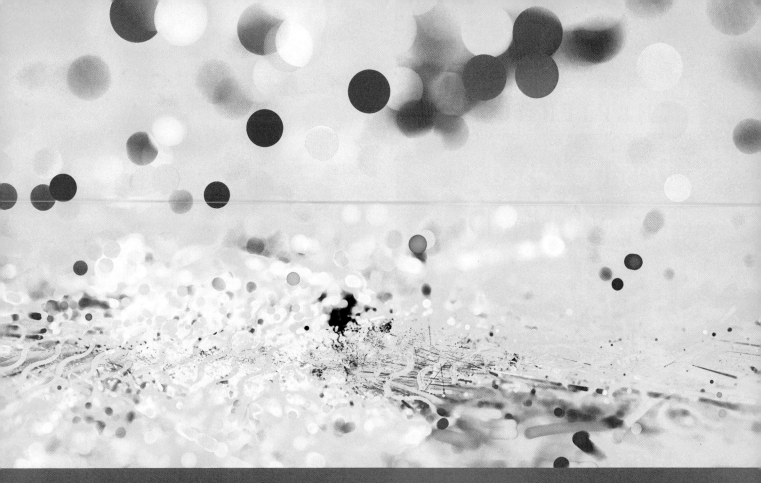

SECTION 7

Dosage Based on Body Weight and Body Surface Area

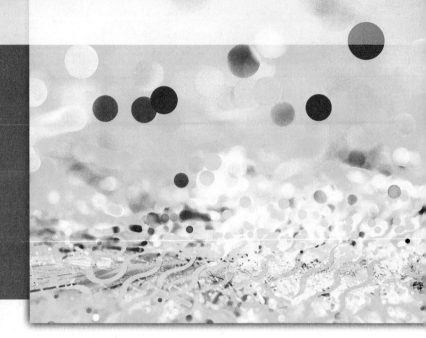

CHAPTER 16

Dosage Based on Body Weight

OBJECTIVES

The learner will:

1. Convert body weight from lb to kg.

2. Convert body weight from kg to lb.

3. Calculate dosages using mcg/mg per kg or mcg/mg per lb.

4. Determine if dosages ordered are within the normal range.

INTRODUCTION

For **adults**, weight is usually measured in **pounds**. For **infants and neonates**, whose ability to metabolize drugs is not fully developed, it is recorded in **kilograms**. To provide an **accurate comparison of changes in weight** in clinical settings, patients' weights are **recorded first thing in the morning, before breakfast**.

🔑 Ordering medications is the responsibility of the physician, and it is often based on body weight.

Individualized dosages may be calculated in terms of mcg or mg per kg or lb per day. The total daily dosage may be administered in divided (more than one) dosages—for example, every 6 hours or every 8 hours.

Familiarity with average dosages is often acquired by staff nurses in clinical specialties, allowing them to **recognize physician or transcription errors** in dosages ordered. However, the **ability to recognize the accuracy of dosages ordered** is beyond the expectations for students, or in fact, for staff nurses.

Day-to-day patient dosages in clinical settings are increasingly prepared by hospital pharmacologists. The **nursing role** in administration is to carefully follow the medication records to **make sure ordered drugs are given and charted on time**, with reporting and charting of an **unusual patient response**, if any is noted.

All of the steps involved in calculating dosages based on body weight **are included** in this chapter, in case your instructor feels it is appropriate to assign them at this time.

CONVERTING lb TO kg

If body weight is recorded in lb, but the drug literature lists dosage per kg, a conversion from lb to kg will be necessary. There are 2.2 lb in 1 kg. This means that **kg body weights are smaller than lb weights**, so **the conversion from lb to kg is made by dividing body weight by 2.2**. For ease of calculation, fractional lb may be converted to the nearest quarter and written as decimal fractions instead of oz: ¼ lb (4 oz) as 0.25, ½ lb (8 oz) as 0.5, and ¾ lb (12 oz) as 0.75. If this kind of accuracy is critical, the prescribing orders should so indicate.

EXAMPLE 1

A child weighs 41 lb 12 oz. Convert to kg.

$$41 \text{ lb } 12 \text{ oz} = 41.75 \div 2.2 = 18.97 = \textbf{19 kg}$$

The kg weight should be a smaller number than 41.75 because you are dividing, and 19 kg is.

EXAMPLE 2

Convert the weight of a 144½ lb adult to kg.

$$144\frac{1}{2} \text{ lb} = 144.5 \div 2.2 = 65.68 = \textbf{65.7 kg}$$

EXAMPLE 3

Convert the weight of a 27¼ lb child to kg.

$$27\frac{1}{4} \text{ lb} = 27.25 \div 2.2 = 12.38 = \textbf{12.4 kg}$$

PROBLEMS 16-1

Convert these body weights. Round to the nearest tenth kg.

1. 58¾ lb   = _____ kg

2. 63½ lb   = _____ kg

3. 163¼ lb   = _____ kg

4. 39¾ lb   = _____ kg

5. 100¼ lb   = _____ kg

6. 134½ lb   = _____ kg

7. 112¾ lb   = _____ kg

8. 73¼ lb   = _____ kg

9. 121½ lb   = _____ kg

10. 92¾ lb   = _____ kg

Answers **1.** 26.7 kg   **2.** 28.9 kg   **3.** 74.2 kg   **4.** 18.1 kg   **5.** 45.6 kg   **6.** 61.1 kg   **7.** 51.3 kg   **8.** 33.3 kg
9. 55.2 kg   **10.** 42.2 kg

CONVERTING kg TO lb

There are 2.2 lb in 1 kg. To convert from kg to lb, **multiply by 2.2**. Because you are multiplying, **the answer in lb will be larger than the kg** being converted. Express weight to the nearest tenth lb.

EXAMPLE 1

A child weighs 23.3 kg. Convert to lb.

$$23.3 \text{ kg} = 23.3 \times 2.2 = 51.26 = \textbf{51.3 lb}$$

The answer must be larger because you are multiplying, and it is.

EXAMPLE 2

Convert an adult weight of 73.4 kg to lb.

$$73.4 \text{ kg} = 73.4 \times 2.2 = 161.48 = \textbf{161.5 lb}$$

EXAMPLE 3

Convert the weight of a 14.2 kg child to lb.

$$14.2 \text{ kg} = 14.2 \times 2.2 = 31.24 = \textbf{31.2 lb}$$

PROBLEMS 16-2

Convert kg to lb. Round to the nearest tenth lb.

1. 21.3 kg   = _____ lb

2. 99.2 kg   = _____ lb

3. 28.7 kg   = _____ lb

4. 71.4 kg   = _____ lb

5. 30.8 kg   = _____ lb

6. 43.7 kg   = _____ lb

7. 63.8 kg   = _____ lb

8. 57.1 kg   = _____ lb

9. 84.2 kg   = _____ lb

10. 34.9 kg   = _____ lb

Answers 1. 46.9 lb   **2.** 218.2 lb   **3.** 63.1 lb   **4.** 157.1 lb   **5.** 67.8 lb   **6.** 96.1 lb   **7.** 140.4 lb   **8.** 125.6 lb **9.** 185.2 lb   **10.** 76.8 lb

CALCULATING DOSAGES FROM DRUG LABEL INFORMATION

Information you will need to calculate dosages from body weight will be on the actual drug label or on the drug package insert.

Calculating the dosage is a two-step procedure. First, calculate the **total daily dosage**. Then, **divide by the number of doses per day** to obtain the actual dose administered at one time.

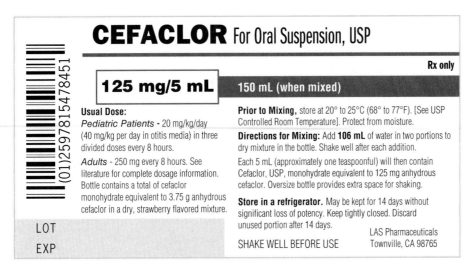

Figure 16-1

Let's start by looking at some oral antibiotic labels that contain the mg/kg/day dosage guidelines.

EXAMPLE 1

Refer to the information written on the left of the sample antibiotic label in **Figure 16-1** for children's dosages. Notice that the dosage is **20 mg/kg/day (or 40 mg/kg/day in otitis media)**. This dosage is to be given in **divided doses every 8 hours**—or a total of 3 doses (24 hr ÷ 8 hr = 3 doses).

Once you have located the dosage information, you can move ahead and calculate the dosage. Let's assume you are checking the dosage ordered for an **18.2 kg** child. Start by calculating the **recommended daily dosage range**.

Lower daily dosage = 20 mg/kg

20 mg × 18.2 kg (weight of child) = **364 mg/day**

Upper daily dosage = 40 mg/kg

40 mg × 18.2 kg = **728 mg/day**

The recommended range for this 18.2 kg child is 364–728 mg/day.

The drug is to be given in three divided doses.

Lower dosage: 364 mg ÷ 3 = **121 mg per dose**

Upper dosage: 728 mg ÷ 3 = **243 mg per dose**

The per-dose dosage range is 121 mg to 243 mg per dose every 8 hours.

Now that you have the dosage range for this child, you are able to assess the accuracy of physician orders. Let's look at some orders and see how you can use the dosage range you just calculated.

1. **If the order is to give 125 mg every 8 hours, is this within the recommended dosage range?**
   Yes, 125 mg is within the average range of 121–243 mg per dose.

2. **If the order is to give 375 mg every 8 hours, is this within the recommended dosage range?**
   No, this is an overdosage. The maximum recommended dosage is 243 mg per dose. The 375 mg dose should not be given; the prescriber must be called and the order questioned.

3. **If the order is for 75 mg every 8 hours, is this an accurate dosage?**
   The recommended lower limit for an 18.2 kg child is 121 mg. Although 75 mg might be **safe**, it will probably be **ineffective**. Notify the prescriber that the dosage appears to be too low.

4. **If the order is for 250 mg every 8 hours, is this accurate?**
Because 243 mg per dose is the recommended upper limit, 250 mg is essentially within the normal range. The drug strength is 125 mg per 5 mL, and a 250 mg dosage is 10 mL. The prescriber has probably ordered this dosage based on the available dosage strength and for ease of preparation.

5. **If the dosage ordered is 125 mg every 4 hours, is this an accurate dosage?**
In this order, the **frequency of administration** does not match the recommended dosage of every 8 hours. The total daily dosage of 750 mg (125 mg × 6 doses = 750 mg) is slightly, but not significantly, higher than the 728 mg maximum. There may be a reason the prescriber ordered the dosage every 4 hours, but call to verify it.

> 🔑 To determine the safety of an ordered dosage, use body weight to calculate the dosage range ordered, and compare this with the recommended dosage range in mg/kg/day (or mg/lb/day). Assessment must also include the frequency of dosage ordered.

The difference between 4 mg and 6 mg is much more critical than the difference between 243 mg and 250 mg because the drug potency is obviously greater.

Additional factors to consider include the patient's age, weight, and medical condition. Although these factors cannot be dealt with at length, keep in mind that **the younger, the older, or the more compromised by illness an individual is, the more critical a discrepancy is likely to be**.

Discrepancies in dosages are much more significant if the number of mg or mcg ordered is small.

CALCULATING DOSAGES FROM DRUG LITERATURE

Parenteral labels are very small, and very few contain suggested dosage ranges. To obtain these dosages, you will have to refer to the **drug package inserts**, the *Physicians' Desk Reference* (*PDR*), or **similar references**. These references will contain extensive details about each drug's chemistry, actions, adverse reactions, recommended administration, and so on, so it will be necessary for you to search for and select the information you need under the heading **Dosage and Administration**. In the following exercises, the searching has been done for you, and only those excerpts necessary for your calculations are shown.

PROBLEMS 16-3

Refer to the cefazolin package insert in **Figure 16-2** to locate the information for pediatric dosages.

1. What is the dosage range in mg/kg/day for mild-to-moderate infections? _____

2. What is the dosage range for mild-to-moderate infections in mg/lb/day? _____

3. The total dosage will be divided into how many doses per day? _____

4. In severe infections, what is the maximum daily dosage recommended in mg/kg? _____

   In mg/lb? _____

CEFAZOLIN SODIUM

FOR INJECTION, USP

PEDIATRIC DOSAGE

In pediatric patients, a total daily dosage of 25
to 50 mg per kg (approximately 10 to 20 mg per
pound) of body weight, divided into 3 or 4 equal
doses, is effective for most mild to moderately
severe infections. Total daily dosage may be
increased to 100 mg per kg (45 mg per pound) of
body weight for severe infections. Since safety for
use in premature infants and in neonates has not
been established, the use of Cefazolin for Injection
in these patients is not recommended.

Figure 16-2

Information from DailyMed; National Institutes of Health.

Answers 1. 25–50 mg   **2.** 10–20 mg   **3.** 3–4 doses per day   **4.** 100 mg/kg; 45 mg/lb

---

PROBLEMS 16-4

Use the information you just obtained from Figure 16-2 to do the calculations for a child
who weighs 35 lb and has a moderately severe infection.

1. What is the lower daily dosage range? _____

2. What is the upper daily dosage range? _____

3. If the medication is given in 4 divided dosages, what will the
   per-dosage range be? _____

4. If a dosage of 125 mg is ordered every 6 hours, will you need to
   question it? _____

Answers 1. 350 mg/day   **2.** 700 mg/day   **3.** 87.5 mg to 175 mg per dose   **4.** No; within normal range

SUMMARY

This concludes the chapter on calculation and assessment of dosages based on body weight. The
important points to remember from this chapter are:

- Dosages are frequently ordered on the basis of weight, especially for children.

- Dosages may be recommended based on mcg or mg per kg or lb per day, usually administered
  in divided doses.

- Body weight may need to be converted from kg to lb or lb to kg to correlate with dosage
  recommendations.

- To convert lb to kg, divide by 2.2; to convert kg to lb, multiply by 2.2.

- Calculating dosage is a two-step procedure: (1) Calculate the total daily dosage for the weight
  then (2) divide by the number of doses to be administered.

- To check the accuracy of a prescriber's order, calculate the correct dosage and compare it with the dosage ordered.

- Dosage discrepancies are much more critical if the dosage range is low, such as 2–5 mg, as opposed to high, such as 250–500 mg.

- Factors that make discrepancies particularly serious include age, low body weight, and severity of medical condition.

- If the drug label does not contain all the necessary information for safe administration, additional information should be obtained from drug package inserts, the *PDR*, drug formularies, or the hospital pharmacist.

SUMMARY SELF-TEST

Read the dosage labels and literature provided to answer the questions.

1. A 43 lb child has an order for oral cefaclor. What is the daily dosage for this child?   _____

2. What is the per-dose dosage?   _____

3. Is an order for 250 mg of cefaclor every 8 hours correct for this child?   _____

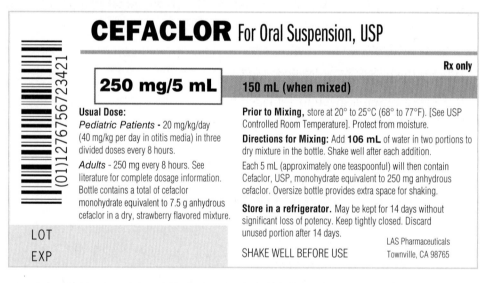

4. Refer to the penicillin V potassium oral solution label and identify the dosage strength in mg.   _____

5. What is the dosage strength in units?   _____

6. This medication is shipped in powdered form. How much diluent is needed for reconstitution?   _____

7. What kind of diluent?   _____

8. What dosage in mg/kg/day is specified for pediatric patients?   _____

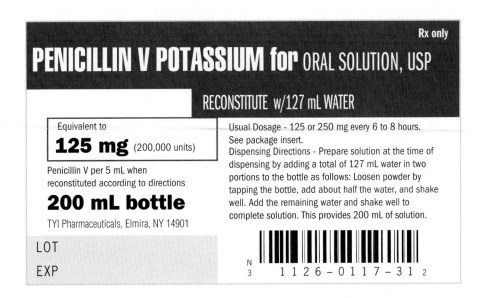

9. Cefaclor oral suspension has been ordered for a child weighing 100 lb.
   Calculate the daily dose. _____

10. What will the per-dose dosage be? _____

11. Would a 5 mL dosage every 8 hours be reasonable for this child? _____

12. How is this oral cefaclor suspension to be reconstituted? _____

13. What precautions did you learn about pouring and administering
    suspensions such as cefaclor? _____

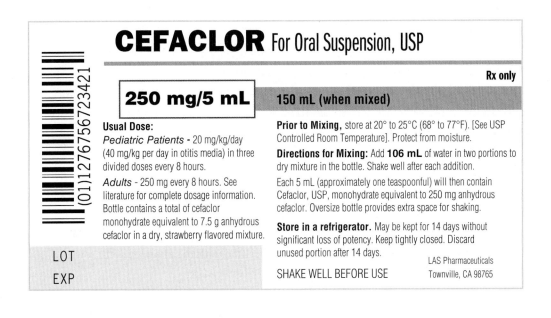

14. Refer to the acyclovir sodium injection insert to locate the adult and adolescent dosages in mg/kg.   _____

15. What will the dosage be per dose for an adult with mucosal herpes simplex who weighs 61.4 kg?   _____

16. What would the dosage be for an adolescent with herpes simplex encephalitis who weighs 180 lb?   _____

17. What mg/kg dosage is recommended for an infant with herpes simplex encephalitis?   _____

18. Read the literature to locate the time period recommended for intravenous infusion.   _____

19. There are bold print precautions regarding parenteral administration on this insert. What are they?   _____

ACYCLOVIR SODIUM

FOR INJECTION, USP

DOSAGE AND ADMINISTRATION

CAUTION—RAPID OR BOLUS INTRAVENOUS INJECTION MUST BE AVOIDED (see WARNINGS and PRECAUTIONS**).**

INTRAMUSCULAR OR SUBCUTANEOUS INJECTION MUST BE AVOIDED (see WARNINGS**).**

Therapy should be initiated as early as possible following onset of signs and symptoms of herpes infections. A maximum dose equivalent to 20 mg/kg every 8 hours should not be exceeded for any patient.

DOSAGE IN HERPES SIMPLEX INFECTION:

Mucosal and Cutaneous Herpes Simplex (HSV-1 and HSV-2) Infections in Immunocompromised Patients

Adults and Adolescents (12 years of age and older): 5 mg/kg infused at a constant rate over 1 hour, every 8 hours for 7 days.

Pediatrics (Under 12 years of age): 10 mg/kg infused at a constant rate over 1 hour, every 8 hours for 7 days.

DOSAGE IN SEVERE INITIAL CLINICAL EPISODES OF HERPES GENITALIS:

Adults and Adolescents (12 years of age and older): 5 mg/kg infused at a constant rate over 1 hour, every 8 hours for 5 days.

DOSAGE IN HERPES SIMPLEX ENCEPHALITIS:

Adults and Adolescents (12 years of age and older): 10 mg/kg infused at a constant rate over 1 hour, every 8 hours for 10 days.

Pediatrics (3 months to 12 years of age): 20 mg/kg infused at a constant rate over 1 hour, every 8 hours for 10 days.

Neonatal Herpes Simplex Virus Infections (Birth to 3 months): 10 mg/kg infused at a constant rate over 1 hour, every 8 hours for 10 days. In neonatal herpes simplex infections, doses of 15 mg/kg or 20 mg/kg (infused at a constant rate over 1 hour every 8 hours) have been used; the safety and efficacy of these doses are not known.

Information from DailyMed; National Institutes of Health.

---

20. Refer to the voriconazole package insert information to locate the IV maintenance dosage in mg/kg every 12 hours (written with the abbreviation q12h, now slated for deletion) for invasive aspergillosis.   _____

21. What would the daily IV dosage be for an individual weighing 92.7 kg?   _____

22. What would the daily oral dosage be for this same 92.7 kg individual? _____

23. What will a single IV maintenance dosage be for the same 92.7 kg individual? _____

24. Locate the voriconazole information on the maximum rate of administration for intravenous administration. _____

25. There is a bold type and capitalized warning for IV administration of voriconazole on this insert. What is it? _____

VORICONAZOLE

FOR INJECTION, USP

DOSAGE AND ADMINISTRATION

Voriconazole for injection requires reconstitution to 10 mg/mL and subsequent dilution to 5 mg/mL or less prior to administration as an infusion, at a maximum rate of 3 mg/kg per hour over 1 to 2 hours.

Infection	Loading dose IV	Maintenance Dose IV	Oral
Invasive Aspergillosis	6 mg/kg q12h for the first 24 hours	4 mg/kg q12h	200 mg q12h
Candidemia in non-neutropenic patients and other deep tissue *Candida* infections	6 mg/kg q12h for the first 24 hours	3 to 4 mg/kg q12h	200 mg q12h
Esophageal Candidiasis	N/A	N/A	200 mg q12h
Scedosporiosis and Fusariosis	6 mg/kg q12h for the first 24 hours	4 mg/kg q12h	200 mg q12h

DO NOT ADMINISTER AS AN IV BOLUS INJECTION.

Information from DailyMed; National Institutes of Health.

---

26. Refer to the fluconazole injection insert to locate the first-day dosage for a child with esophageal candidiasis. _____

27. What is the dosage recommendation for subsequent days? _____

28. How long must treatment for this condition be continued? _____

29. What will the first dose be for a child weighing 18.2 kg? _____

30. What will the subsequent dosage be for this same 18.2 kg child? _____

31. How often will this dosage be administered? _____

32. What is the maximum mg/kg dosage recommended if the child has a particularly severe infection? _____

33. What would the first dose of fluconazole be for a child weighing 72 lb? _____

FLUCONAZOLE INJECTION
FOR INTRAVENOUS INFUSION ONLY

DOSAGE AND ADMINISTRATION IN CHILDREN

The following dose equivalency scheme should generally provide equivalent exposure in pediatric and adult patients:

Pediatric Patients	Adults
3 mg/kg	100 mg
6 mg/kg	200 mg
12 * mg/kg	400 mg

*Some older children may have clearances similar to that of adults. Absolute doses exceeding 600 mg/day are not recommended. Experience with fluconazole in neonates is limited to pharmacokinetic studies in premature newborns. (See CLINICAL PHARMACOLOGY.) Based on the prolonged half-life seen in premature newborns (gestational age 26 to 29 weeks), these children, in the first two weeks of life, should receive the same dosage (mg/kg) as in older children, but administered every 72 hours. After the first two weeks, these children should be dosed once daily. No information regarding fluconazole pharmacokinetics in full-term newborns is available.

Oropharyngeal candidiasis: The recommended dosage of fluconazole for oropharyngeal candidiasis in children is 6 mg/kg on the first day, followed by 3 mg/kg once daily. Treatment should be administered for at least 2 weeks to decrease the likelihood of relapse.

Esophageal candidiasis: For the treatment of esophageal candidiasis, the recommended dosage of fluconazole in children is 6 mg/kg on the first day, followed by 3 mg/kg once daily. Doses up to 12 mg/kg/day may be used based on medical judgment of the patient's response to therapy. Patients with esophageal candidiasis should be treated for a minimum of three weeks and for at least 2 weeks following the resolution of symptoms.

Systemic Candida infections: For the treatment of candidemia and disseminated Candida infections, daily doses of 6 to 12 mg/kg/day have been used in an open, noncomparative study of a small number of children.

Cryptococcal meningitis: For the treatment of acute cryptococcal meningitis, the recommended dosage is 12 mg/kg on the first day, followed by 6 mg/kg once daily. A dosage of 12 mg/kg once daily may be used, based on medical judgment of the patient's response to therapy. The recommended duration of treatment for initial therapy of cryptococcal meningitis is 10 to 12 weeks after the cerebrospinal fluid becomes culture negative. For suppression of relapse of cryptococcal meningitis in children with AIDS, the recommended dose of Fluconazole Injection is 6 mg/kg once daily.

Information from DailyMed; National Institutes of Health.

Answers

1. 390 mg
2. 130 mg/dose
3. no, too high
4. 125 mg/5 mL
5. 200,000 units/5 mL
6. 127 mL
7. water
8. 125 or 250 mg every 6–8 hours
9. 910 mg/day
10. 303 mg/dose
11. yes
12. Add 106 mL water in 2 portions. Shake well after each addition until mixed.
13. Shake well to mix completely before pouring; administer immediately to prevent settling out.
14. 5 mg/kg
15. 307 mg
16. 818 mg
17. 20 mg/kg
18. 1 hour
19. no rapid or bolus injection; no intramuscular or subcutaneous injection
20. 4 mg/kg
21. 742 mg daily
22. 400 mg daily
23. 371 mg/dose
24. 3 mg/kg per hour over 1–2 hours
25. not for IV bolus injection
26. 6 mg/kg
27. 3 mg/kg
28. minimum of 3 weeks and at least 2 weeks following resolution of symptoms
29. 109 mg
30. 55 mg
31. once daily
32. 12 mg/kg/day
33. 196 mg

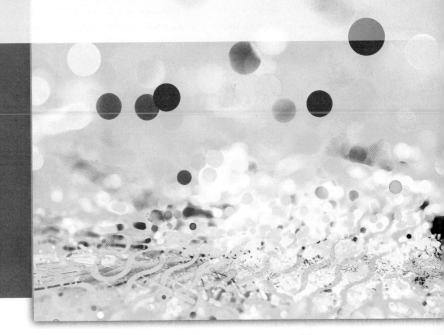

CHAPTER 17

Dosage Based on Body Surface Area (BSA)

OBJECTIVES

The learner will:

1. Recognize that body surface area (BSA) is calculated using formulas for weight and height.

2. Use BSA to calculate dosage.

3. Assess the accuracy of dosages prescribed using BSA.

INTRODUCTION

Body surface area (BSA or SA) is a major factor in calculating dosages for a number of drugs, because **many of the body's physiologic processes are more closely related to body surface than they are to weight alone**. Body surface is used extensively to calculate dosages of antineoplastic agents for cancer chemotherapy, and for patients with severe burns. However, an increasing number of other drugs is also calculated using BSA.

> ⚷ Ordering medications based on BSA is the responsibility of the physician, often determined in consultation with clinical pharmacologists.

While familiarity with the accuracy of dosages may be acquired by staff nurses in clinical specialties, determining the **accuracy of dosages based on BSA** is beyond the expectations for students using this text and, in fact, for staff nurses.

At this point in your learning, it is sufficient for you to have a sense of how sophisticated BSA calculation is, because those patients' whose medications are ordered based on it are often critically ill infants or children.

The complete "how to do" set of BSA calculations is included in this text for optional assignment by your instructor. It will also be an excellent library reference should you need to return to this information in your graduate career.

Body surface is calculated in **square meters (m²)** using the patient's **weight and height** and a calculator that has **square root** ($\sqrt{\ }$) capabilities. Two formulas are used by physicians and pharmacists: one using kg and cm measurements, and another using lb (pound) and in. (inch) measurements. We'll look at these separately.

CALCULATING BSA FROM kg AND cm

The safest way to calculate BSA is by using a time-tested formula with kilogram and centimeter measurements:

$$\text{BSA} = \sqrt{\frac{\text{wt (kg)} \times \text{ht (cm)}}{3600}}$$

EXAMPLE 1

Calculate the BSA of a man who weighs **104 kg** and whose height is **191 cm**. Express BSA to the nearest hundredth.

$$\sqrt{\frac{104 \text{ (kg)} \times 191 \text{ (cm)}}{3600}}$$
$$= \sqrt{5.517}$$
$$= 2.348 = \mathbf{2.35 \ m^2}$$

Calculators vary in the way a square root must be obtained. Here is how the BSA was calculated in this example and throughout the chapter:

$$104. \times 191. \div 3600. = 5.517, \text{ then immediately enter } \sqrt{\ }$$

Practice with your own calculator to determine how to calculate a square root. Be careful to **insert periods after all whole numbers** or you may obtain a wrong answer from preset decimal placement.

The m² BSA is rounded to hundredths. Answers may vary slightly depending on how your calculator is set. Consider answers within 2–3 hundredths to be correct. Fractional weights and heights are also used in calculations. Refer to Examples 2 and 3.

EXAMPLE 2

Calculate the BSA of an adolescent who weighs **59.1 kg** and is **157.5 cm** in height. Express BSA to the nearest hundredth.

$$\sqrt{\frac{59.1 \text{ (kg)} \times 157.5 \text{ (cm)}}{3600}}$$
$$= \sqrt{2.585}$$
$$= 1.607 = \mathbf{1.61 \ m^2}$$

EXAMPLE 3

A child is **96.2 cm** tall and weighs **15.17 kg**. What is his BSA in m² to the nearest hundredth?

$$\sqrt{\frac{15.17 \text{ (kg)} \times 96.2 \text{ (cm)}}{3600}}$$
$$= \sqrt{0.4053}$$
$$= 0.636 = \mathbf{0.63 \ m^2}$$

PROBLEMS 17-1

Calculate the BSA in m². Express answers to the nearest hundredth.

1. An adult weighing 59 kg whose height is 160 cm _____

2. A child weighing 35.9 kg whose height is 63.5 cm _____

3. A child weighing 7.7 kg whose height is 40 cm _____

4. An adult weighing 92 kg whose height is 178 cm _____

5. A child weighing 46 kg whose height is 102 cm _____

Answers **1.** 1.62 m²   **2.** 0.8 m²   **3.** 0.29 m²   **4.** 2.13 m²   **5.** 1.14 m²

CALCULATING BSA FROM lb AND in

The formula for calculating BSA from lb and in. measurements is equally easy to use. **The only difference is the denominator, which is 3131**.

$$\text{BSA} = \sqrt{\frac{\text{wt (lb)} \times \text{ht (in.)}}{3131}}$$

EXAMPLE 1

Calculate BSA to the nearest hundredth for a child who is **24 in**. tall and weighs **34 lb**.

$$\sqrt{\frac{34 \text{ (lb)} \times 24 \text{ (in.)}}{3131}}$$
$$= \sqrt{0.260}$$
$$= 0.510 = \mathbf{0.51 \ m^2}$$

EXAMPLE 2

Calculate BSA to the nearest hundredth for an adult who is **61.3 in**. tall and weighs **142.7 lb**.

$$\sqrt{\frac{142.7 \text{ (lb)} \times 61.3 \text{ (in.)}}{3131}}$$
$$= \sqrt{2.793}$$
$$= 1.671 = \mathbf{1.67 \ m^2}$$

EXAMPLE 3

A child weighs **105 lb** and is **51 in**. tall. Calculate BSA to the nearest hundredth.

$$\sqrt{\frac{105 \text{ (lb)} \times 51 \text{ (in.)}}{3131}}$$
$$= \sqrt{1.710}$$
$$= 1.307 = \mathbf{1.31 \ m^2}$$

PROBLEMS 17-2

Determine the BSA. Express answers to the nearest hundredth.

1. A child weighing 92 lb who measures 35 in. _____

2. An adult who weighs 175 lb and who is 67 in. tall _____

3. An adult who is 70 in. tall and weighs 194 lb _____

4. A child who weighs 72.4 lb and is 40.5 in. tall _____

5. A child who measures 26 in. and weighs 36 lb _____

Answers **1.** $1.01\ m^2$ **2.** $1.94\ m^2$ **3.** $2.08\ m^2$ **4.** $0.97\ m^2$ **5.** $0.55\ m^2$

DOSAGE CALCULATIONS BASED ON BSA

Once you know the BSA in m^2, dosage calculation involves only straight multiplication.

EXAMPLE 1

The dosage recommended is **5 mg per m^2**. The child has a BSA of **1.1 m^2**.

$$1.1\ (m^2) \times 5\ mg = \textbf{5.5 mg}$$

EXAMPLE 2

The recommended child's dosage is 25–50 mg/m^2. The child has a BSA of **0.76 m^2**.

Lower dosage: 0.76 $(m^2) \times 25\ mg = 19\ mg$
Upper dosage: 0.76 $(m^2) \times 50\ mg = 38\ mg$
The dosage range is 19–38 mg

PROBLEMS 17-3

Determine the dosage for the following drugs. Express answers to the nearest whole number.

1. The recommended child's dosage is 5–10 mg/m^2.
   The BSA is 0.43 m^2. _____

2. A child with a BSA of 0.81 m^2 is to receive a drug with a
   recommended dosage of 40 mg/m^2. _____

3. Calculate the recommended dosage of 20 mg/m^2 for a child with
   a BSA of 0.51 m^2. _____

4. An adult is to receive a drug with a recommended dosage of
   20–40 $units/m^2$. The BSA is 1.93 m^2. _____

5. The adult recommended dosage is 3–5 mg/m^2.
   Calculate dosage for 2.08 m^2. _____

Answers **1.** 2–4 mg **2.** 32 mg **3.** 10 mg **4.** 39–77 units **5.** 6–10 mg

ASSESSING ORDERS BASED ON BSA

In situations where you have to check a dosage against m² recommendations, you will be referring to drug package inserts, medication protocols, or the *Physicians' Desk Reference (PDR)* to determine what the dosage should be.

EXAMPLE 1

Refer to the vinblastine information insert in **Figure 17-1** and calculate the **first dose** for an adult whose BSA is **1.66 m²**. Calculations are to the nearest whole number.

Recommended first dose $= 3.7$ mg/m²

1.66 (m²) $\times 3.7$ mg $= 6.14 = $ **6 mg**

STERILE VINBLASTINE SULFATE

FOR INJECTION, USP

DOSAGE AND ADMINISTRATION

Caution—It is extremely important that the intravenous needle or catheter be properly positioned before any vinblastine sulfate is injected. Leakage into surrounding tissue during intravenous administration of vinblastine sulfate may cause considerable irritation. If extravasation occurs, the injection should be discontinued immediately and any remaining portion of the dose should then be introduced into another vein. Local injection of hyaluronidase and the application of moderate heat to the area of leakage will help disperse the drug and may minimize discomfort and the possibility of cellulitis.

There are variations in the depth of the leukopenic response that follows therapy with vinblastine sulfate. For this reason, it is recommended that the drug be given no more frequently than once every seven days.

It is wise to initiate therapy for adults by administering a single intravenous dose of 3.7 mg/m² of body surface area (bsa). Thereafter, white blood cell counts should be made to determine the patient's sensitivity to vinblastine sulfate.

A simplified and conservative incremental approach to dosage at weekly intervals may be outlined as follows:

	Adults	Children
First dose	3.7 mg/m² bsa	2.5 mg/m² bsa
Second dose	5.5 mg/m² bsa	3.75 mg/m² bsa
Third dose	7.4 mg/m² bsa	5 mg/m² bsa
Fourth dose	9.25 mg/m² bsa	6.25 mg/m² bsa
Fifth dose	11.1 mg/m² bsa	7.5 mg/m² bsa

The above-mentioned increases may be used until a maximum dose not exceeding 18.5 mg/m² bsa for adults is reached. The dose should not be increased after that dose which reduces the white cell count to approximately 3,000 cells/mm³. In some adults, 3.7 mg/m² bsa may produce this leukopenia; other adults may require more than 11.1 mg/m² bsa; and, very rarely, as much as 18.5 mg/m² bsa may be necessary. For most adult patients, however, the weekly dosage will prove to be 5.5 to 7.4 mg/m² bsa.

Figure 17-1

Information from DailyMed; National Institutes of Health.

EXAMPLE 2

A child with a BSA of 0.96 m^2 is to receive her **fourth dose** of vinblastine.

Recommended fourth dose = 6.25 mg/m^2

0.96 (m^2) × 6.25 mg = **6 mg**

PROBLEMS 17-4

Calculate the following dosages of vinblastine to the nearest whole number from the information available in Figure 17-1.

1. Calculate the dosage for an adult's third dose. The patient's BSA is 1.91 m^2. _____

2. Calculate the child's first dose for a patient with a BSA of 1.2 m^2. _____

3. Calculate the adult's fifth dose. The BSA is 1.53 m^2. _____

4. Calculate the child's second dose for a BSA of 1.01 m^2. _____

5. Calculate the adult's second dose for a BSA of 2.12 m^2. _____

Answers 1. 14 mg   **2.** 3 mg   **3.** 17 mg   **4.** 4 mg   **5.** 12 mg

PROBLEMS 17-5

Refer to Figure 17-2 for carmustine to locate the following information. Express all dosages to the nearest whole number.

1. What is the dosage per m^2 if the drug is to be given in a single dose? _____

2. If the patient has a BSA of 1.91 m^2, what will the daily dosage range be? _____

3. If the order for this patient is a single dosage of 325 mg, is there any need to question it? _____

4. If the dosage ordered is 450 mg, is there any need to question it? _____

CARMUSTINE

FOR INJECTION, USP

DOSAGE AND ADMINISTRATION

The recommended dose of carmustine for injection, USP as a single agent in previously untreated patients is 150 to 200 mg/m^2 intravenously every 6 weeks. Administer as a single dose or divided into daily injections such as 75 to 100 mg/m^2 on two successive days. Lower the dose when carmustine for injection, USP is used with other myelosuppressive drugs or in patients in whom bone marrow reserve is depleted. Administer carmustine for injection, USP for the duration according to the established regimen. Premedicate each dose with anti-emetics.

Figure 17-2

Information from DailyMed; National Institutes of Health.

Answers 1. 150–200 mg/m^2 **2.** 287–382 mg   **3.** No   **4.** Yes, too high

PROBLEMS 17-6

Refer to the package insert for the antineoplastic medication bleomycin in **Figure 17-3** to answer the following questions.

    1. Locate the dosage information on Hodgkin's disease and identify the dosage per m^2.   _____

    2. This insert also identifies the dosage per kg. What is this dosage?   _____

    3. Calculate the unit dosage based on m^2 for an adult with a BSA of 1.73 m^2.   _____

    4. How often is dosage recommended?   _____

BLEOMYCIN

FOR INJECTION, USP

DOSAGE AND ADMINISTRATION (HODGKIN'S DISEASE)

Because of the possibility of an anaphylactoid reaction, lymphoma patients should be treated with 2 units or less for the first 2 doses. If no acute reaction occurs, then the regular dosage schedule may be followed.

The following dose schedule is recommended:

Squamous cell carcinoma, non-Hodgkin's lymphoma, testicular carcinoma–0.25 to 0.5 units/kg (10 to 20 units/m^2) given intravenously, intramuscularly, or subcutaneously weekly or twice weekly.

Hodgkin's Disease–0.25 to 0.5 units/kg (10 to 20 units/m^2) given intravenously, intramuscularly, or subcutaneously weekly or twice weekly. After a 50% response, a maintenance dose of 1 unit daily or 5 units weekly intravenously or intramuscularly should be given.

Pulmonary toxicity of Bleomycin for Injection, USP appears to be dose-related with a striking increase when the total dose is over 400 units. Total doses over 400 units should be given with great caution.

Note: When Bleomycin for Injection, USP is used in combination with other antineoplastic agents, pulmonary toxicities may occur at lower doses.

Improvement of Hodgkin's disease and testicular tumors is prompt and noted within 2 weeks. If no improvement is seen by this time, improvement is unlikely. Squamous cell cancers respond more slowly, sometimes requiring as long as 3 weeks before any improvement is noted.

Malignant Pleural Effusion– 60 units administered as a single dose bolus intrapleural injection (see **ADMINISTRATION, INTRAPLEURAL**).

Figure 17-3

Information from DailyMed; National Institutes of Health.

Answers **1.** 10–20 units/m^2 **2.** 0.25–0.5 unit/kg   **3.** 17–35 units   **4.** Weekly or twice weekly

PROBLEMS 17-7

Refer to the mitomycin package insert information in **Figure 17-4** to answer the following questions.

    1. This preparation is a combination of two drugs. It is shipped in powdered form. How much diluent must be added to prepare a mitomycin 40 mg and mannitol 80 mg dosage strength?   _____

    2. What kind of diluent is specified?   _____

3. What dosage is required in m²? _____

4. What mitomycin dosage will be required for an individual with a BSA of 1.73 m²? _____

5. How will this be administered? _____

MITOMYCIN

FOR INJECTION, USP

DOSAGE AND ADMINISTRATION

Parenteral drug products should be inspected visually for particulate matter and discoloration prior to administration whenever solution and container permit.

Mitomycin should be given intravenously only, using care to avoid extravasation of the compound. If extravasation occurs, cellulitis, ulceration, and slough may result.

Each vial contains mitomycin 20 mg and mannitol 40 mg or mitomycin 40 mg and mannitol 80 mg. To administer, add Sterile Water for Injection, 40 mL or 80 mL respectively. Shake to dissolve. If product does not dissolve immediately, allow to stand at room temperature until solution is obtained.

After full hematological recovery (see guide to dosage adjustment) from any previous chemotherapy, the following dosage schedule may be used at 6 to 8 week intervals:

20 mg/m² intravenously as a single dose via a functioning intravenous catheter.

Because of cumulative myelosuppression, patients should be fully reevaluated after each course of mitomycin, and the dose reduced if the patient has experienced any toxicities. Doses greater than 20 mg/m² have not been shown to be more effective, and are more toxic than lower doses.

Figure 17-4

Information from DailyMed; National Institutes of Health.

Answers 1. 80 mL **2.** Sterile Water for Injection **3.** mitomycin 20 mg/m² **4.** 35 mg **5.** Intravenously as a single dose via a functioning intravenous catheter

SUMMARY

This concludes the chapter on dosage calculation based on BSA. The important points to remember from this chapter are:

- The BSA in m² is calculated from a patient's weight and height.

- BSA is more important than weight alone in calculating some drug dosages, because many physiologic processes are more closely related to surface area than they are to weight.

- BSA is calculated in square meters (m²) using a formula.

- Two formulas for calculation of BSA are available:

$$\text{Using kg and cm:} \sqrt{\frac{\text{wt (kg)} \times \text{ht (cm)}}{3600}}$$

$$\text{Using lb and in.:} \sqrt{\frac{\text{wt (lb)} \times \text{ht (in.)}}{3131}}$$

- After the BSA has been obtained, it can be used to calculate specific drug dosages and assess the accuracy of physician orders.

SUMMARY SELF-TEST

Use the formula method to calculate the following BSAs. Express m² to the nearest hundredth.

1. The weight is 58 lb and the height is 36 in.   _____

2. An adult weighing 74 kg and measuring 160 cm   _____

3. A child who is 14.2 kg and measures 64 cm   _____

4. An adult weighing 69 kg whose height is 170 cm   _____

5. An adolescent who is 55 in. and 103 lb   _____

6. A child who is 112 cm and weighs 25.3 kg   _____

7. An adult who weighs 55 kg and measures 157.5 cm   _____

8. An adult who weighs 65.4 kg and is 132 cm in height   _____

9. A child whose height is 58 in. and whose weight is 26.5 lb   _____

10. A child whose height is 60 cm and weight is 13.6 kg   _____

Read the drug insert information provided in Figure 17-5 to answer the following questions. Calculate dosages to the nearest whole number.

ANTIBIOTIC

DOSAGE AND ADMINISTRATION

DOSAGE SHOULD BE INDIVIDUALIZED ACCORDING TO THE NEEDS AND THE RESPONSE OF THE PATIENT.

Each tablet contains 4 mg of antibiotic.

PEDIATRIC PATIENTS

Age 2 to 6 years-The total daily dosage for pediatric patients may be calculated on the basis of body weight or body area using approximately 0.25 mg/kg/day or 8 mg per square meter of body surface (8 mg/m²). The usual dose is 2 mg (1/2 tablet) two or three times a day, adjusted as necessary to the size and response of the patient. The dose is not to exceed 12 mg a day.

Age 7 to 14 years-The usual dose is 4 mg (1 tablet) two or three times a day, adjusted as necessary to the size and response of the patient. The dose is not to exceed 16 mg a day.

Adults-The total daily dose for adults should not exceed 0.5 mg/kg/day.

The therapeutic range is 4 to 20 mg a day, with the majority of patients requiring 12 to 16 mg a day. An occasional patient may require as much as 32 mg a day for adequate relief. It is suggested that dosage be initiated with 4 mg (1 tablet) three times a day and adjusted according to the size and response of the patient.

Figure 17-5

Information from DailyMed; National Institutes of Health.

11. Read the information on children's dosage to calculate the daily dosage for a 6-year-old child whose BSA is 0.78 m².   _____

12. If a dosage of 4 mg is ordered for this 6-year-old child, would you question it?   _____

13. What would the daily dosage be for a 4-year-old child whose BSA is 0.29 m²?   _____

14. What would the daily dosage be for a 5-year-old child with a BSA of 0.51 m²?   _____

Refer to **Figure 17-6** to answer the following questions.

CARBOplatin

FOR INJECTION, USP

DOSAGE AND ADMINISTRATION

NOTE: Aluminum reacts with carboplatin, USP causing precipitate formation and loss of potency, therefore, needles or intravenous sets containing aluminum parts that may come in contact with the drug must not be used for the preparation or administration of carboplatin injection.

Single Agent Therapy

Carboplatin injection as a single agent, has been shown to be effective in patients with recurrent ovarian carcinoma at a dosage of 360 mg/m^2 IV on day 1 every 4 weeks (alternatively see **FORMULA DOSING**). In general, however, single intermittent courses of carboplatin injection should not be repeated until the neutrophil count is at least 2,000 and the platelet count is at least 100,000.

Combination Therapy with Cyclophosphamide

In the chemotherapy of advanced ovarian cancer, an effective combination for previously untreated patients consists of:

Carboplatin injection 300 mg/m^2 IV on day 1 every 4 weeks for 6 cycles (alternatively see **FORMULA DOSING**).

Cyclophosphamide 600 mg/m^2 IV on day 1 every 4 weeks for 6 cycles. For directions regarding the use and administration of cyclophosphamide, please refer to its package insert (see **CLINICAL STUDIES**).

Intermittent courses of carboplatin injection in combination with cyclophosphamide should not be repeated until the neutrophil count is at least 2,000 and the platelet count is at least 100,000.

Figure 17-6

Information from DailyMed; National Institutes of Health.

---

15. A patient is to be treated with the drug carboplatin for ovarian carcinoma. Her BSA is 1.61 m^2. What will her dosage be? _____

16. Another patient with ovarian cancer, who weighs 130 lb and measures 62 in., is to receive carboplatin. What is her BSA? _____

17. What dosage of carboplatin will she require? _____

18. Carboplatin is given in conjunction with cyclophosphamide. What is the recommended m^2 dosage for this drug? _____

19. Calculate the BSA of a third patient who is receiving therapy for ovarian cancer. She weighs 53.2 kg and measures 150.3 cm. _____

20. What will the companion dosage of cyclophosphamide be for this patient? _____

Answers

1. 0.82 m^2	**6.** 0.89 m^2	**11.** 6 mg per day	**16.** 1.6 m^2
2. 1.81 m^2	**7.** 1.55 m^2	**12.** Yes; too low	**17.** 576 mg
3. 0.50 m^2	**8.** 1.55 m^2	**13.** 2 mg per day	**18.** 600 mg
4. 1.81 m^2	**9.** 0.70 m^2	**14.** 4 mg	**19.** 1.49 m^2
5. 1.35 m^2	**10.** 0.48 m^2	**15.** 580 mg	**20.** 894 mg

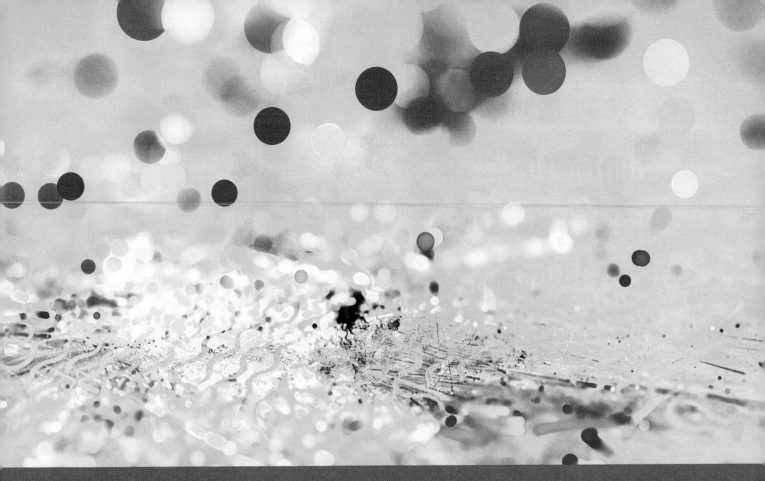

SECTION 8
Pediatric Medication Considerations

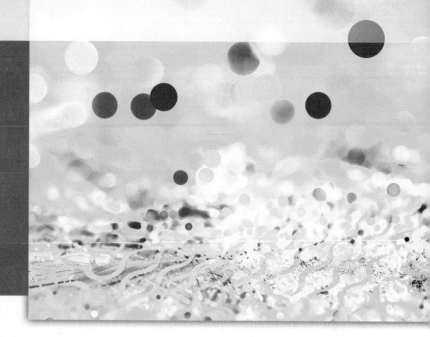

CHAPTER 18

Pediatric Oral and Parenteral Medications

OBJECTIVES

The learner will:

1. Explain how suspensions are measured and administered.

2. Calculate pediatric oral dosages.

3. List the precautions of IM and subcutaneous injection in infants and children.

4. Calculate pediatric IM and subcutaneous dosages.

INTRODUCTION

Two differences between adult and pediatric dosages are immediately apparent: **Most oral drugs are prepared as liquids** because infants and small children cannot be expected to swallow tablets easily, if at all, and **dosages are dramatically smaller**. The oral route is used whenever possible with pediatric patients, but when a child cannot swallow or the drug is ineffective given orally, drugs will be administered by a parenteral route.

Both the subcutaneous and intramuscular routes may be used depending on the type of drug to be administered. However, the smaller size of infants and children limits the use of both routes, as does the nature of the drug being used. For example, many antibiotics are administered intravenously rather than intramuscularly.

ORAL MEDICATIONS

Most oral pediatric drugs are prepared as liquids to facilitate ease in swallowing. If the child is old enough to cooperate, these dosages may be measured in a medication cup. Solutions are also frequently measured using oral syringes, such as the ones shown in **Figure 18-1**. Notice that oral syringes have the same metric calibrations as hypodermic syringes, but they may also include household measures—for example, tsp. **Oral syringes have different-sized tips** to prevent their use with hypodermic needles.

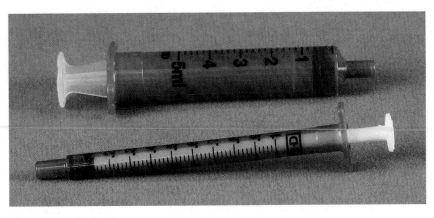

Figure 18-1 Oral syringes.

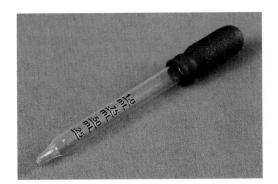

Figure 18-2 Calibrated dropper.

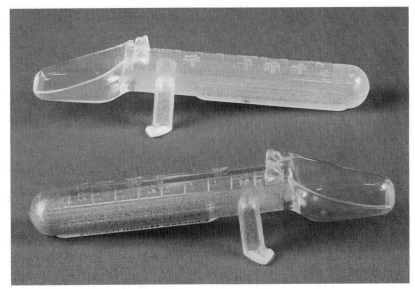

Figure 18-3 Animal-shaped measures.

On some oral syringes, the **tip is positioned off-center (*eccentric*)** to further distinguish them from hypodermic syringes, or they may be **amber-colored**, as in Figure 18-1.

If oral syringes are not available, hypodermic syringes (**without the needle**) can also be used for dosage measurement. In addition to accuracy, syringes provide an excellent method of administering oral liquid drugs to infants and small children. Some oral liquid preparations incorporate a calibrated medication dropper as an integral part of the medication bottle. These may be **calibrated in mL** like the dropper shown in **Figure 18-2** or in the **actual dosage**—for example, 25 mg or 50 mg. Animal-shaped measures such as those shown in **Figure 18-3** are also helpful in enticing reluctant toddlers to take necessary medications. In each instance, the goal is to ensure that the infant or child actually swallows the total dosage.

Care must be taken with liquid oral drugs to identify those prepared as **suspensions**. A **suspension consists of an insoluble drug in a liquid base**, as with the cefaclor oral suspension shown in **Figure 18-4**. The drug in a suspension settles to the bottom of the bottle between uses, and **thorough mixing immediately prior to pouring** is mandatory. Suspensions must also be administered to the child promptly after measurement to prevent the drug from settling out again and an incomplete dosage being administered.

⚷ Suspensions must be thoroughly mixed before measurement and promptly administered to prevent the settling out of their insoluble drugs.

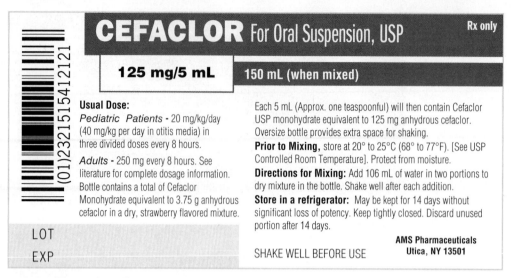

CEFACLOR For Oral Suspension, USP

Rx only

125 mg/5 mL | 150 mL (when mixed)

Usual Dose:
Pediatric Patients - 20 mg/kg/day (40 mg/kg per day in otitis media) in three divided doses every 8 hours.

Adults - 250 mg every 8 hours. See literature for complete dosage information. Bottle contains a total of Cefaclor Monohydrate equivalent to 3.75 g anhydrous cefaclor in a dry, strawberry flavored mixture.

LOT

EXP

Each 5 mL (Approx. one teaspoonful) will then contain Cefaclor USP monohydrate equivalent to 125 mg anhydrous cefaclor. Oversize bottle provides extra space for shaking.

Prior to Mixing, store at 20° to 25°C (68° to 77°F). [See USP Controlled Room Temperature]. Protect from moisture.

Directions for Mixing: Add 106 mL of water in two portions to dry mixture in the bottle. Shake well after each addition.

Store in a refrigerator: May be kept for 14 days without significant loss of potency. Keep tightly closed. Discard unused portion after 14 days.

SHAKE WELL BEFORE USE

AMS Pharmaceuticals
Utica, NY 13501

Figure 18-4

When a tablet or capsule is administered, carefully check the child's mouth to be certain the medication has actually been swallowed. If swallowing is a problem, some tablets can be crushed and given in a small amount of applesauce, ice cream, or juice if the child has no dietary restrictions.

⚷ Enteric-coated and timed-release tablets or capsules cannot be crushed because this would destroy the coating that allows them to function on a delayed-action basis.

INTRAMUSCULAR AND SUBCUTANEOUS MEDICATIONS

The drugs most often given subcutaneously are insulin and immunizations that specifically require the subcutaneous route. Any site with sufficient subcutaneous tissue may be used, with the upper arm being the site of choice for immunizations. The intramuscular route is used most frequently for preoperative and postoperative medications for sedation and pain, and for immunizations such as DPT (diphtheria, pertussis, tetanus), which must be administered deep IM. **The intramuscular site of choice for infants and small children is the vastus lateralis or rectus femoris of the thigh because the gluteal muscles do not develop until a child has learned to walk**. Usually, not more than 1 mL is injected per site, and sites are rotated regularly.

Dosage calculation is the same as for adults, except **dosages are sometimes calculated to the nearest hundredth and measured using a tuberculin (TB) syringe**. There is less margin for error in pediatric dosages, and calculations and measurements must be carefully double-checked.

SUMMARY

This concludes the introduction to pediatric oral, IM, and subcutaneous medication administration. The important points to remember from this chapter are:

■ Take care when administering oral drugs to ensure that the child has actually swallowed the dosage.

■ If liquid medications are prepared as suspensions, mix the suspension thoroughly prior to measurement, and administer it promptly to prevent the settling out of insoluble drugs.

■ Be careful not to confuse oral syringes, which are unsterile, with hypodermic syringes, which are sterile.

■ The IM site of choice for infants and small children is the vastus lateralis or rectus femoris of the thigh.

- Usually not more than 1 mL is injected per IM or subcutaneous site, and sites are rotated regularly.

- Pediatric parenteral dosages are frequently calculated to the nearest hundredth and measured using a TB syringe.

SUMMARY SELF-TEST

For Part 1, use the pediatric medication labels provided to measure the following dosages. Indicate in the second column if the medication is a suspension.

Part 1   mL   Suspension

1. Prepare a 20 mg dosage of fluoxetine.   _____   _____

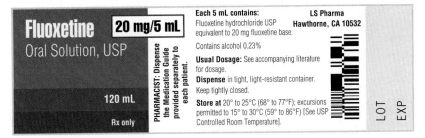

2. Prepare a 125 mg dosage of penicillin V potassium.   _____   _____

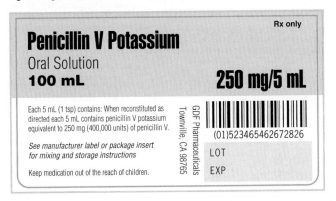

3. Prepare 100 mg of amoxicillin.   _____   _____

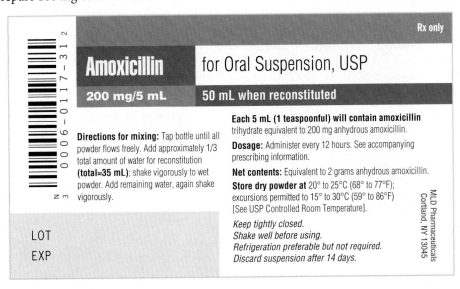

	mL	Suspension

4. Prepare 100 mg of cefpodoxime proxetil.   _____   _____

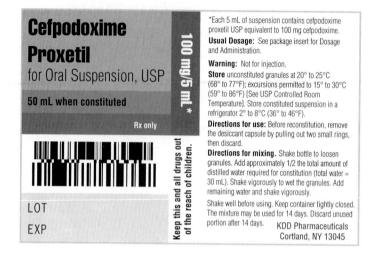

5. Prepare 374 mg of cefaclor.   _____   _____

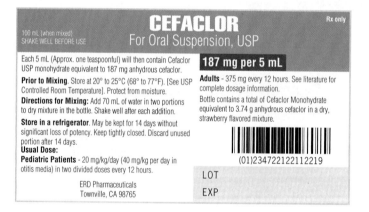

6. Prepare valproic acid 375 mg.   _____   _____

7. Prepare valproic acid 125 mg.   _____   _____

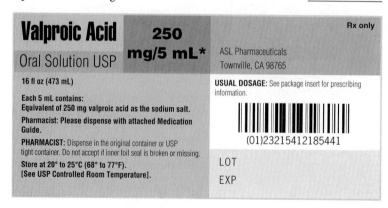

mL   Suspension

_____   _____

8. Prepare 120 mg of acetaminophen.

Rx only

Acetaminophen Oral Suspension

4 FL OZ (118 mL)

• **Fever reducer** • **Pain reliever**
Alcohol Free/Aspirin Free/Ibuprofen Free

Do not use
• With any other acetaminophen containing products. This may lead to an overdose, which may cause liver damage. (see overdose warning)

When using this product
• Do not exceed recommended dosage (see overdose warning)

Keep this and all drugs out of the reach of children.

Overdose Warning: Taking more than the recommended dose (overdose) could cause serious health problems, including liver damage. In case of accidental overdose, seek professional assistance or contact a Poison Control Center immediately. Quick medical attention is critical even if you do not notice any signs or symptoms.

TAMPER EVIDENT: DO NOT USE IF PRINTED SAFETY SEAL ON THE BOTTLE IS BROKEN OR MISSING.

Stop use and ask a doctor if
• New symptoms occur
• Redness or swelling is present
• Pain gets worse or lasts for more than 5 days
• Fever gets worse or lasts for more than 3 days

Other information
• Dosage cup provided
• Store at controlled room temperature

LAD Pharmaceuticals
Townville, CA 98765

LOT

EXP

Drug Facts

Active ingredient (in each 5 mL teaspoonful)　　　　　**Purpose**

Acetaminophen   160 mg.. Pain reliever/fever reducer

Uses temporarily: • Reduces fever • Relieves minor aches and pains due to:
　　　　• The common cold • Flu • Headaches • Sore throat • Immunizations
　　　　• Toothaches

Warnings
Sore throat warning: If sore throat is severe, persists for more than 2 days, is accompanied or followed by fever, headache, rash, nausea, or vomiting, consult a doctor promptly.

Directions
• **Do not exceed recommended dosage (see overdose warning)**
• Shake well before using
• Find right dose on chart below. If possible, use weight to dose; otherwise, use age.
• If needed, repeat dose every 4 hours
• Do not use more than 5 times in 24 hours
• Only use enclosed measuring cup

Weight (lb)	Age (yr)	Dose (tsp or mL)
under 36	under 4	do not use
36-48	4-6	do not use unless directed by a doctor
49-59	7-8	2 tsps or 10 mL
60-71	9-10	2 1/2 tsps or 12.5 mL
72-95	11	3 tsps or 15 mL

N 3   1 2 3 6 – 0 1 1 7 – 3 1 2

9. Prepare 561 mg of cefaclor.

_____   _____

CEFACLOR

Rx only

For Oral Suspension, USP

187 mg/5 mL

100 mL (when mixed)

Prior to Mixing, store at 20° to 25°C (68° to 77°F). [See USP Controlled Room Temperature]. Protect from moisture.

Directions for Mixing: Add 70 mL of water in two portions to dry mixture in the bottle. Shake well after each addition.
Each 5 mL (Approx. one teaspoonful) will then contain Cefaclor USP monohydrate equivalent to 187 mg anhydrous cefaclor. Oversize bottle provides extra space for shaking.

Store in a refrigerator; May be kept for 14 days without significant loss of potency. Keep tightly closed. Discard unused portion after 14 days. Shake well before use

Usual Dose:
Pediatric Patients - 20 mg/kg/day (40 mg/kg per day in otitis media) in two divided doses every 12 hours.
Adults - 375 mg every 12 hours. See literature for complete dosage information.

Bottle contains a total of Cefaclor Monohydrate equivalent to 3.74 g anhydrous cefaclor in a dry, strawberry flavored mixture.
LKK Pharmaceuticals
Syosset, NY 11773

(01)23215151121111

LOT

EXP

mL

Suspension
_____   _____

10. Prepare a 20 mg dosage of meperidine.

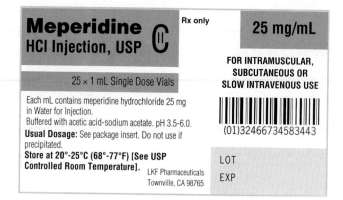

11. A dosage of morphine 10 mg has been ordered.

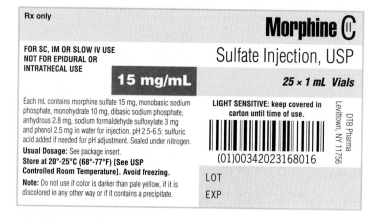

12. Draw up a 200 mg dosage of clindamycin.

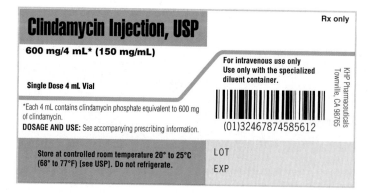

mL   Suspension

13. Prepare a 40 mg dosage of meperidine.   _____   _____

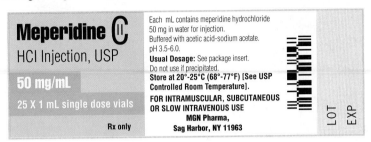

14. A dosage of phenytoin 60 mg has been ordered.   _____   _____

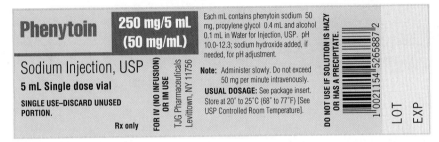

15. Prepare a 6 mg dosage of morphine.   _____   _____

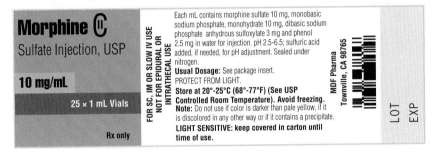

Answers

1. 5 mL; no	**5.** 10 mL; suspension	**9.** 15 mL; suspension	**13.** 0.8 mL; no
2. 2.5 mL; no	**6.** 7.5 mL; no	**10.** 0.8 mL; no	**14.** 1.2 mL; no
3. 2.5 mL; suspension	**7.** 2.5 mL; no	**11.** 0.7 mL; no	**15.** 0.6 mL; no
4. 5 mL; suspension	**8.** 3.8 mL; suspension	**12.** 1.3 mL; no	

CHAPTER 19

Pediatric IV Medications

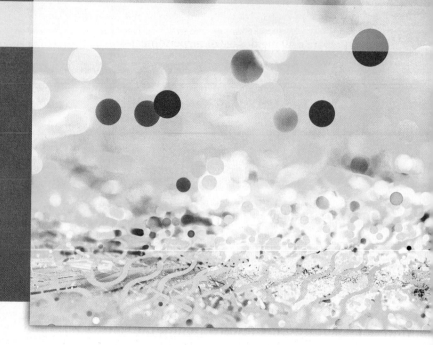

INTRODUCTION

Pediatric nursing is an advanced nursing discipline. This chapter includes some important basic information—a first baby step in preparation for pediatric nursing responsibilities. It gives you a general orientation to pediatric dosages, but you may forego completion of all calculations unless your instructor specifically assigns them.

Pediatric IV medication administration involves a multifaceted challenge and responsibility. Infants and children, particularly under the age of 4, are **incompletely developed physiologically, and drug tolerance, absorption, and excretion are ongoing concerns**. In addition, infants and acutely ill children can tolerate only a **narrow range of hydration**, making administration of IV drugs, which are diluted for administration, a critical and exact skill. Drug dilution protocols may specify a range for dilution, and on many occasions, the smallest possible volume may have to be used so as not to overhydrate a child. Dosage and dilution decisions may have to be made on a day-to-day or even a dose-to-dose basis, and require a team effort involving the nurse, physician, and pharmacist. In addition, the suitability of any flow rate calculated for administration must be made on an individual basis. For example, a calculated flow rate of 100 gtt/min for a 2-year-old child is too high a rate to administer.

The **fragility of infants' and children's veins**, and the irritating nature of many medications, mandate careful site inspection for signs of inflammation and infiltration. This should be done immediately before, during, and after each infusion. Signs of inflammation include redness, heat, swelling, and tenderness. Signs of infiltration include swelling, coolness, pain or discomfort, and lack of blood return in the IV tubing. Either complication necessitates discontinuing the IV and restarting the infusion at a new site.

IV medication guidelines are always used to determine drug dosages, dilutions, and administration rates.

Let's start by looking at the different methods of IV medication administration.

METHODS OF IV MEDICATION ADMINISTRATION

Intravenous medications may be administered over a period of several hours or on an **intermittent** basis involving several dosages in a 24-hour period. When ordered to infuse over several hours, medications are usually added to an IV solution bag. Adding the drug to the IV bag may be a hospital pharmacy or nurse responsibility. The steps for adding the drug to the solution are as follows:

Step 1: **Locate the type and volume of IV solution ordered.**

Step 2: **Measure the dosage of drug to be added.**

Step 3: **Use strict aseptic technique to add the drug to the solution bag through the medication port.**

Step 4: **Mix the drug thoroughly in the solution.**

Step 5: **Label the IV solution bag with the name and dosage of the drug added.**

Step 6: **Add your initials and the time and date you added the drug.**

Step 7: **Hang the IV and then set the flow rate for the infusion. Chart the administration when it has completed.**

For intermittent administrations, the medication may also be prepared in small-volume solution bags, or using a calibrated burette such as the one illustrated in **Figure 19-1**. Because the total capacity of burettes is between 100 and 150 mL, calibrated in 1 mL increments, the exact measurement of small volumes is possible.

Regardless of the method of intermittent administration, the medication infusion is **routinely followed by a flush** to make sure the medication has cleared the tubing and that the total dosage has been administered. The volume of the flush will vary depending on the length of IV tubing from the medication source—that is, the burette or syringe—to the infusion site. If a primary line exists, the medication may be administered by IVPB (IV piggyback) via a secondary line. If no IV is infusing, a saline or heparin lock (heplock) is frequently in place and used for intermittent administration.

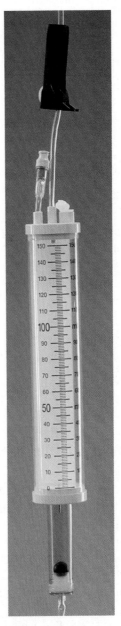

Figure 19-1
Calibrated burette.

When IV medications are diluted for administration, it is necessary to determine hospital policy on **inclusion of the medication volume as part of the volume specified for dilution**. For example, if 20 mg has a volume of 2 mL, and it is to be diluted in 30 mL, does this mean you must add 28 mL of diluent to the burette or 30 mL?

Hospital policies may vary, but in all examples and problems in this chapter, **the drug volume will be treated as part of the total diluent volume**. The sequencing of medication and flush administration for burette use, covered earlier in the text, is also representative of the procedure that might be followed for IVPB administrations.

MEDICATION ADMINISTRATION VIA BURETTE

When a burette is used for medication administration, the entire preparation is usually done by nurses. Volumetric and syringe pumps are used extensively to administer intermittent IV medications to infants and children. When these devices are used, the alarm will sound each time the burette or syringe empties to signal when each successive step is necessary. For example, an alarm will sound when the medication has infused and the flush must be started, and again when the flush is completed.

Let's look at some example orders and go step by step through one procedure that may be used with their administration.

EXAMPLE 1

A dosage of **250 mg in 15 mL** of D5 1/2NS is to be infused in **30 min**. It is to be followed with a **5 mL D5 1/2NS flush**. A volumetric pump will be used, and the tubing is a **microdrip** burette.

Step 1: **Read the drug label to determine what volume the 250 mg dosage is contained in. Let's assume this is 1 mL.**

Step 2: **The dilution is to be 15 mL. Run a total of 14 mL of D5 1/2NS into the burette, then add the 1 mL containing the medication dosage of 250 mg. This gives the ordered volume of 15 mL. Roll the burette between your hands to mix the drug thoroughly with the solution.**

Step 3: **Calculate the flow rate for this microdrip using dimensional analysis.**

$$\text{Total volume} = \textbf{15 mL} \qquad \text{Infusion time} = \textbf{30 min}$$

$$\frac{\text{mL}}{\text{hr}} = \frac{\text{15 mL}}{\text{30 min}} \times \frac{\text{60 min}}{\text{1 hr}} = \textbf{30 mL/hr}$$

Step 4: **Set the pump to infuse 30 mL/hr.**

Step 5: **Label the burette to identify the drug and dosage added. Attach a label that states "medication infusing." This makes it possible for others to know the status of the administration if you are not present when the infusion is complete and the pump alarms.**

Step 6: **When the medication has infused, add the 5 mL D5 1/2NS flush. Remove the "medication infusing" label and attach a "flush infusing" label. Continue to infuse at the 30 mL/hr rate until the burette empties for the second time.**

Step 7: **When the flush has been completed, restart the primary IV or disconnect from the saline/heparin lock. Remove the "flush infusing" label. Chart the dosage and time.**

EXAMPLE 2

An antibiotic dosage of **125 mg in 1 mL** is to be **diluted in 20 mL** of D5 1/4NS and infused over **30 min**. A **flush of 15 mL** D5 1/4NS is to follow. A volumetric pump will be used.

Step 1: **A dosage of 125 mg has a volume of 1 mL. Add 19 mL of D5 1/4NS to the burette, add the 1 mL of medication, and mix thoroughly.**

Step 2: **Calculate the mL/hr flow rate using dimensional analysis.**

$$\text{Total volume} = \textbf{20 mL} \qquad \text{Infusion time} = \textbf{30 min}$$

$$\frac{\text{mL}}{\text{hr}} = \frac{20 \text{ mL}}{30 \text{ min}} \times \frac{60 \text{ min}}{1 \text{ hr}} = \textbf{40 mL/hr}$$

Step 3: **Set the pump to infuse 40 mL/hr.**

Step 4: **Label the burette with the drug and dosage, and attach a "medication infusing" label.**

Step 5: **When the medication has infused, start the 15 mL flush. Remove the "medication infusing" label and add the "flush infusing" label.**

Step 6: **When the flush has completed, restart the primary IV or disconnect from the saline lock. Remove the "flush infusing" label. Chart the dosage and time.**

⌖ If a 60 gtt/mL calibrated burette is used without a pump, the gtt/min rate will be the same as the mL/hr rate.

EXAMPLE 3

An antibiotic dosage of **50 mg** has been ordered diluted in **20 mL** of D5W to infuse over **20 min**. A **15 mL flush** of D5W is to follow. A **microdrip** will be used, but an infusion control device will not be used.

Step 1: **Read the medication label to determine what volume contains 50 mg. You determine that 50 mg is contained in 2 mL.**

Step 2: **Run 18 mL of D5W into the burette and add the 2 mL containing 50 mg of drug. Roll the burette between your hands to mix the solution thoroughly.**

Step 3: **Calculate the flow rate in gtt/min necessary to deliver the medication.**

$$\text{Total volume} = \textbf{20 mL} \qquad \text{Infusion time} = \textbf{20 min}$$

$$\frac{\text{gtt}}{\text{min}} = \frac{60 \text{ gtt}}{1 \text{ mL}} \times \frac{20 \text{ mL}}{20 \text{ min}} = \textbf{60 gtt/min}$$

Step 4: **The mL/hr and gtt/min rates are identical for a microdrip. Set the rate at 60 gtt/min.**

Step 5: **Label the burette with the drug name and dosage, and attach a "medication infusing" label.**

Step 6: **When the medication has cleared the burette, add the 15 mL D5W flush. Continue to run at 60 gtt/min. Remove the "medication infusing" label and replace it with a "flush infusing" label.**

Step 7: **When the burette empties for the second time, restart the primary IV or disconnect from the saline lock. Remove the "flush infusing" label. Chart the dosage and time administered.**

EXAMPLE 4

An IV medication dosage of **100 mcg** has been ordered diluted in **35 mL** of NS and infused in **50 min**. A **10 mL** flush is to follow. A **microdrip** burette will be used.

Step 1: **Read the medication label to determine what volume contains 100 mcg: 100 mcg = 1.5 mL**

Step 2: **Run 33.5 mL of NS into the burette, and add the 1.5 mL of medication. Roll the burette between your hands to mix the solution thoroughly.**

Step 3: **Calculate the gtt/min flow rate.**

$$\frac{\text{gtt}}{\text{min}} = \frac{60 \text{ gtt}}{1 \text{ mL}} \times \frac{35 \text{ mL}}{50 \text{ min}} = \textbf{42 gtt/min}$$

Step 4: **Set the flow rate at 42 gtt/min.**

Step 5: **Label the burette with the drug name and dosage and a "medication infusing" label.**

Step 6: **When the medication has cleared the burette, add the 10 mL flush. Continue to run at 42 gtt/min. Replace the "medication infusing" label with a "flush infusing" label.**

Step 7: **When the burette empties all of the flush solution, restart the primary IV or disconnect from the saline lock. Remove the "flush infusing" label, and chart the dosage and time administered.**

PROBLEMS 19-1

Determine the volume of solution that must be added to a burette to mix the following IV drugs. Then calculate the flow rate in gtt/min for each administration using a microdrip, and indicate the mL/hr setting for a pump.

1. An IV medication of 75 mg in 3 mL is ordered diluted to 55 mL to infuse over 45 min.
   Dilution volume _____   gtt/min _____   mL/hr _____

2. A dosage of 100 mg in 2 mL is diluted to 30 mL of D5W to infuse in 20 min.
   Dilution volume _____   gtt/min _____   mL/hr _____

3. The volume of a 10 mg dosage of medication is 1 mL. Dilute to 40 mL and administer over 50 min.
   Dilution volume _____   gtt/min _____   mL/hr _____

4. A dosage of 15 mg with a volume of 3 mL is to be diluted to 70 mL and administered in 50 min.
   Dilution volume _____   gtt/min _____   mL/hr _____

5. A medication of 1 g in 4 mL is to be diluted to 60 mL and infused over 90 min.
   Dilution volume _____   gtt/min _____   mL/hr _____

Answers 1. 52 mL; 73 gtt/min; 73 mL/hr   **2.** 28 mL; 90 gtt/min; 90 mL/hr   **3.** 39 mL; 48 gtt/min; 48 mL/hr
4. 67 mL; 84 gtt/min; 84 mL/hr   **5.** 56 mL; 40 gtt/min; 40 mL/hr

COMPARING IV DOSAGES ORDERED WITH AVERAGE DOSAGES

Questioning a physician order is extremely rare. This exercise is geared to your deeper understanding of how dosages are calculated, and determining if they are correct gives you a goal in doing them.

> Dosages of IV medications are calculated on the basis of body weight or body surface area (BSA).

Average dosages may be listed in terms of mg, mcg, or units per day or per hour. BSA in m^2 is most often used to calculate doses of chemotherapeutic drugs, which are administered only by certified nursing staff. The following examples will demonstrate how to use average dosage to check dosages ordered.

EXAMPLE 1

A child weighing **22.6 kg** has an order for **500 mg** of medication in **100 mL** of D5W **every 12 hours**. The normal dosage range is **40–50 mg/kg/day**. Determine whether the dosage ordered is within the normal range.

Step 1: **Calculate the normal daily dosage range for this child.**

40 mg/day × 22.6 kg = **904 mg**
50 mg/day × 22.6 kg = **1130 mg**

Step 2: **Calculate the dosage infusing in 24 hr.**

500 mg in 12 hr = **1000 mg in 24 hr**

Step 3: **Assess the accuracy of the dosage ordered.**

The 500 mg in 12 hr is within the 904–1130 mg/day dosage range.

EXAMPLE 2

A child with a body weight of **18.4 kg** is to receive a medication with a dosage range of **100–150 mg/kg/day**. The order is for **600 mg** in **75 mL** of D5W **every 6 hours**. Determine whether the dosage is within the normal range.

Step 1: **Calculate the normal daily dosage range.**

100 mg/day × 18.4 kg = **1840 mg/day**
150 mg/day × 18.4 kg = **2760 mg/day**

Step 2: **Calculate the daily dosage ordered.**

The dosage ordered is 600 mg every 6 hours (4 doses/24 hours):

600 mg × 4 = **2400 mg/day**

Step 3: **Assess the accuracy of the dosage ordered.**

The dosage ordered, 2400 mg/day, is within the normal range of 1840–2760 mg/day.

EXAMPLE 3

A child who weighs **17.7 kg** is receiving an IV of **250 mL** of D5W that contains **2000 units** of medication, which is to infuse at **50 mL/hr**. The dosage range is **10–25 units/kg/hr**. Assess the accuracy of this dosage.

Step 1: **Calculate the dosage range per hour.**

$$10 \text{ units/kg/hr} \times 17.7 \text{ kg} = \textbf{177 units/hr}$$
$$25 \text{ units/kg/hr} \times 17.7 \text{ kg} = \textbf{442.5 units/hr}$$

Step 2: **Calculate the dosage infusing per hour.**

$$\frac{\text{units}}{\text{hr}} = \frac{2000 \text{ units}}{250 \text{ mL}} \times \frac{50 \text{ mL}}{1 \text{ hr}} = \textbf{400 units/hr}$$

Step 3: **Assess the accuracy of the dosage ordered.**

The IV is infusing at a rate of 50 mL per hour, which is 400 units/hr. The normal dosage range is 177–442.5 units/hr. The dosage is within normal range.

EXAMPLE 4

A child who weighs **32.7 kg** has an IV of **250 mL** of D5 1/4S containing **400 mcg** of medication to infuse in **5 hours**. The normal range for this drug is **1–3 mcg/kg/hr**. Determine whether this dosage is within the normal dosage range.

Step 1: **Calculate the hourly dosage range.**

$$1 \text{ mcg/kg/hr} \times 32.7 \text{ kg} = \textbf{32.7 mcg/hr}$$
$$3 \text{ mcg/kg/hr} \times 32.7 \text{ kg} = \textbf{98.1 mcg/hr}$$

Step 2: **Calculate the dosage infusing per hour.**

$$400 \text{ mcg} \div 5 \text{ hr} = \textbf{80 mcg/hr}$$

Step 3: **Assess the accuracy of the dosage ordered.**

The dosage of 80 mcg/hr infusing is within the normal range of 32.7–98.1 mcg/hr.

PROBLEMS 19-2

Calculate the normal dosage range to the nearest tenth and the dosage being administered for the following medications. Assess the dosages ordered.

1. A child who weighs 24.4 kg has an IV of 250 mL of D5W containing 2500 units of a drug. The dosage range for this drug is 15–25 units/kg/hr. The pump is set to deliver 50 mL/hr.

   Dosage range per hr _____   Dosage infusing per hr _____

   Assessment _____

2. A solution of D5W containing 25 mg of a drug is to infuse in 30 min. The dosage range is 4–8 mg/kg/day every 6 hours. The child weighs 18.7 kg.

   Dosage range per day _____   Daily dosage ordered _____

   Assessment _____

3. An IV solution containing 125 mg of medication is infusing. The dosage range is 5–10 mg/kg/dose, and the child weighs 14.2 kg.

   Dosage range per dose _____   Assessment _____

4. A child who weighs 14.3 kg is to receive an IV drug with a dosage range of 50–100 mcg/kg/day in two divided doses. An infusion of 50 mL of D5W containing 400 mcg to run 30 min has been ordered.

   Daily dosage range _____   Daily dosage ordered _____

   Assessment _____

5. A dosage of 4 mg (4000 mcg) of drug in 500 mL of D5 1/2S is to infuse in 4 hours. The dosage range of the drug is 24–120 mcg/kg/hr, and the child weighs 16.1 kg.

   Dosage range per hr _____   Dosage infusing per hr _____

   Assessment _____

6. A child who weighs 20.9 kg is to receive a medication with a normal dosage range of 80–160 mg/kg/day in divided doses every 6 hours. The IV ordered contains 500 mg.

   Dosage range per day _____   Daily dosage ordered _____

   Assessment _____

7. A child who weighs 22.3 kg is to receive 750 mL of D5 1/4S containing 6 g of a drug, which is to run for 24 hours. The dosage range of the drug is 200–300 mg/kg/day.

   Dosage range per day _____   Assessment _____

8. An IV of 50 mL of D5W containing 55 mcg of a drug is infusing in a 30-min period. The child weighs 14.9 kg and the dosage range is 6–8 mcg/kg/day, every 12 hours.

   Dosage range per day _____   Daily dosage ordered _____

   Assessment _____

9. A child who weighs 27.1 kg is to receive a medication with a normal range of 0.5–1 mg/kg/dose. An IV containing 20 mg of medication has been ordered.

   Dosage per dose _____   Assessment _____

10. An IV medication of 60 mcg in 200 mL is ordered to infuse in 2 hr. The normal dosage range is 1.5–3 mcg/kg/hr. The child weighs 16.7 kg.

    Dosage range per hr _____   Dosage infusing per hr _____

    Assessment _____

Answers 1. 366–610 units/hr; 500 units/hr; normal range   **2.** 74.8–149.6 mg/day; 100 mg/day; normal range   **3.** 71–142 mg/dose; normal range   **4.** 715–1430 mcg/day; 800 mcg; normal range   **5.** 386.4–1932 mcg/hr; 1000 mcg; normal range   **6.** 1672–3344 mg/day; 2000 mg; normal range   **7.** 4460–6690 mg/day; normal range   **8.** 89.4–119.2 mcg/day; 110 mcg; normal range   **9.** 13.6–27.1 mg/dose; normal range   **10.** 25.1–50.1 mcg/hr; 30 mcg; normal range

SUMMARY

This concludes the chapter on administration of IV drugs to infants and children. The important points to remember from this chapter are:

- IV medications may be ordered to infuse in several hours or minutes.

- IV medications are diluted for administration, and it is important to determine the hospital's policy on inclusion of the medication volume as part of the total dilution volume.

- A flush is used following medication administration to make sure the medication has cleared the tubing and the total dosage has been administered.

- The volume of flush solution on intermittent infusions will vary depending on the amount needed to clear the infusion line.

- Average dosage ranges are used to assess dosages ordered.

- Pediatric IV medication administration requires constant assessment of the child's ability to tolerate dosage, dilution, and rate of administration.

- Children's veins are very fragile, and intravenous sites must be checked for inflammation and infiltration immediately before, during, and after each medication administration.

SUMMARY SELF-TEST

Determine the volume of solution that must be added to a calibrated burette to mix the following IV drugs. The medication volume is included in the total dilution volume. Calculate the flow rate in gtt/min for each infusion. A microdrip with a calibration of 60 gtt/mL is used.

	Volume of Diluent	gtt/min Rate
1. An IV antibiotic of 750 mg in 3 mL has been ordered diluted to a total of 25 mL of D5W to infuse in 40 minutes.	_____	_____
2. A dosage of 500,000 units of a penicillin preparation with a volume of 4 mL has been ordered diluted to 50 mL D5 1/2NS to infuse in 60 min.	_____	_____
3. A dosage of 1.5 g/2 mL of an antibiotic is to be diluted to a total of 40 mL of D5W and administered in 40 min.	_____	_____
4. An antibiotic dosage of 200 mg in 4 mL is to be diluted to 50 mL and administered in 70 min.	_____	_____
5. A dosage of 20 mg in 2 mL has been ordered diluted to 30 mL to be infused in 35 min.	_____	_____
6. A dosage of 25 mg in 5 mL has been ordered diluted to 40 mL and administered in 50 min.	_____	_____
7. A 10 mg in 2 mL dosage has been ordered diluted to 20 mL to infuse in 30 min.	_____	_____
8. A medication dosage of 800 mg in 4 mL is to be diluted to 60 mL and infused in 80 min.	_____	_____
9. A dosage of 0.5 g in 2 mL is to be diluted to 40 mL and run in 30 min.	_____	_____
10. A medication of 1000 mg in 1 mL is to be diluted to 15 mL and administered in 20 min.	_____	_____

The following IV drugs are to be administered using a volumetric or syringe pump. Determine the amount of diluent to be added and the flow rate in mL/hr at which to set the pumps.

	Volume of Diluent	mL/hr Rate
11. A dosage of 40 mg in 4 mL is to be diluted to 50 mL and administered in 90 min.	_____	_____
12. A 2 g in 5 mL dosage has been ordered diluted to a total of 90 mL and administered in 45 min.	_____	_____
13. An 80 mg dosage with a volume of 2 mL is to be diluted to 80 mL and administered in 60 min.	_____	_____
14. A 60 mg dosage with a volume of 4 mL is ordered diluted to 30 mL and run in 20 min.	_____	_____
15. A 5 mg per 2 mL dosage is to be diluted to 80 mL and administered in 50 min.	_____	_____
16. The dosage ordered is 0.75 g in 3 mL to be diluted to 30 mL and infused in 40 min.	_____	_____
17. A medication of 100 mg in 2 mL is ordered diluted to 30 mL and run in 25 min.	_____	_____
18. The dosage ordered is 100 mg in 1 mL to be diluted to 50 mL and infused in 45 min.	_____	_____
19. A 30 mg dosage in 1 mL has been ordered diluted to 10 mL to infuse in 10 min.	_____	_____
20. A dosage of 250 mg in 5 mL has been ordered diluted to 40 mL and infused in 60 min.	_____	_____

Calculate the normal dosage range to the nearest tenth and the dosage being administered for the following medications. Assess the dosages ordered.

21. A child who weighs 15.4 kg is to receive a dosage with a range of 5–7.5 mg/kg/dose. The solution bag is labeled 100 mg.

   Dosage range _____   Assessment _____

22. The order is for 200 units in 75 mL. The child weighs 13.1 kg, and the dosage range is 15–20 units/kg per dose.

   Dosage range _____   Assessment _____

23. A dosage of 1.5 mg in 20 mL has been ordered. The normal dosage range is 0.1–0.3 mg/kg/day in two divided doses. The child's weight is 12.4 kg.

   Dosage range per day _____

   Daily dosage ordered _____   Assessment _____

24. A dosage of 400 mg in 75 mL of medication is to be infused every 8 hours. The normal range is 15–45 mg/kg/day, and the child weighs 27.9 kg.

   Dosage range per day _____

   Daily dosage ordered _____   Assessment _____

25. A child who weighs 15.7 kg is to receive a medication with a normal hourly range of 3–7 mcg/kg. A 250 mL solution bag containing 350 mcg is infusing at a rate of 50 mL/hr.

    Dosage range per hr _____   Dosage infusing per hr _____

    Assessment _____

26. A child who weighs 19.6 kg is to receive a medication with a normal dosage range of 60–80 mg/kg/day. A 90 mL infusion containing 375 mg has been ordered every 6 hours.

    Dosage range per day _____   Daily dosage ordered _____

    Assessment _____

27. Two infusions of 250 mL each containing 300 mg of medication are to infuse continuously over a 24-hr period. The child receiving the infusion weighs 11.7 kg, and the normal dosage range of the drug is 50–100 mg/kg/day.

    Dosage range per day _____

    Daily dosage ordered _____   Assessment _____

28. The order is for 100 mL of D5W containing 150 mg of medication to infuse every 8 hours. The normal dosage range is 3–12 mg/kg/day, and the child weighs 40.1 kg.

    Dosage range per day_____   Daily dosage ordered _____

    Assessment _____

29. A child has an infusion of 250 mL containing 500 units of medication to run at 50 mL/hr. The normal dosage range is 10–25 units/kg/hr. The child weighs 10.3 kg.

    Dosage range per hr _____   Dosage infusing per hr _____

    Assessment _____

30. The normal dosage range of a drug is 0.5–1.5 units/kg/hr. A child who weighs 10.7 kg has a 150 mL volume of solution containing 45 units infusing at a rate of 20 mL/hr.

    Normal dosage range per hr _____   Dosage infusing per hr _____

    Assessment _____

31. A child who weighs 12.5 kg is receiving an IV of 2500 units of medication in 250 mL of D5W at 40 mL/hr. The normal dosage range is 10–25 units/kg/hr.

    Normal dosage range per hr _____

    Dosage infusing per hr _____   Assessment _____

32. A child who weighs 10 kg is to receive a medication with a normal dosage range of 60–80 mg/kg/day. The order is for 200 mg every 6 hours.

    Normal dosage range per hr _____

    Daily dosage ordered _____   Assessment _____

33. The order is for 0.5 g in 100 mL of D5W every 6 hours. The normal dosage range is 100–200 mg/kg/day. The child weighs 15 kg.

    Normal dosage range per hr _____

    Daily dosage ordered_____   Assessment _____

34. A continuous IV of 500 mL with 20 mEq KCl is infusing at 30 mL/hr. The dosage for potassium chloride is not to exceed 40 mEq/day.

    Dosage infusing per hr _____

    Dosage infusing per day _____   Assessment _____

35. A 24 kg child is receiving 116 mg of medication via IV 3 times each day (every 8 hours). The dosage range for this drug is 10–20 mg/kg/day.

    Normal dosage range per day ——————

    Dosage received after 3 doses ——————   Assessment ——————

36. A child who weighs 15 kg has an order for 40 mcg of medication in 75 mL D5W to infuse every 12 hours. The normal dosage range is 8–10 mcg/kg/day.

    Normal dosage per day ——————

    Dosage ordered ——————   Assessment ——————

37. The usual dosage for children is 50 mg/kg/24 hr in equally divided doses. The order is to infuse 50 mL with 290 mg every 6 hours. The child weighs 51 lb.

    Normal dosage per day ——————

    Daily dosage ordered ——————   Assessment ——————

38. Order: 500 mL D5RL with 30 mEq KCl to infuse at 40 mL/hr. A maximum of 10 mEq/hr of KCl should not be exceeded, and the total 24-hr dosage should not exceed 40 mEq/day.

    Dosage infusing per hr ——————   Dosage infusing per day ——————

    Assessment ——————

39. A child who weighs 30 kg has an IV of 100 mL of D5W containing 600 mcg of medication to infuse in 2 hours. The normal range for this drug is 2–4 mcg/kg/hr.

    Normal dosage range per hr ——————

    Dosage infusing per hr ——————   Assessment ——————

40. A 150 mL solution with 18 mg of medication is ordered to infuse in 10 hours. The normal range for this drug is 0.2–0.6 mg/kg/hr. The child weighs 9 kg.

    Normal dosage range per hr ——————

    Dosage infusing per hr ——————   Assessment ——————

Answers

1. 22 mL; 38 gtt/min
2. 46 mL; 50 gtt/min
3. 38 mL; 60 gtt/min
4. 46 mL; 43 gtt/min
5. 28 mL; 51 gtt/min
6. 35 mL; 48 gtt/min
7. 18 mL; 40 gtt/min
8. 56 mL; 45 gtt/min
9. 38 mL; 80 gtt/min
10. 14 mL; 45 gtt/min
11. 46 mL; 33 mL/hr
12. 85 mL; 120 mL/hr
13. 78 mL; 80 mL/hr
14. 26 mL; 90 mL/hr
15. 78 mL; 96 mL/hr
16. 27 mL; 45 mL/hr

17. 28 mL; 72 mL/hr
18. 49 mL; 67 mL/hr
19. 9 mL; 60 mL/hr
20. 35 mL; 40 mL/hr
21. 77–115.5 mg/dose; normal
22. 196.5–262 units/dose; normal
23. 1.2–3.7 mg/day; 3 mg; normal
24. 418.5–1255.5 mg/day; 1200 mg; normal
25. 47.1–109.9 mcg/hr; 70 mcg; normal
26. 1176–1568 mg/day; 1500 mg; normal

27. 585–1170 mg/day; 600 mg; normal
28. 120.3–481.2 mg/day; 450 mg; normal
29. 103–257.5 units/hr; 100 units/hr; too low
30. 5.4–16.1 units/hr; 6 units/hr; normal
31. 125–312.5 units/hr; 400 units/hr; too high
32. 600–800 mg/day; 800 mg; normal
33. 1500–3000 mg/day; 2000 mg; normal

34. 1.2 mEq/hr; 28.8 mEq/day; normal
35. 240–480 mg/day; 348 mg; normal
36. 120–150 mcg/day; 80 mcg/day; too low
37. 1160 mg/day; 1160 mg; normal
38. 2.4 mEq/hr; 58 mEq/day; too high
39. 60–120 mcg/hr; 300 mcg; too high
40. 1.8–5.4 mg/hr; 1.8 mg; normal

ISMP's List of *Error-Prone Abbreviations, Symbols,* and *Dose Designations*

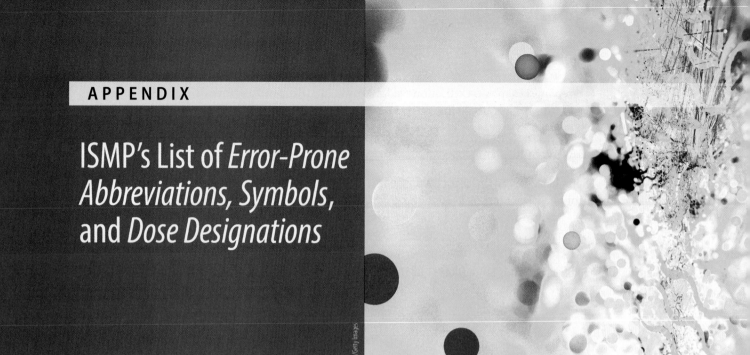

Institute for Safe Medication Practices

ISMP's List of *Error-Prone Abbreviations, Symbols,* and *Dose Designations*

The abbreviations, symbols, and dose designations found in this table have been reported to ISMP through the ISMP National Medication Errors Reporting Program (ISMP MERP) as being frequently misinterpreted and involved in harmful medication errors. They should **NEVER** be used when communicating medical information. This includes internal communications, telephone/verbal prescriptions, computer-generated labels, labels for drug storage bins, medication administration records, as well as pharmacy and prescriber computer order entry screens.

Abbreviations	Intended Meaning	Misinterpretation	Correction
μg	Microgram	Mistaken as "mg"	Use "mcg"
AD, AS, AU	Right ear, left ear, each ear	Mistaken as OD, OS, OU (right eye, left eye, each eye)	Use "right ear," "left ear," or "each ear"
OD, OS, OU	Right eye, left eye, each eye	Mistaken as AD, AS, AU (right ear, left ear, each ear)	Use "right eye," "left eye," or "each eye"
BT	Bedtime	Mistaken as "BID" (twice daily)	Use "bedtime"
cc	Cubic centimeters	Mistaken as "u" (units)	Use "mL"
D/C	Discharge or discontinue	Premature discontinuation of medications if D/C (intended to mean "discharge") has been misinterpreted as "discontinued" when followed by a list of discharge medications	Use "discharge" and "discontinue"
IJ	Injection	Mistaken as "IV" or "intrajugular"	Use "injection"
IN	Intranasal	Mistaken as "IM" or "IV"	Use "intranasal" or "NAS"
HS	Half-strength	Mistaken as bedtime	Use "half-strength" or "bedtime"
hs	At bedtime, hours of sleep	Mistaken as half-strength	
IU**	International unit	Mistaken as IV (intravenous) or 10 (ten)	Use "units"
o.d. or OD	Once daily	Mistaken as "right eye" (OD-oculus dexter), leading to oral liquid medications administered in the eye	Use "daily"
OJ	Orange juice	Mistaken as OD or OS (right or left eye); drugs meant to be diluted in orange juice may be given in the eye	Use "orange juice"
Per os	By mouth, orally	The "os" can be mistaken as "left eye" (OS-oculus sinister)	Use "PO," "by mouth," or "orally"
q.d. or QD**	Every day	Mistaken as q.i.d., especially if the period after the "q" or the tail of the "q" is misunderstood as an "i"	Use "daily"
qhs	Nightly at bedtime	Mistaken as "qhr" or every hour	Use "nightly"
qn	Nightly or at bedtime	Mistaken as "qh" (every hour)	Use "nightly" or "at bedtime"
q.o.d. or QOD**	Every other day	Mistaken as "q.d." (daily) or "q.i.d. (four times daily) if the "o" is poorly written	Use "every other day"
q1d	Daily	Mistaken as q.i.d. (four times daily)	Use "daily"
q6PM, etc.	Every evening at 6 PM	Mistaken as every 6 hours	Use "daily at 6 PM" or "6 PM daily"
SC, SQ, sub q	Subcutaneous	SC mistaken as SL (sublingual); SQ mistaken as "5 every;" the "q" in "sub q" has been mistaken as "every" (e.g., a heparin dose ordered "sub q 2 hours before surgery" misunderstood as every 2 hours before surgery)	Use "subcut" or "subcutaneously"
ss	Sliding scale (insulin) or ½ (apothecary)	Mistaken as "55"	Spell out "sliding scale;" use "one-half" or "½"
SSRI	Sliding scale regular insulin	Mistaken as selective-serotonin reuptake inhibitor	Spell out "sliding scale (insulin)"
SSI	Sliding scale insulin	Mistaken as Strong Solution of Iodine (Lugol's)	
i/d	One daily	Mistaken as "tid"	Use "1 daily"
TIW or tiw	3 times a week	Mistaken as "3 times a day" or "twice in a week"	Use "3 times weekly"
U or u**	Unit	Mistaken as the number 0 or 4, causing a 10-fold overdose or greater (e.g., 4U seen as "40" or 4u seen as "44"); mistaken as "cc" so dose given in volume instead of units (e.g., 4u seen as 4cc)	Use "unit"
UD	As directed ("ut dictum")	Mistaken as unit dose (e.g., diltiazem 125 mg IV infusion "UD" misinterpreted as meaning to give the entire infusion as a unit [bolus] dose)	Use "as directed"
Dose Designations and Other Information	Intended Meaning	Misinterpretation	Correction
Trailing zero after decimal point (e.g., 1.0 mg)**	1 mg	Mistaken as 10 mg if the decimal point is not seen	Do not use trailing zeros for doses expressed in whole numbers
"Naked" decimal point (e.g., .5 mg)**	0.5 mg	Mistaken as 5 mg if the decimal point is not seen	Use zero before a decimal point when the dose is less than a whole unit
Abbreviations such as mg. or mL. with a period following the abbreviation	mg mL	The period is unnecessary and could be mistaken as the number 1 if written poorly	Use mg, mL, etc. without a terminal period

Institute for Safe Medication Practices

ISMP's List of *Error-Prone Abbreviations, Symbols,* and *Dose Designations* (continued)

Dose Designations and Other Information	Intended Meaning	Misinterpretation	Correction
Drug name and dose run together (especially problematic for drug names that end in "l" such as Inderal40 mg; Tegretol300 mg)	Inderal 40 mg Tegretol 300 mg	Mistaken as Inderal 140 mg Mistaken as Tegretol 1300 mg	Place adequate space between the drug name, dose, and unit of measure
Numerical dose and unit of measure run together (e.g., 10mg, 100mL)	10 mg 100 mL	The "m" is sometimes mistaken as a zero or two zeros, risking a 10- to 100-fold overdose	Place adequate space between the dose and unit of measure
Large doses without properly placed commas (e.g., 100000 units; 1000000 units)	100,000 units 1,000,000 units	100000 has been mistaken as 10,000 or 1,000,000; 1000000 has been mistaken as 100,000	Use commas for dosing units at or above 1,000, or use words such as 100 "thousand" or 1 "million" to improve readability

Drug Name Abbreviations	Intended Meaning	Misinterpretation	Correction
To avoid confusion, do not abbreviate drug names when communicating medical information. Examples of drug name abbreviations involved in medication errors include:			
APAP	acetaminophen	Not recognized as acetaminophen	Use complete drug name
ARA A	vidarabine	Mistaken as cytarabine (ARA C)	Use complete drug name
AZT	zidovudine (Retrovir)	Mistaken as azathioprine or aztreonam	Use complete drug name
CPZ	Compazine (prochlorperazine)	Mistaken as chlorpromazine	Use complete drug name
DPT	Demerol-Phenergan-Thorazine	Mistaken as diphtheria-pertussis-tetanus (vaccine)	Use complete drug name
DTO	Diluted tincture of opium, or deodorized tincture of opium (Paregoric)	Mistaken as tincture of opium	Use complete drug name
HCl	hydrochloric acid or hydrochloride	Mistaken as potassium chloride (The "H" is misinterpreted as "K")	Use complete drug name unless expressed as a salt of a drug
HCT	hydrocortisone	Mistaken as hydrochlorothiazide	Use complete drug name
HCTZ	hydrochlorothiazide	Mistaken as hydrocortisone (seen as HCT250 mg)	Use complete drug name
MgSO4**	magnesium sulfate	Mistaken as morphine sulfate	Use complete drug name
MS, MSO4**	morphine sulfate	Mistaken as magnesium sulfate	Use complete drug name
MTX	methotrexate	Mistaken as mitoxantrone	Use complete drug name
NoAC	novel/new oral anticoagulant	No anticoagulant	Use complete drug name
PCA	procainamide	Mistaken as patient controlled analgesia	Use complete drug name
PTU	propylthiouracil	Mistaken as mercaptopurine	Use complete drug name
T3	Tylenol with codeine No. 3	Mistaken as liothyronine	Use complete drug name
TAC	triamcinolone	Mistaken as tetracaine, Adrenalin, cocaine	Use complete drug name
TNK	TNKase	Mistaken as "TPA"	Use complete drug name
TPA or tPA	tissue plasminogen activator, Activase (alteplase)	Mistaken as TNKase (tenecteplase), or less often as another tissue plasminogen activator, Retavase (reteplase)	Use complete drug names
ZnSO4	zinc sulfate	Mistaken as morphine sulfate	Use complete drug name

Stemmed Drug Names	Intended Meaning	Misinterpretation	Correction
"Nitro" drip	nitroglycerin infusion	Mistaken as sodium nitroprusside infusion	Use complete drug name
"Norflox"	norfloxacin	Mistaken as Norflex	Use complete drug name
"IV Vanc"	intravenous vancomycin	Mistaken as Invanz	Use complete drug name

Symbols	Intended Meaning	Misinterpretation	Correction
ℨ ♏	Dram Minim	Symbol for dram mistaken as "3" Symbol for minim mistaken as "mL"	Use the metric system
x3d	For three days	Mistaken as "3 doses"	Use "for three days"
> and <	More than and less than	Mistaken as opposite of intended; mistakenly use incorrect symbol; "< 10" mistaken as "40"	Use "more than" or "less than"
/ (slash mark)	Separates two doses or indicates "per"	Mistaken as the number 1 (e.g., "25 units/10 units" misread as "25 units and 110" units)	Use "per" rather than a slash mark to separate doses
@	At	Mistaken as "2"	Use "at"
&	And	Mistaken as "2"	Use "and"
+	Plus or and	Mistaken as "4"	Use "and"
°	Hour	Mistaken as a zero (e.g., q2° seen as q 20)	Use "hr," "h," or "hour"
Φ or ⌀	zero, null sign	Mistaken as numerals 4, 6, 8, and 9	Use 0 or zero, or describe intent using whole words

**These abbreviations are included on The Joint Commission's "minimum list" of dangerous abbreviations, acronyms, and symbols that must be included on an organization's "Do Not Use" list, effective January 1, 2004. Visit www.jointcommission.org for more information about this Joint Commission requirement.

ISMP
INSTITUTE FOR SAFE MEDICATION PRACTICES
www.ismp.org

Index

Note: Page numbers followed by *f* denote material in figures.